A Clinician's Guide to Nuclear Medicine

Andrew Taylor, MD
Professor of Radiology and Co-Director of Nuclear Medicine
Emory University School of Medicine
Atlanta, GA

David M. Schuster, MD
Assistant Professor of Radiology, Medical Director
Center for Positron Emission Tomography
Emory University School of Medicine
Atlanta, GA

Naomi Alazraki, MD
Professor of Radiology and Co-Director of Nuclear Medicine
Emory University School of Medicine
Chief of Nuclear Medicine
Veterans Affairs Medical Center
Atlanta, GA

Society of Nuclear Medicine, Inc.
1850 Samuel Morse Drive, Reston, VA 20190-5316

2nd printing, January 2003

Made in the United States of America

Library of Congress Cataloging-in-Publication Data

Taylor, Andrew, 1942-
   A clinician's guide to nuclear medicine/Andrew T. Taylor, Jr., David M. Schuster,
Naomi Alazraki.
      p. ; cm.
   Includes bibliographical references and index.
   ISBN 0-932004-72-5
   1. Nuclear medicine. 2. Radioisotopes in medical diagnosis. I. Schuster, David M.,
   1962- II. Alazraki, Naomi P. III. Title.
   [DNLM: 1. Nuclear Medicine–methods. WN 440 T238c 2000]
   R895 .T39 2000
   616.07'575–dc21

                                                                    00-032987

Table of Contents

How to Use This Book

This book is written to aid physicians who take care of patients. Its goal is to guide the clinician, resident, intern and medical student in the use of diagnostic and therapeutic nuclear medicine procedures. In what way can nuclear medicine aid in the diagnosis and management of common medical and surgical diseases? What tests are available? What are their advantages; what are their limitations? When should they be used? Are they cost-effective? What are the alternative tests, and how do they compare with the nuclear medicine procedures? What should the patient expect when he or she comes to the nuclear medicine department? Are there special medication, diet or hydration requirements? Are there radiation risks to patients or their families? What radionuclide therapy options are available, and when should these be considered?

To accomplish its task, this book is organized to address the common clinical questions that arise in patient management, particularly those that can be addressed by nuclear medicine procedures. Most of the chapters are arranged by organ system and begin with a brief introduction. The introduction is followed by three lists called "Scans and Primary Clinical Indications," "Clinical Questions" and "Patient Information," which are cross-referenced by page number to the subsequent discussion in the chapter. To allow the clinician to quickly find the desired information, chapters are further subdivided into sections called "Scans," "Clinical Questions," "Worth Mentioning," and "Patient Information." Selected images are included in the text to illustrate common clinical conditions. Chapters or sections dealing with uncommon procedures have been abbreviated. Each chapter concludes with a short list of pertinent literature. The book closes with a table listing the cost of common nuclear medicine procedures and a standard index.

SCANS

This section is subdivided into the following six subheadings to allow the clinician to quickly locate the desired information.

A. Background

The background briefly sets the clinical stage for the discussion that follows in the subsequent subheadings.

B. Radiopharmaceuticals

This section reviews the diagnostic or therapeutic radiopharmaceuticals used for each particular scan or procedure. The full name of the radiopharmaceuticals, as well as their common name or abbreviation, are given in this section.

C. How the study is performed

This section describes what will happen to the patient in the nuclear medicine department, how long the study will take and what instrumentation will be used.

D. Patient preparation

Some scans require patient preparation. There may be hydration, diet or medication requirements or restrictions. These are described briefly along with the rationale for the specific requirements or restrictions.

E. Understanding the report

This section explains any terms or measurements that may be included in the final report, places them in the appropriate clinical context and emphasizes the clinical focus of the report.

F. Potential problem

This section addresses any potential problems that may interfere with the performance or interpretation of the study or procedure.

CLINICAL QUESTIONS

This section sequentially reviews each of the clinical questions listed at the beginning of the chapter and discusses the advantages and limitations of nuclear medicine procedures compared with other diagnostic or therapeutic options.

WORTH MENTIONING

This brief section includes information that does not fit into the format of the rest of the chapter and mentions new areas of clinical or basic research that may become clinically applicable.

PATIENT INFORMATION

Patients want to know what to expect when they are referred for a "nuclear" test. To meet this need, the book provides a summary, written for the patient, that outlines the test procedure, the radiation risks and any special hydration, diet or medication requirements for most of the common nuclear medicine diagnostic studies. These summaries may be copied from the book, reviewed by the nuclear medicine practitioner, modified if necessary, incorporated into the physician letterhead and given to patients when the test is scheduled. This approach will allow patients to plan appropriately for their study, minimize unnecessary delays and suboptimal examinations, and alleviate patient anxiety.

Radionuclide therapy may need to be individualized and should be discussed directly with the patient by the physician administering the therapy. For this reason, patient summaries for therapeutic procedures rarely are included. Patient summaries for low-volume procedures have also been omitted.

REFERENCES
The references contain selected readings that review the subject area in more detail, expand on specific topics and support the positions expressed in the chapters.

COST
Cost plays an increasingly important role in the choice of diagnostic tests and therapies. Cost, however, is not equivalent to charge. The charge for any given test or procedure may vary widely. To allow the reader to place costs in a balanced perspective, a table is provided at the end of the book that lists the costs of common nuclear medicine studies as well as the cost of common alternative tests and procedures. These costs are expressed in terms of 1999 Medicare reimbursements.

INDEX
The book concludes with a standard index.

Acknowledgments

We are indebted to the Education and Research Foundation of the Society of Nuclear Medicine for the vision and financial support that made this book possible. We particularly wish to thank Jonathan Masor, MD, for reviewing the book in its entirety and providing us with his insightful and valuable critique. We also are indebted to B. David Collier, MD and Edward B. Silberstein, MD, for their detailed and thoughtful review of multiple chapters and to Kenneth A. McKusick, MD, who prepared the cost analysis in Chapter 29. Finally, we also want to thank the following clinicians and nuclear medicine experts who generously gave their time and expertise to review and critique individual chapters: John Aarsvold, PhD; M. Donald Blaufox, MD, PhD; Eva Dubovsky, MD, PhD; William Fajman, MD; John Froggatt, MD; Julie Furdyna, MD; James Galt, PhD; Raghuveer Halkar, MD; Robert Hendel, MD; Muta Issa, MD; Michael Kipper, MD; Massoud Majd, MD; Hani Nabi, MD; Joe V. Nally, MD; Maria Ribeiro, MD; A. Maziar Zaffari, MD; and Jack Ziffer, MD, PhD. Medicine and nuclear medicine are rapidly evolving fields. During the 2 yr we have been writing this book, we have revised and updated chapters frequently on the basis of new material appearing in the literature and comments from reviewers. The reviewers' suggestions were immensely valuable, but the final chapters have been reviewed only by the authors, and we are responsible for any errors that may be present.

Additional financial support was provided by MedImage Inc.

Dedication

Andrew Taylor and Naomi Alazraki: We would like to dedicate this book to the physicians, scientists, technologists, residents and students with whom we have worked and who have contributed so much to our education.

David M. Schuster: This book is dedicated to my family; to my teachers, including all the technologists and other support staff I have ever worked with; to Nancy for understanding so much; and to all loved and dear ones—past, present, and future.

1
Cardiovascular Diseases

There have been remarkable advances in cardiovascular nuclear medicine during the past 25 yr. The body of literature documenting those advances is probably the most abundant and rich of any clinical imaging field. Techniques to measure and quantitate myocardial perfusion, left ventricular ejection fraction (EF), wall motion and myocardial viability are used widely for diagnosis of coronary artery disease (CAD), significance of anatomic stenosis, myocardial viability and prognosis.

SCANS AND PRIMARY CLINICAL INDICATIONS

I. Myocardial perfusion imaging Page 2

- To diagnose (or exclude) CAD in patients at intermediate or low-intermediate risk for CAD

- To diagnose or exclude CAD for patients at low risk for CAD who have an abnormal or inconclusive stress electro-caridiograph (ECG) examination

- To diagnose CAD in patients presenting in the emergency room (ER) with acute chest pain and are found to have a normal or inconclusive ECG

- To assess cardiac risk for preoperative patients having major surgery who are at risk for CAD

- To determine hemodynamic significance of borderline coronary stenosis and appropriateness of revascularization in patients who have had coronary angiography

1

CLINICAL QUESTIONS

PATIENT INFORMATION

SCANS

I. MYOCARDIAL PERFUSION IMAGING

A. Background

Myocardial perfusion images show the distribution of radiopharmaceuticals, which are extracted rapidly from the coronary artery blood into myocardium in proportion to myocardial perfusion (Fig. 1). Combined with exercise or pharmacologic stress, myocardial perfusion imaging (stress and rest) is the most widely used nuclear cardiology procedure. Exercise increases myocardial oxygen demand; in response, cardiac output increases, and the coronary vessels dilate to satisfy the myocardium's increased oxygen needs by allowing coronary artery blood flow to increase. If there is significant coronary artery stenosis due to atherosclerosis, the diseased vessel cannot dilate adequately as do the normal vessels. Therefore, during stress physiology, the myocardium supplied by a stenosed vessel does not receive as much perfusion as the myocardium supplied by normal vessels, and images show relative count deficiency, reflecting relatively decreased perfusion of the myocardial region supplied by the diseased coronary artery. The location of a myocardial defect usually correlates to the predictable vascular anatomy, although vascular anatomic variations are not uncommon.

Thallium myocardial perfusion imaging was performed for many years using planar imaging, but today single-photon emission computed tomography (SPECT) has become the dominant imaging technology because of its superior image contrast and better localization of perfusion abnormalities. Algorithms to perform electrocardiographic gated SPECT imaging are widely available; images displayed as a cine show myocardial wall motion or wall thickening and can be processed to calculate left ventricular ejection fraction (LVEF).

B. Radiopharmaceuticals

1. Thallium-201 chloride. Thallium-201, injected intravenously, is extracted efficiently from the blood into myocardial cells (extraction fraction ~80%) by active transport mechanisms dependent on metabolic integrity of the sodium-postassium–adenosine triphosphatase pump. Only about 3–6% of the injected dose accumulates in the myocardium, depending on whether the study is conducted in a stressed or resting patient. If thallium is injected during maximum stress (i.e., treadmill exercise), its distribution on images started 5 min after injection reflects myocardial perfusion (therefore, coronary artery blood flow) at the time of injection (maximum stress). With time, thallium washes out of cells, while simultaneously continuing to be actively transported from the blood into the myocardium, resulting in the process known as redistribution. The behavioral characteristics of thallium make it an excellent agent for perfusion and the preferred SPECT agent for viability imaging (discussed later).

2. Technetium-99m sestamibi (Cardiolite) and tetrofosmin (Myoview). These are the technetium-labeled myocardial perfusion-imaging radiopharmaceuticals available in the United States. A third radiopharmaceutical, ^{99m}Tc-Teboroxime, is not available commercially in the United States at this time (2000). Sestamibi and tetrofosmin do not wash out from myocardial cells rapidly as does thallium, but enter the myocardial cells where they remain relatively fixed for hours, providing an image of myocardial perfusion at the time of the injection. The efficiency of extraction from blood by myocardial cells is lower for sestamibi or tetrofosmin

1

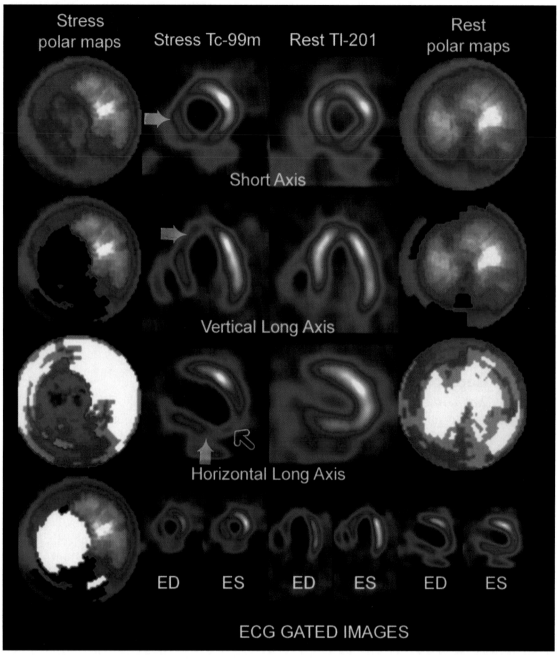

Figure 1.

than for thallium, but because higher doses can be administered with no more radiation to the patient than from a much smaller thallium dose, many more counts are imaged with technetium, giving superior images. Gating the images to the ECG is easily done for viewing as a cine of the beating myocardium.

Figure 1. Dual-isotope stress/rest myocardial perfusion study. SPECT images (two central vertical rows labeled stress technetium [Tc]-99m and rest thallium [Tl]-201) are shown in three projections: short axis (top), vertical long axis (middle) and horizontal long axis (bottom). Images show stress perfusion defects (arrows) involving the septal (short axis), anteroseptal (vertical long axis), apical and inferior walls (horizontal long axis). The perfusion defects normalize on rest thallium images, indicating ischemia. The polar maps,* also called bull's eye plots (first column is stress, and fourth column is rest), show the same stress perfusion deficits that are seen on images. The stress raw data (top left), black-out (second from top left) and standard deviation maps (third from top left) indicate severe count (perfusion) deficits, and the reversibility (white-out of the defect) map (bottom, first column) indicates complete normalization (reversibility) of the defect at rest. The rest polar maps (fourth column) are normal. Bottom row shows gated images of end diastolic (ED) and end systolic (ES) frames from each image set: short axis, horizontal long axis and vertical long axis. There is minimal hypokinesis of the septal and apical walls, consistent with ischemic myocardium. The measured global ejection fraction for this patient was 50% (normal). The technetium agents used for stress images, sestamibi and tetrofosmin, would provide comparable images.

  *Polar maps, or bull's eye plots, are two-dimentional displays of the counts recorded at each pixel location corresponding to a precise anatomic location in the left ventricular myocardium. In the polar map display, the apex is at the center and myocardium is arranged in concentric circles (short axis slices) progressing from the apex to the base. The counts are color-coded (white is the highest count-pixel, and green-black is the lowest count-pixel). The black-out map blackens each pixel in which the counts detected fall below the mean value of the comparable pixel in a gender-matched file of normal individuals, called the normal file, by more than 2.5 standard deviation units. The standard deviation map color-codes each pixel to show the number of standard deviation units below the mean normal. The reversibility map shows white at each pixel that was black on the black-out map if significant normalization of counts occurred on the rest images at that pixel location.

---

3. Rubidium-82. This positron emitter has a 2-min physical half-life; it can be imaged only by a positron emission tomography (PET) instrument. It is supplied from a generator that is purchased monthly and is expensive ($26,000 per month). Stress imaging can be done only with pharmacologic stress.

C. How myocardial perfusion imaging is performed

Exercise testing is usually performed with treadmill exercise. Patients who are unable to use the treadmill or unable to achieve 85% of maximum predicted heart rate on the treadmill are given pharmacologic stress using intravenous (IV) dipyridamole or adenosine, which dilate the coronary arteries and pharmacologically increase myocardial blood flow. Stenotic vessels are unable to dilate and are detected as areas of relative hypoperfusion. In cases in which pharmacologic stress agents are inappropriate because of restrictive lung diseases such as asthma (dipyridamole and adenosine may cause or exacerbate bronchoconstriction in patients who are wheezing) or an inability to tolerate withdrawal of theophylline for 2 days (theophylline interferes with vasodilatation by adenosine or dipyridamole), dobutamine stress can be performed. The radionuclide is administered at peak stress. Dipyridamole infusion is generally over a 5-min period, with thallium or technetium administered immediately after the dipyridamole infusion; adenosine is infused over 3–6 min, and the radiopharmaceutical is given at 2–3 min by separate IV access. Dobutamine is administered in a stepwise fashion, increasing the dose from 5 μg/kg to a maximum of 50 μg/kg in 3-min stages. Atropine may be used to further increase heart rate.

  Common protocols used for myocardial perfusion imaging are listed and described below.

> 1) Thallium stress—redistribution, followed by reinjection rest thallium
> 2) Technetium stress—technetium rest
> 3) Dual isotope: Thallium rest—technetium stress

      4) Rest thallium—delayed rest thallium (up to 24 hr)
      5) Rest rubidium—pharmacologic stress rubidium (PET)

*1. Thallium stress—redistribution, followed by reinjection rest thallium (as warranted).*The patient exercises on a treadmill and thallium is injected at peak stress followed in 5–10 min by imaging that takes about 12–25 min. The patient returns 2.5–3 hr later for redistribution imaging or for rest reinjection of thallium (smaller dose than before), followed 30 min later by the second imaging. Some centers perform reinjection only if redistribution images show fixed defects. Total time (maximum) for the patient is approximately 4 hr. The patient is free to eat or leave the department during the 2.5 hr between the stress examination and the rest scan. The reinjection of thallium at rest enhances the counts in the image, representing resting perfusion, and usually shows filling-in of a stress perfusion defect if the affected myocardium is ischemic and not infarcted. Sometimes it takes many hours of redistribution for thallium uptake in severely hypoxic but viable myocardium (i.e., hibernating or stunned myocardium) to be visualized on images, and delayed imaging of thallium up to 24 hr may be useful in confirming viability of myocardium.

2. Technetium (sestamibi or tetrofosmin) stress—technetium rest. Intravenous injections are performed at peak stress and at rest, each followed by imaging. The time required for the study is about 1 hr less than the thallium protocol above. Stress and rest images can be gated to give LVEF, wall motion and wall thickening. All stress technetium gated-perfusion protocols (also 3, below) have been described as one-stop shopping, i.e., they provide assessment of left ventricular function as well as perfusion.

3. Dual isotope: thallium rest—technetium stress. Rest thallium is followed by stress sestamibi or tetrofosmin. The total time required is approximately 2 hr shorter for this protocol than for the thallium protocol above. The technetium agents are gated easily to the ECG so that wall motion, wall thickening, and LVEF can be determined as well as myocardial perfusion. Recently, some programs for thallium gated acquisition have become available.

4. Rest thallium—delayed rest (redistribution) thallium (up to 24 hr). The best SPECT imaging protocol for assessing myocardial viability is thallium imaging at 30 min after rest injection, followed by delayed imaging at several hours, up to 24 hr (see viability discussion, FDG metabolic scans, below, and Clinical Question 5).

5. Rest rubidium—pharmacologic stress rubidium (PET). A rest injection of rubidium followed by rapid imaging takes about 2–4 min. Emission rubidium imaging is preceded by a transmission image (about 3–20 min) to map tissue attenuation parameters used to correct rubidium images for tissue attenuation. Pharmacologic stress rubidium (using dipyridamole or adenosine) requires less patient time than SPECT myocardial perfusion studies (thallium or technetium). Dipyridamole or adenosine infusion (about 5–6 min) and rubidium injection are immediately followed with a rapid emission acquisition (2–4 min) by the PET camera. Thus, total patient time is about 30–40 min.

D. Patient preparation

1) Patients need to be carefully instructed to fast from midnight before the examination (water is permitted).
2) Patients should refrain from caffeine-containing food and drink for 24 hr because he or she may require dipyridamole or adenosine stress.
3) Withhold theophylline-containing medications for 2 days, if possible. (The caffeine and theophylline restrictions apply to patients who are having pharmacologic stress because caffeine and theophylline negate the vasodilatory action of dipyridamole and adenosine. However, those scheduled for exercise stress testing also should avoid caffeine/theophylline because they may be unable to reach their predicted maximum heart rate on treadmill stress and may require pharmacologic stress.)
4) Beta-blockers and nitrates should be withheld unless the purpose of the test is to assess the ability of the beta-blocker or the nitrates to control symptoms at the levels of treadmill stress achieved during the test.
5) If left bundle branch block (LBBB) exists, pharmacologic stress is preferred over treadmill stress to minimize artifactual appearance of ischemia in the septal wall.
6) Patients should avoid taking Viagra (sildenafil) for 48 hr before the study in case nitroglycerin is needed to counteract ischemia resulting from the stress examination. Nitroglycerin given to patients on Viagra can cause serious (even fatal) hypotension.

E. Understanding the report

The report may summarize the patient's clinical problems that led to the request for the nuclear medicine test and describe the myocardial perfusion imaging procedure, including the radiopharmaceutical used, the dose, the physiologic conditions of the patient at the time of injection and the route of injection. The report may also summarize treadmill or pharmacologic stress, blood pressure, heart rate and presence of chest pain or discomfort. Although a separate stress ECG report often is issued, the nuclear medicine report frequently summarizes those results, including ECG abnormalities, reactions to pharmacologic agents and interventions administered. The number of stress perfusion defects, the size (extent), the severity and the anatomic distribution of each defect are reported, and findings such as transient ischemic dilation, increased uptake of the tracer in the lungs and others that indicate that the patient is at high risk for subsequent cardiac events (see Clinical Question 10) are noted. When ECG gating has been done, the report will indicate left ventricular regional and global function analysis. In summary, the report is an integration of all the findings, recognizing artifacts and concluding with a diagnostic impression.

F. Potential problems

1. False-positive and false-negative results: is there a gold standard? Sensitivity and specificity of the myocardial perfusion study historically has been based on whether a coronary artery stenosis ($\geq$50% as seen on a coronary arteriogram) may or may not cause hemodynamic deficits at physiologic stress levels. If the scan is normal, it may be labeled "false negative" when in fact it is telling a physiologic truth, while the arteriogram is telling an anatomic truth. In addition, there are recognized problems of interobserver variability in determining the exact percent stenosis on an arteriogram; because only the internal border of the artery is seen with no marker of the outside margin, percent stenosis can be misjudged. Furthemore, in clinical practice, patients are sometimes referred for stress myocardial perfusion imaging after catheterization to determine if a 45–65% stenosis is hemodyamically significant, thereby using the physiologic test to judge the anatomic test's significance. Therefore, "false positive" and "false negative" may sometimes be misleading labels. Finally, a myocardial perfusion deficit reflects perfusion at the cellular level, which may or may not be related to a 50% stenosis of the relevant coronary artery. Other causes for mismatches between the perfusion images and arteriography include stress-induced coronary artery spasm, diffuse coronary artery narrowing, cardiomyopathic disease, anomalies such as coronary artery bridging, small-vessel disease (not seen on arteriograms) and technical artifacts such as attenuation and motion.

2. Selection/verification bias falsely decreases specificity. Specificity can be falsely diminished by the bias in patient selection. This occurs when results from the nuclear scan influence access to the gold standard (catheterization), which in turn, is used to verify the results of the nuclear scan. Because the gold standard is the coronary arteriogram, only those patients who are referred for coronary arteriography are included in studies to determine the accuracy (sensitivity and specificity) of the myocardial perfusion study. For example, 1000 patients have myocardial perfusion studies. Of them, 500 have normal scans, and 500 have abnormal scans leading to cardiac catheterization. Of the 500 who have catheterization, 400 have coronary artery stenosis >50%. Using only the catheterization results as the gold standard, the specificity—TN $\div$ (TN + FP), where TN = true negative and FP = false positive—of the perfusion scan would be 0 $\div$ (0 + 100), or 0%. If the 500 who did not undergo catheterization because they were presumed normal had been included as normal, the specificity would improve to 83%, 500 $\div$ (500 + 100).

To address this problem of selection/verification bias, some investigators have used a normalcy rate, i.e., specificity is based on a population with <5% probability of CAD that did not have cardiac catheterization, but had myocardial perfusion scans. The normalcy rate for SPECT myocardial perfusion studies is reported to range from 85% to 95%. Test verification bias also artifactually increases sensitivity. Using the above example of 1000 patients, the measured sensitivity would be TP ÷ (TP + FN) = 400/400 = 100%, where TP = true positive and FN = false negative.

3. Submaximal stress. If the patient does not achieve 85% of maximum predicted heart rate during treadmill stress, the sensitivity of the myocardial perfusion study may be reduced compared with maximal stress. The study can be converted to pharmacologic stress using dipyridamole or adenosine. Patients who cannot stress on a treadmill or who have lung disease and cannot tolerate discontinuing theopylline can be stressed using dobutamine.

4. Patient motion. Motion during the study may cause artifacts, necessitating repeat imaging or reducing the specificity of the scan interpretation.

5. Attenuation artifacts from diaphragm in men and from breasts in women. Photon attenuation by soft tissues (breasts overlying the anterior wall myocardium in women and diaphragm interfering with the inferior wall counts in men) has been the major source of artifacts in SPECT myocardial perfusion studies. Hardware and software algorithms to correct for soft-tissue attenuation have been introduced by manufacturers, but they continue to be further refined and validated. Quantitative software that compares the patient's counts to a normal file also can assist the interpreter in distinguishing attenuation from coronary disease. One advantage of PET imaging is that attenuation correction is widely available for PET.

II. FDG METABOLIC SCANS
A. Background
Myocardial cells metabolize fatty acid and glucose, but ischemic myocardium preferentially uses glucose as an energy substrate. Therefore, the glucose analog, fluorodeoxyglucose (FDG) is effective for imaging the ischemic myocardium of patients with CAD. Additional information about FDG can be found in chapter 15, Introduction to Cancer and FDG Imaging.

B. Radiopharmaceuticals
Fluorine (F)-18 FDG is a glucose analog labeled with cyclotron-produced ^{18}F, which has a 118-min physical half-life. FDG is transported from the blood to myocardial cells where it is phosphorylated; it is not further metabolized and is trapped in the myocardial cells, which allows imaging to proceed without significant changes in radiotracer levels in the heart muscle during the image acquisition. The images reflect glucose use (uptake) by myocardial cells; glucose

uptake requires cellular metabolic integrity, which indicates viable myocardium. Thallium-201 rest/delayed redistribution imaging (see discussion above) is also used widely to assess viability.

C. How the FDG scan is performed

The patient is given either an oral glucose load to stimulate insulin secretion or a standardized infusion of glucose, insulin and potassium based on body weight. Insulin inhibits the release of fatty acids from adipose tissue and reduces the level of fatty acids in the plasma, and this stimulates the heart to use glucose rather than fatty acids as an energy substrate. Following the glucose load, the patient receives an IV injection of 6–12 mCi (172–444 MBq) of FDG. Imaging begins approximately 45 min to 1 hr later, so that FDG myocardial uptake can reach a favorable level.

FDG can be imaged by conventional PET, SPECT cameras equipped with special high-energy collimators or coincidence SPECT cameras. Total patient time including equilibration can range from 1.5 to 2.5 hr for an FDG heart scan.

There is a protocol to image sestamibi or tetrofosmin stress perfusion and resting FDG metabolism simultaneously, using a SPECT camera with high-energy collimation. This protocol requires specially designed collimators and is not widely available.

D. Patient preparation

The patient needs to be fasting (water is permitted) after midnight before the FDG study. Caffeine products should be discontinued for 24 hr, and theophylline discontinued for 2 days so that pharmacologic stress perfusion imaging can be performed in addition to the metabolic FDG scan, if ordered.

E. Understanding the report

The report describes the procedure used for FDG imaging. Because FDG is the imaging gold standard for myocardial viability, absent or markedly reduced myocardial FDG uptake (<50% relative to a normal region of myocardium) indicates nonviability. The applicable perfusion pattern (Fig. 2, Table 1) is described in the report.

F. Potential problems

1. Serum glucose levels and myocardial cell accumulation of glucose. Uptake of FDG by myocardial cells may be altered misleadingly if serum glucose is not at the desired level (~120 mg/dl). Diabetic patients present problems for titrating the serum glucose levels adequately. Thus, the protocol for FDG imaging may not be optimal in diabetic patients. Use of the hyperinsulinemic-euglycemic clamp or pretreatment with nicotinic acid derivatives may improve image quality and viability assessment for diabetic patients. Pretreatment with nicotinic acid also may result in requirement for increased insulin.

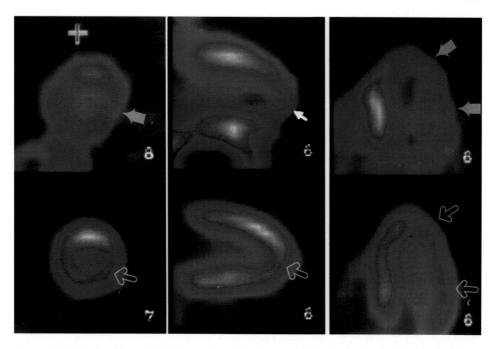

Figure 2. Rubidium perfusion and FDG metabolism PET viability study. Rubidium images (top row), performed with dipyridamole stress, show a perfusion deficit in the apex and lateral wall (arrows). FDG images (bottom row) show normal metabolism in those regions (open arrows) indicating myocardial viability. This pattern is consistent with hibernating or stunned myocardium. It also can be seen with uncomplicated ischemic myocardium.

2. Heterogeneity of FDG myocardial uptake. In healthy volunteers, heterogeneous myocardial FDG uptake has been described, depending on their fasting versus fed status. Regional myocardial variations in glucose metabolism can be a potential problem for interpretation.

Table I. Evaluation of Viability Based on Paired Perfusion (Rb, Tl, Tc) and Metabolism (FDG) Imaging

	Perfusion	Metabolism	Viability
Normal (matched)	Normal	Normal	Yes
Scar (matched)	Reduced	Reduced	Yes, if mild reduction No, depending on severity
Ischemia/Stunning/ Hibernating (mismatched)	Reduced	Normal or increased	Yes

3. Borderline FDG myocardial uptake. A quantitative (or semiquantitative) estimate of FDG in the abnormal myocardium helps assess likelihood of viability. A
borderline 50% level of FDG (compared with the most normal region of FDG
uptake in the left ventricle [LV] wall) indicates some viability but restoration of
LV function after revascularization can't be predicted with confidence when
there is borderline FDG uptake.

III. MUGA OR GATED BLOOD POOL IMAGING

A. Background

The MUGA scan (also commonly known as radionuclide ventriculography) is
considered the gold standard for calculation of LVEF. The MUGA scan consists
of gamma camera images of the labeled blood within the chambers of the heart
gated to the patient's ECG. The images are viewed as a cine on the computer
screen, giving the viewer information about wall motion. Quantification of EF
assumes that changes in chamber volume are comparable to changes in counts
detected by the camera (Fig. 3). Myocardial infarct, pericardial effusion, ventricular apical aneurysm, posterior basal wall aneurysm, endothelial thrombi
mass or left atrial myxoma defect sometimes can be identified on MUGA images
(see First Pass Angiocardiography, background, below).

B. Radiopharmaceuticals

Technetium-99m autologous red blood cells are labeled by in vitro (kit), in
"vivtro" or in vivo methods. In vivo means that a sample of the patient's blood
is withdrawn from a vein, labeled to technetium in a test tube and reinjected. In
vivtro is a combination of in vivo and in vitro: The patient's blood is withdrawn
from a vein into a syringe that contains technetium and the chelating agent,
which attaches to the red cells so that they can bind the technetium. After a brief
incubation period, the labeled blood is reinjected from the syringe. In vivo labeling of the red cells is achieved by injecting the chelating agent intravenously (to
complex with red blood cells), followed a few minutes later by injecting ^{99m}Tc.
The in vivo labeling method is the simplest and easiest but the in vitro kit gives
the best labeling and image quality; the in vivtro method is intermediate in
labeling efficiency and image quality.

C. How the gated blood pool scan is performed

After the patient's red cells are labeled with 10–20 mCi (370–740 MBq, adult
dose) technetium, images are acquired with ECG gating. The electrocardio-
graph R-to-R interval is divided into 8 to 24 frames; each frame becomes an
image of $\frac{1}{8}$ to $\frac{1}{24}$ of the cardiac cycle and is formed from the summation of multiple beats over a 5- to 7-min period; the successive frames can be displayed as a

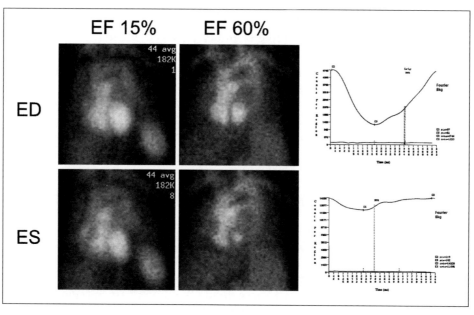

Figure 3. Gated blood pool study. Two gated blood pool studies are shown in left anterior oblique projections, including an end diastolic (ED) frame (top row) and an end systolic (ES) frame (bottom row). The patient, whose images are shown in the right column, is normal (EF 60%); note the symmetrically contracted left ventricle (LV) chamber of the end systolic frame. In contrast, the patient, whose images are shown in the left column, is abnormal (EF 15%), showing global severe hypokinesis and ventricular dilation, particularly of the LV. These images show blood pool in the cardiac chambers, aorta and pulmonary artery (seen well in right column). Note the enlarged spleen in the abnormal patient (left column). Gated blood pool count histograms (far right column), plot of counts (y-axis) versus time (x-axis) over one composite cardiac cycle (approximately 1 min for 60 bpm), plotted at 40-msec intervals are shown at far right. The count histogram (ECG volume curve equivalent) shows a normal EF 60% (top) and abnormal EF 15% (bottom) corresponding to the gated blood pool images.

cine of the beating heart. Patients may be imaged in several projections. The procedure takes about 30–40 min.

D. Patient preparation

There is no special patient preparation needed for this test. The test is usually done at rest, but it is possible to do this test during supine bicycle or treadmill stress if special equipment is available. In that case, the patient should be fasting for about 4 hr prior to the study.

E. Understanding the report

The important information provided by a resting MUGA includes the following: 1) the EF, which can be performed serially to monitor cardiac function; 2) regional wall motion impairment, which usually correlates with regional myocardial damage or infarction; 3) the size of the LV and right ventricle (RV); and 4) overall quality of contractions of the chambers. If done during stress and rest, an increase of 5–7 percentage points in LVEF at stress provides strong evidence against CAD.

F. Potential problems

1. Chamber enlargements. Multiple chamber enlargement may result in overlapping of chamber blood pools on the images in all projections, diminishing the accuracy of the EF measurements. This can be minimized by adjustments to the camera projection and tilt.

2. Commercial software for EF calculations. It is advisable to follow serial EFs for a given patient using the same equipment and software to eliminate the variabilities introduced into the EF determination by equipment and software differences.

IV. FIRST PASS ANGIOCARDIOGRAPHY

A. Background

First pass angiocardiography is a dynamic series of images of the tracer as it flows sequentially from the vena cava into the right atrium, RV, pulmonary arteries and lungs, left atrium, LV, aorta and great vessels. The LV can be temporally separated from overlapping activity in other chambers. A region of interest (ROI) is mapped over the LV, and a background ROI is placed lateral to the LV. Background corrected counts in the LV end diastolic (LVED) and LV end systolic (LVES) images are then determined. EF is calculated for both first pass and MUGA studies according to the following formula: LVEF = (LVED counts – LVES counts)/LVED counts.

In the pediatric population, congenital anomalous vascular pathways can be identified, as well as shunts. Left-to-right shunts can be calculated from a count-based Qp:Qs (pulmonary to systemic flow ratio), which is extracted from the appearance and disappearance of the tracer as it passes through an ROI placed over the lungs. Using gamma variate curve fitting algorithms, Qp and Qs are determined.

B. Radiopharmaceuticals

Technetium-99m diethylenetriamine pentaacetic acid (DTPA), a glomerular filtered renal imaging agent, is the most widely used agent, although there are many appropriate ^{99m}Tc radiopharmaceuticals that can be used for a first pass cardiac study.

C. How the first pass scan is performed

The technetium radiopharmaceutical (10–20 mCi [370–740 MBq] adult dose) is injected as a bolus through a peripheral vein and is typically imaged at 40 frames per second as it passes through the heart and lungs.

D. Patient preparation

There is no special patient preparation needed for this test. There are no dietary or medication restrictions for a resting study. It is possible to do this test during bicycle or treadmill stress if special equipment is available. In that case, some recommend that the patient should be fasting for about 4 hr prior to the study.

E. Understanding the report

This report provides the LVEF. Because the first pass study typically is acquired in only one view, information on wall motion is not as complete as with gated SPECT or MUGA. The first pass study can provide the same information as the gated blood pool study, but specialized, high-count efficient instrumentation (multicrystal camera) is preferred to perform first pass studies reliably. The first pass study is quicker to perform and process. If it is a resting study, the patient can leave the department within about 10 min of starting the procedure. The test is performed successfully during bicycle or treadmill stress with multicrystal scintillation cameras capable of ultra-high counting rates and motion corrections by tracking anatomic locations pixel by pixel during multiple-image frame acquisitions while the patient stresses.

F. Potential problems

1. RVEF. Although there is considerable experience with first pass LVEF determinations, there is much less experience with RVEF determinations. The test may not be available, and accuracy is lower.

2. Stress first pass requires specialized equipment. See Patient Preparation, above.

CLINICAL QUESTIONS

1. Does an asymptomatic patient with multiple risk factors have CAD?

The first test is ECG. Additional screening tests for patients with risk factors for CAD include a stress ECG examination, an ultra-fast computed tomography (CT) scan to identify the presence of coronary calcifications that are associated with CAD, a myocardial perfusion imaging study, or a stress/dobutamine echocardiogram. A positive finding on either of the first two tests often leads to a stress myocardial perfusion examination to identify CAD and, if present, to determine the extent, severity and anatomic location of CAD and the patient's prognostic assessment. Patients who are unable to stress adequately on a treadmill, including women who may have less reliable stress ECG performance, can be referred for a myocardial perfusion pharmacologic stress examination instead of the routine stress ECG.

Ultrafast CT (electron beam CT). Sensitivity for coronary calcification detected by ultrafast CT exceeds 90%; specificity is 40–50%. Older people often have calcific deposits without CAD, and detection of smaller calcific deposits, more likely present in younger men and women who may have CAD, is more problemat-

1

ic to quantitate accurately. Overall, the presence and amount of calcium detected on electron beam CT (EBCT) appears to correlate with the presence and associated amount of atherosclerotic plaque. But the variability in detected calcium quantity is such that serial measurements to assess an individual's progression or regression of disease are unreliable. EBCT is not available widely, and therefore, its applicability is limited.

Stress echocardiography. Stress two-dimensional (2D) echocardiography is used to detect CAD by eliciting a wall-motion abnormality. LVEF usually is estimated but can be measured using an area-length measurement at end diastole and end systole; however, in the absence of a contrast agent, it is difficult to see the LV endocardial borders.

Stress is performed by dobutamine pharmacologic stress or treadmill exercise. Wall-motion abnormality indicates ischemia; images are obtained during peak stress (dobutamine) or afterward (treadmill exercise). The 2D echocardiogram images are obtained soon after termination of the treadmill exercise because patient motion during exercise interferes with image quality. If treadmill exercise is used, there is likely underestimation of extent and severity of ischemia because the measurement (imaging) actually is made after a sudden decrease in the double product achieved during exercise.

The sensitivity of exercise and dobutamine 2D echocardiography is somewhat lower than that of SPECT myocardial perfusion imaging, especially for accurate characterization of multi-vessel disease and diagnosis of CAD for patients with single-vessel disease. Cost of the echocardiography procedure is lower than that of myocardial perfusion imaging, although addition of new echocardiography contrast agents will increase the costs. In addition to CAD, echocardiography gives information on valvular anatomy and diastolic dysfunction to guide use of drugs (for example, calcium channel blockers for diastolic dysfunction and angiotensin-converting enzyme [ACE] for most other valvular abnormalities). Echocardiography also can guide the need for surgery for aortic stenosis/insufficiency and mitral stenosis/regurgitation, as well as the need for bacterial endocarditis prophylaxis.

Coronary angiography. Coronary angiography, the gold standard for CAD detection, is expensive, invasive and provides anatomic, not physiologic, information about the disease. There is no incremental prognostic gain over the stress myocardial perfusion study from a coronary angiogram for the present or the short-term (6–12 mo) future. The coronary angiogram is necessary for planning the most appropriate revascularization procedure, either as bypass surgery or percutaneous angioplasty. The presence of luminal irregularities, which are not hemodynamically significant, is a risk factor and may be a potential forerunner for progression to serious CAD; these are diagnosed only by angiography.

Clinical cost-effectiveness studies show that particularly for patients with pretest low–intermediate level probabilities for CAD, the stress myocardial perfusion study should be done and followed by coronary angiography (cardiac catheterization) only if warranted by an abnormal perfusion study. Stress myocardial perfusion imaging is appropriate for preoperative assessment of cardiac risk (see below) and to alleviate concerns of patients with risk factors who are experiencing atypical chest pain. Asymptomatic patients with risk factors and some patients with atypical chest pain can be screened using stress ECG, or ultra-fast CT, if available. The stress ECG test is associated with generally lower sensitivities for detecting CAD, ranging from 35–40% for single-vessel disease to 62–67% for two-vessel disease and to 73–86% for three-vessel disease. If abnormal, these screening tests should be followed by a stress myocardial perfusion study.

2. Does a patient presenting with atypical chest pain have CAD?

Patients presenting with atypical chest pain should be evaluated with careful history and physical examination. A gastrointestinal cause for atypical chest pain may be apparent without need for cardiac workup. Presence of risk factors for CAD (hyperlipidemia, hypertension, etc.) enhance the need for further testing. In any case, if the patient's anxiety is sufficiently high or disruptive, noninvasive testing to provide peace of mind if CAD is absent, as usually is the case, or appropriate therapy if indeed CAD is present, is more compelling. An ECG would be followed by either a stress ECG test, an ultra-fast CT scan for coronary calcification (if available) or a stress myocardial perfusion study. If either of the first two tests is abnormal, a stress myocardial perfusion scan or dobutamine stress echocardiogram would follow.

3. Is a patient with acute chest pain but nondiagnostic ECG having an infarct?

In acute chest pain patients, prognostic-outcomes data show that normal or near normal myocardial perfusion scans are associated with a subsequent event rate of about 1% per year and zero deaths over the ensuing 30 days. Patients with known CAD and prior revascularization procedures have low risk for cardiac events if their perfusion scans are normal. In contrast, abnormal perfusion scans with ischemic stress defects (which reverse at rest) have high incidences of subsequent cardiac events during the following year. (See Clinical Question 10).

Nuclear imaging can cost-effectively assist in the triage of patients with acute chest pain presenting in the ER. If the myocardial perfusion scan shows a perfusion deficit, the patient should be admitted with a diagnosis of CAD and possible evolving myocardial infarct. If the scan is normal, the patient can be discharged to outpatient care, saving the costs of an unnecessary hospital admission. The patient is injected with the radiotracer in the ER while chest pain is present; at some centers, doses can be prepared and stored for ER use at any time. The patient will be stabilized and imaged later, if necessary, because the technetium images show perfusion in myocardium at the time of the injection for up to several hours, but usually the scan is completed within 1–2 hr of presentation in the ER. Serum markers, e.g., troponin, do not become significantly elevated in 100% of true infarctions until >6 hr after an event, which compromises or delays effective thrombolytic therapeutic intervention. At 4 hr, only 50% of acute myocardial infarction (MI) patients have significantly elevated troponin, and increased creatine kinase or phosphokinase; myoglobin serum levels take much longer to become elevated. Cost-effectiveness studies show that savings of $757–$883 per patient were realized when the myocardial perfusion scan was used to decide on hospital admission versus discharge to home.

If the patient has suffered an MI in the past, a perfusion defect also may be present from that remote infarction. If the location of the previous infarct is known, this will assist in distinguishing a new defect in another location. Later rest imaging, or later troponin serum marker results, may assist in evaluating the significance of a myocardial defect in a patient with a prior MI. An acute ischemic defect that has not progressed to infarct will reverse (normalize) on a resting scan performed at a later time in the absence of ischemic chest pain.

Patients who present in the ER with chest pain and normal or nondiagnostic ECG should have a myocardial perfusion scan with sestamibi or tetrofosmin. If the scan is normal, the patient can be discharged; if the scan is abnormal, the patient needs to be admitted for appropriate therapy for CAD and possible evolving infarct.

4. How do I evaluate and cost-effectively manage my patient with stable angina?

There is wide variation in practice patterns for evaluating patients with stable angina. The major options include noninvasive diagnostic workup (treadmill ECG, stress myocardial perfusion imaging or dobutamine echocardiography) followed by cardiac catheterization and revascularization, versus direct cardiac catheterization and revascularization. A large prospective study of >11,000 consecutive stable angina patients recently showed that an initial stress myocardial perfusion imaging strategy followed by selective cardiac catheterization, compared with the direct cardiac catheterization strategy, resulted in 30–40% lower costs of care for patients at all levels of pretest clinical risk (low, intermediate and high) over a 3-yr period. Outcomes measures of cardiac death and MI over 3 yr of follow-up were the same for both groups. This study indicates that the less invasive, lower morbidity, less expensive diagnostic evaluation strategy for the individual patient with stable angina also saves health care dollars on a larger scale.

5. Is a borderline coronary artery stenosis hemodynamically significant (i.e., likely to be responsible for or contributing to the patient's symptoms)?

Coronary angiograms (performed at rest) show anatomic narrowing of vessels that may or may not correlate with true flow impairments at stress. The hemodynamic significance of a lesion can be demonstrated by stress-induced reversible myocardial perfusion deficit in the region corresponding to the stenosed vessel's myocardial territory. If no stress perfusion deficit is elicited, the lesion is not hemodynamically significant, i.e., does not warrant revascularization, and the prognosis is good (cardiac event rate of <1% per year, which is the same as in age-matched asymptomatic controls).

6. Surgical risk: Is the patient's cardiac status adequate to tolerate major surgery?

Patients who are scheduled for major surgery and who have a family history for CAD and/or other risk factors, even if asymptomatic, may be at high risk for a cardiac event. A large stress perfusion defect that normalizes at rest (Fig. 1) on a myocardial perfusion scan carries a high risk of perisurgical event. Depending on extent, severity and location of a defect, the patient may be sent for cardiac catheterization and revascularization before the scheduled surgery (presuming it is nonemergent).

Published data indicate a positive predictive value of thallium studies of 30%, as correlated with cardiac events, and a negative predictive value of 98%. Thus, a negative (normal) scan is an excellent indicator of very low likelihood of perioperative cardiac events, whereas an abnormal scan greatly increases the risk for cardiac events, even though most patients with positive scans escape having a cardiac event. Noninvasive screening (myocardial perfusion, dobutamine echocardiography) is incrementally cost-effective compared with no preoperative risk assessment for patients 60 yr of age or older.

7. Myocardial viability: Will revascularization restore function?

Patients with an LVEF of 30% or lower are high surgical risks and should not be subjected to the risk of revascularization if the myocardium supplied by stenotic vessels is not viable. For this reason, it is important to distinguish between nonviable and viable (hibernating or stunned) myocardium.

Hibernating myocardium is a chronic state of diminished myocardial perfusion, presumably a type of defense mechanism of the myocardium to minimize its work and energy expenditure and preserve myocardial viability. Stunning is a more acute form of decreased perfusion and function, a reaction to a shock-inducing event such as one or multiple episodes of ischemia (Fig. 2); stunning occurs despite restoration of myocardial blood flow. Hibernating or stunned myocardium can mimic nonviability by showing severe hypokinesis and perfusion deficit that appears to be fixed on conventional rest imaging. Rest thallium with delayed (24 hr) imaging is almost as accurate (~90% concordance) as the gold standard, FDG imaging, and usually can answer the viability question, if FDG is unavailable.

8. Congestive heart failure: Is CAD the cause?

CAD is the underlying cause of congestive heart failure in 80% of patients. Patients presenting with congestive heart failure should be evaluated with a noninvasive imaging study to assess LVEF, i.e., gated blood pool, gated technetium myocardial perfusion study or echocardiography. Echocardiography measures the LV long axis and short axis to calculate the volume of an ellipse at end systole and end diastole. An accurate measurement of LVEF can be compromised because visualization of the endocardial walls is often difficult or incomplete, and the LV chamber shape is not always shaped like an ellipse. Furthemore, adequate echocardiographic visualization of the LV may be impossible in patients with hyperaerated lungs, i.e., chronic obstructive pulmonary disease, asthma, etc. Use of echocardiographic contrast agents, after U.S. Food and Drug Administration approval, will help with visualization of endocardial walls, at some increase in the cost. As mentioned in Clinical Question 1, above, echocardiography also gives information about valvular function, which may be relevant for patients with congestive failure.

Of the three tests discussed, the gated blood pool and echocardiography are lower in cost. But, because CAD is present so often, the myocardial perfusion study, providing perfusion and functional data, as well as prognosis, is a powerful tool to assess patients with congestive heart failure.

9. Cardiomyopathy: Is CAD present?

Idiopathic and ischemic cardiomyopathy may be clinically indistinguishable, but management and prognosis may be quite different. Both groups of patients have dilatation of the LV and are likely to have perfusion defects on myocardial perfusion images. Thallium and/or technetium stress-rest imaging is an excellent tool to determine if ischemia is complicating cardiomyopathy. Perfusion imaging may be abnormal in patients with nonischemic cardiomyopathy, but the abnormalities tend to be much more extensive in patients with cardiomyopathic defects due to ischemia. Patients with ischemic patterns on perfusion imaging should have coronary angiography, and if CAD is confirmed, myocardial viability determination in regions with fixed defects may be warranted using 24-hr thallium or FDG imaging.

10. What is the prognostic value of myocardial perfusion scans?

These tests provide important prognostic information. Only about 1% per year of patients with normal stress myocardial perfusion scans suffer subsequent events (death or MI), even in patients with known CAD and prior revascularization procedures. In a European study of patients with an intermediate pretest probablility of CAD, patients with normal stress sestamibi studies had only 0.2% annualized mortality rate. In contrast, greater extent and severity of perfusion deficits is highly correlated with risk of subsequent cardiac events (death or MI). Other signs evident on scans associated with poor prognosis include left ventricular enlargement, particularly if greater on stress images (so called transient ischemic dilatation), increased lung counts on stress thallium studies, as well as reversibility of stress defects at rest. Abnormal increased lung uptake of the tracer and transient dilatation of the LV are findings associated with severe CAD, usually multivessel CAD and heart failure.

Stress myocardial perfusion imaging adds incremental prognostic value for patients with low-to-intermediate probability (10–80%) of CAD, for patients prior to vascular surgery, for the elderly, for patients with non–insulin dependent asymptomatic diabetes and for patients who have had revascularization procedures, even though they may be asymptomatic. Significant additive prognostic value is evident in high-risk patients with non–insulin dependent diabetes unable to exercise, the risk of death being 7–8 times higher when a large perfusion defect is present. Exercise dual-isotope myocardial perfusion SPECT effectively risk-stratifies patients over age 65: Those with normal scans have <1% event rate over the first year of follow-up, and the procedure adds incremental prognostic information over non-nuclear examinations. Myocardial perfusion imaging reduces the overall cost of testing per patient.

Patients with unstable angina need cardiac catheterization to plan immediate therapy. This chapter does not address the issues of management of patients with acute coronary syndromes.

11. Is a chemotherapy patient developing cardio-toxicity?

For patients having chemotherapy with cardiotoxic agents (i.e., adriamycin), detection of a fall in LVEF—the earliest sign of cardiotoxicity—is critical. A baseline MUGA (Fig. 3) or first pass EF should be obtained at the start of chemotherapy and repeated before each new round of cardiotoxic drugs. A change in EF of more than 5–7% EF units (i.e., 50% to 43%) is considered significant. Changes of <5–7% are within the range of expected variability from one study to the next. If EF falls below 40%, caution is advised and oncologists may choose to discontinue using cardiotoxic agents or wait until the EF recovers before additional chemotherapy is administered.

PATIENT INFORMATION

I. MYOCARDIAL PERFUSION IMAGING
A. Test/Procedure

Your doctor has requested that you have a heart scan to detect coronary disease. This scan gives your doctor information about the function of your heart and the extent and severity of any abnormality related to blood flow to your heart muscle. A small amount of a radioactive material (e.g., thallium or technetium) is injected into a vein (usually in the forearm) and goes to your heart; pictures are taken of your heart with a special camera. The intravenous injection is sometimes performed while you are exercising on a treadmill to make your heart work harder. Often, coronary disease can be diagnosed only during

1

physical stress when the heart needs to work hard. If you are unable to exercise on a treadmill, a drug that causes the coronary arteries to dilate (enlarge) can be used instead to mimic what happens when your heart works harder. Under these conditions the picture of your heart helps the doctors to determine if you have coronary disease and to assess its severity. The study requires two sets of pictures of the heart. One image is obtained immediately after exercise, and the other is a resting image. The whole study (both images) takes 2–5 hr depending on the protocol used and the need for extra pictures, if any. Your nuclear medicine department can tell you more precisely how long you need to stay.

B. Preparation

Diet. You need to be fasting (water is permitted) after midnight before the study, and you must not ingest anything containing caffeine (coffee, tea, cola drinks) for 24 hr before the study. Caffeine may interfere with the drugs that dilate coronary arteries.

Medications. Medicines given for asthma or lung-airway diseases also can interfere, and you should discuss whether to discontinue those for 2 days before the study with your doctor. If you are taking beta-blocker or nitrate medicines, you should discuss with your doctor whether to discontinue those drugs. If you are taking Viagra, you should stop taking it for 2 days.

C. Radiation risks

The amount of radiation used is similar to that given by some other diagnostic x-ray tests. The radiation exposure to your whole body from this test is about the same as the dose the average person living in the United States receives during 10–15 yr from cosmic rays and naturally occurring background radiation sources. The radiation dose is about 50–100% of the yearly dose considered safe for doctors and technologists who work with radiation. You can be around other people and use a bathroom normally without risk to others.

D. Pregnancy

If you think you are pregnant, or might be pregnant, please inform your doctor so that this can be discussed with the nuclear medicine physician.

II. FDG SCAN USING PET/COINCDENCE/ SPECT

A. Test/Procedure

This is a heart scan to examine the health of your heart. The test is done by administering into a vein a small amount of a radioactive form of sugar called FDG, usually in your arm. The pictures taken by a special camera, called a PET or coincidence camera, tell the doctors how well your heart metabolizes, or uses, sugar. To get the best results from this test, your blood sugar level needs to be in the appropriate range for the heart to absorb the radioactive sugar. This may require giving you some insulin or nonradioactive sugar solution to drink before the radioactive material is administered.

As part of this heart scan, you also may receive a small amount of another radioactive isotope (rubidium or technetium), which can tell the doctors if your heart is getting enough blood through your coronary arteries.

The study takes 2–4 hr depending on how many pictures are needed.

B. Preparation

Diet. You need to be fasting after midnight before the study (small amounts of water are permitted). If you also are to have a rubidium or technetium heart scan to show how effectively your heart muscle is getting its blood supply, you must not ingest anything containing caffeine (coffee, tea, cola drinks) for 24 hr before the study. Caffeine may interfere with the drugs that dilate coronary arteries needed to test the heart's blood supply.

Medications. Medicines given for asthma or lung-airway diseases also can interfere, and you should discuss whether to discontinue those or not with your doctor. No other special preparation is needed.

C. Radiation risk

The amount of radiation used is small and similar to that given by other diagnostic x-ray tests. The radiation exposure to your whole body from this test is about the same as the dose the average person living in the United States receives each year from cosmic rays and naturally occurring background radiation sources. The radiation dose from FDG is about 7% of the yearly dose considered safe for doctors and technologists who work with radiation. You can be around other people and use a bathroom normally without risk to others.

D. Pregnancy

If you think you are pregnant, or might be pregnant, please inform your doctor so that this can be discussed with the nuclear medicine physician.

III. GATED BLOOD POOL IMAGING (MUGA)

A. Test/Procedure

Your doctor has requested that you have this heart scan (called MUGA or gated blood pool study) to examine how well your heart is functioning in terms of the strength of each heartbeat and the amount of blood being pumped with each heartbeat. The test is done by attaching a small amount of a radioactive isotope to your red blood cells. Usually, a small amount (about 2 teaspoons) of blood is taken from a vein (usually in your arm), treated and readministered into your vein. A few minutes later the camera can begin taking pictures of your heart while you lie still. Your electrocardiogram is also recorded. The pictures are displayed as a movie of your beating heart, and computer analysis provides the doctors with important information about the function of your heart.

The pictures take about 30 min. This is preceded by treating your blood so that some of your red blood cells are labeled with the radioactive tracer, which takes another 30 min. Total time is about 1 hr.

B. Preparation

Diet. No special preparation is needed, except for fasting after midnight or for 4 hr before the study (small quantities of water are permitted).

Medications. There are no medication restrictions.

C. Radiation risks

The amount of radiation used is small and similar to that given by other diagnostic x-ray tests. The radiation exposure to your whole body from this test is about the same as the dose the average person living in the United States receives each year from cosmic rays and naturally occurring background radiation sources. The radiation dose is about 7% of the yearly dose considered safe for doctors and technologists who work with radiation. You can be around other people and use a bathroom normally without risk to others.

D. Pregnancy

If you think you are pregnant, or might be pregnant, please inform your doctor so that this can be discussed with the nuclear medicine physician.

References

1. Zaret BL, Wackers FJT. Nuclear Cardiology. *N Engl J Med* 1993;329:775–783, 855–863.
2. Bonow RO. Identification of viable mycardium. *Circulation* 1996;94:2674–2680.
3. Ritchie JL, Bateman TM, Bonow RO, et al. Guidelines for clinical use of cardiac radionuclide imaging: a report of the American College of Cardiology/American Heart Association Task Force collaboration with the American Society of Nuclear Cardiology. *J Nucl Cardiol* 1995;2(2 Pt 1):172–192.
4. Berman DS, Kiat H, Freidman J, et al. Separate acquisition rest-thallium-201/stress Tc-99m sestamibi dual isotope myocardial perfusion SPECT: a clinical validation study. *J Am Coll Cardiol* 1993;23:1455–1464.
5. Berman DS, Kiat H, van Train K, et al. Myocardial perfusion imaging with technetium-99m-sestamibi: comparative analysis of available imaging protols. *J Nucl Med* 1994;35:683–688.
6. Schwaiger M. Myocardial perfusion imaging with PET. *J Nucl Med* 1994;35:693–698.
7. DePuey EG, Rozanski A. Using gated technetium-99m-sestamibi SPECT to characterize fixed myocardial defects as infarct or artifact. *J Nucl Med* 1995;36:952–955.
8. Leppo JA. Dipyridamole myocardial perfusion imaging. *J Nucl Med* 1994;35:730–733.

9. Shaw LJ, Hachamovitch R, Berman DS, et al. The economic consequences of available diagnostic and prognostic strategies for the evaluation of stable angina patients: an observational assessment of the value of pre-catheterization ischemia. *J Am Coll Cardiol* 1999;33:661–669.

10. Soman P, Parsons A, Lahiri N, Lahiri A. The prognostic value of normal Tc-99m sestamibi SPECT study in suspected coronary disease. *J Nucl Cardiol* 1999;6:252–256.

11. Marwick TH, Shaw LJ, Lauer MS, et al. The noninvasive prediction of cardiac mortality in men and women with known or suspected coronary artery disease. *Am J Med* 1999; 106:172–178.

2
Pulmonary System and Thromboembolism

Pulmonary embolism (PE) is a major health problem with considerable controversy surrounding the diagnostic approaches and their interpretation. Approximately 600,000 patients per year have clinically significant PE, and 120,000 of them die annually from this disease in the United States without being diagnosed. Deep vein thrombosis (DVT) is the third most common cardiovascular disease after coronary artery disease and stroke; it affects 2 million in the United States per year and gives rise to PE in an estimated 25–30% of affected individuals.

The problems in diagnosis of pulmonary embolism (PE) relate to the nonspecificity of clinical signs and symptoms and to the relatively invasive nature and high costs associated with the most definitive diagnostic procedure, pulmonary angiography. The radionuclide lung scan is used widely because it is safe, readily available, easily performed and highly sensitive for diagnosis of PE. Spiral CT has an increasingly important role in the diagnosis of PE; the radionuclide ventilation/perfusion lung scan (often called the V/Q scan or V/P scan), however, is still considered the first line diagnostic test. This is based on 35 yr of reliable clinical experience in the diagnoses of PE, an abundance of data that have led to the revised PIOPED (Prospective Investigation of Pulmonary Embolism Diagnosis) criteria for interpretation, the almost nonexistent morbidity and the relatively low cost of the V/P scan.

2

SCANS AND PRIMARY CLINICAL INDICATIONS

CLINICAL QUESTIONS

PATIENT INFORMATION

SCANS

I. VENTILATION/PERFUSION LUNG SCAN

A. Background

The abundant published literature and clinical familiarity with the radionuclide ventilation/perfusion lung scan have led to the following conclusions that are accepted by most pulmonary medicine physicians, angiographers and nuclear medicine physicians: (a) a normal perfusion scan indicates no clinically significant emboli; (b) an abnormal perfusion scan alone is a nonspecific indicator of emboli, but a ventilation/perfusion study showing mismatched abnormalities indicates high probability for pulmonary emboli; and (c) the perfusion scan can guide the selection of sites for angiography or for particular attention on the spiral CT study.

Although the lung perfusion scan (without a ventilation scan) is sensitive for pulmonary embolic disease, its specificity is low. Pulmonary embolus causes segmental perfusion defects, but chronic obstructive pulmonary disease can result in similar findings. The ventilation scan improves the specificity of the lung perfusion scan. Ventilation imaging is most likely to be helpful in patients if existing airway disease involves <50% of the lungs. Interpretation criteria based on mismatched and matched perfusion defects have been established for very low, low, intermediate and high probabilities for PE by two widely quoted authorities: Biello (1979) and PIOPED (1990, revised 1995). In acute PE, the ventilation scan is almost always normal, unless there is superimposed parenchymal or airway abnormality. In chronic PE, there may be secondary ventilation abnormality resulting from the long-standing perfusion deprivation.

B. Radiopharmaceuticals

1. Technetium-99m-macroaggregated albumin (MAA). Technetium-99m-MAA is used for lung perfusion imaging. These particles are too large (mean size 20-40 μm) to pass through a capillary. They are trapped in the capillary bed of the pulmonary arterial circulation, which is the first capillary bed they encounter after peripheral intravenous injection. Usually, about 200,000–700,000 particles of ^{99m}Tc-MAA are injected into a peripheral vein, causing embolization of a small fraction of 1% of the pulmonary capillaries fed from the pulmonary arterial system. These particles are removed within hours by enzymatic and macrophage activity, restoring full perfusion/function to the ^{99m}Tc-MAA embolized regions. In patients with PE, the scan demonstrates an area of decreased radioactivity corresponding to the decreased flow to the embolized lung. Areas of decreased radioactivity are not specific for PE; they also occur in patients with pneumonia, effusions and emphysema, as well as other lung parenchymal and airway abnormalities.

2. Technetium-99m-DTPA aerosol or xenon-133 gas. Technetium-99m-DTPA aerosol or ^{133}Xe gas is used for the ventilation scan. The xenon is more physi-

2

ologic, and early images show the wash-in phase, followed by its gradual wash-out from the lungs on the delayed images. Only wash-in (equivalent of a first or single breath of xenon) is obtained with an aerosolized particulate material. The advantage of aerosolized ventilation delivery is that lung ventilation can be imaged in multiple projections, whereas xenon is usually limited to the posterior projection. Xenon's advantage is that it adds wash-out information, which cannot be obtained using the ^{99m}Tc-DTPA aerosol. The use of either xenon or aerosol is an institutional preference, and both are considered clinically effective.

C. How the lung V/P scan is performed

The perfusion lung scan is performed by injecting the ^{99m}Tc-radiolabeled particles (2–5 mCi [80—180 MBq] adult dose) into a peripheral vein and then imaging the lungs in multiple projections. The ventilation lung scan usually precedes the perfusion scan; the patient breathes a small amount of a radioactive gas (^{133}Xe, 5–20 mCi [200–750 MBq] adult dose) while being imaged, or the patient inhales ^{99m}Tc-DTPA–labeled aerosol (~1 mCi [37 MBq] adult dose) and is imaged immediately afterward. The patient usually is imaged while lying supine but may sit upright (after the injection of the perfusion tracer). The V/P scan is performed with conventional scintillation camera planar imaging. A few centers have used the tomographic camera technology of SPECT for perfusion scans to depict the lung anatomic segmental volumes, but no substantive advantages have been documented. The ventilation and perfusion procedures take about 30–60 min.

Quantitative lung scan. The quantitative lung scan is performed exactly as a conventional lung scan, except that the images are computer processed by drawing regions of interest over each lung and over regions corresponding to the lobes within each lung. Ventilation images also can be quantitated, if desired, or the quantitative study may be limited to the perfusion images.

D. Patient preparation

The patient first has a chest x-ray performed to identify pathology that may obviate a much more expensive test; furthermore, the chest x-ray is needed for correlation with the V/P scan. After obtaining the chest x-ray, there is no special preparation for lung V/P studies. The patient can eat and drink fluids, as usual. If the patient has a large pleural effusion, tapping off fluid will result in a better look at the underlying lung, but there should be no undue delays imposed to obtain a needed V/P study.

E. Understanding the report

The report may describe the specific signs and symptoms that triggered the request of a lung scan by the clinician and the patient's risk factors with a clinical estimate of pretest probability for PE, if suspicion of PE is the reason for the test. In the report, the nuclear medicine physician describes the procedure, including the radiopharmaceutical dose, the imaging procedure, the findings and locations of perfusion defects and whether there are matching or mismatching ventilation defects or chest x-ray abnormalities. The impression describes the probability of PE as high (Fig. 1), intermediate, low or very low and may incorporate modulation of the scan probability on the bases of clinical pretest assessment, if provided by the clinician (see Table 1).

1. Mismatched or matched V/P scan. The terms "mismatched" or "matched" V/P scan refer to an assessment of any region of perfusion abnormality vis a vis its ventilation. A region of lung with abnormal (decreased) perfusion may show normal ventilation (mismatched V/P) or abnormal ventilation (matched V/P). Ventilation is abnormal if images show decreased counts on the initial wash-in images (i.e., slow to wash-in) or increased counts on the wash-out images (i.e., slow to wash-out). Although wash-in images are obtained with all ventilation imaging agents, wash-out images can be obtained only with xenon gas.

2. Understanding probabilities of PE. Ventilation/perfusion scans for PE are interpreted as normal or in terms of probabilities (high probability for PE, intermediate [indeterminate] probability or low probability). If the scan is normal, the likelihood of PE approaches zero. The degree of abnormality and the probability is based on the presence of mismatched or matched V/P abnormalities, their sizes and their numbers. Patients with near normal or very low probability scans are least likely to have PE (0–5%), whereas some patients called low probability, particularly patients with underlying lung parenchymal problems (limited to <50% of lung parenchyma), may have a probability of PE ranging from 10% to 20%. High probability indicates 80–100% of patients will have PE (see Table 1). All scans that do not meet criteria for high or low probability interpretations are called indeterminate probability for PE. The clinical estimates of probability of PE can be altered markedly by the V/P scan interpretation: for example, 83% of patients thought to have a low clinical probability for PE actually have PE if they had high probability V/P scans (Table 1).

3. Quantitative lung scan. The report describes the percent contribution to global perfusion of each lung. Combined with pulmonary function tests, these quantitative regional lung function studies allow the clinician to predict how much lung function will remain after proposed surgical excision of an entire lung or a part of one. Ventilation can be quantitated similarly.

F. Potential problems

1. False-positives. Conditions that can mimic high probability PE scans include vasculitis, other rarer conditions such as pulmonary arterial anomalies, i.e., hypoplasias and stenoses, as well as fat emboli. Vasculitis is associated most often with collagen vascular diseases and recent radiation therapy to the chest.

2

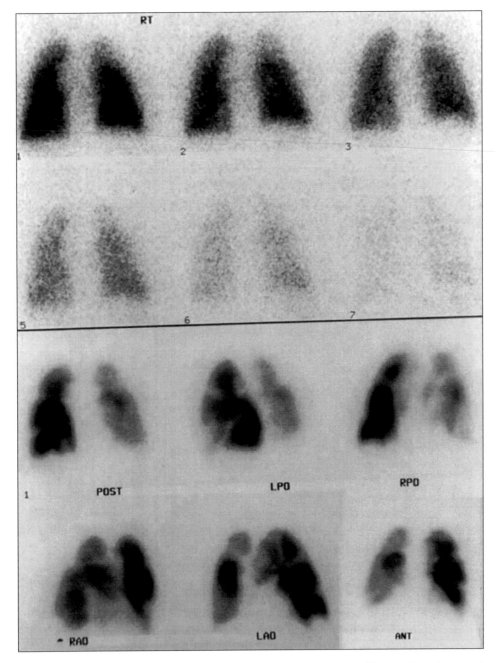

Figure 1. High probability V/P scan. Ventilation images (above) were performed using ^{133}Xe gas. They show normal first breath (wash-in, upper left image), except for limited right apical slowed wash-in. The remaining five images show generally homogeneous wash-out of activity from both lungs. The perfusion images (below) performed with ^{99m}Tc-MAA particles show multiple perfusion defects throughout both lungs, many of which are wedge-shaped and segmental. The perfusion defects are mismatched by normal ventilation.

Table 1. Percentages of Patients with PE Correlated to V/P Scan Interpretations and Clinical Prescan Risk Assessments

V/P scan probability for PE	Clinical Prescan Probability		
	High	Intermediate	Low
High	95%	85%	83%
Intermediate	71%	29%	14%
Low	43%	16%	4%
Normal and near normal	0%*	7%	2%

*Based on 5 patients of the total of 887 of which 90 had clinical high pretest probability.

Based on the PIOPED study. (See discussion under Clinical Question 3.) (Reproduced with permission of Ralph D. Pulmonary embolism: the implications of prospective investigation of PE diagnosis. *Radiol Clin North Am* 1994;32:679–687.)

2. Clinical pretest probability of PE. The clinician's estimate of pretest probability of PE can be useful for deriving the post-test probability, but it may be difficult to obtain a valid quantitative or semiquantitative clinical pretest probability because standardized criteria for clinical pretest probability for PE do not exist.

3. Interpretations of defect sizes. Interpretations of size of a defect as "moderate" or "small" may at times be difficult and subjective. Differences in estimating sizes of defects may lead to differences in the interpretation of the probability of PE. A high probability scan is defined as two unmatched moderate or large perfusion defects or, if the patient has prior cardiopulmonary disease, four mismatched defects. A defect of "moderate" size means 25–75% of the area of a lung segment. A "large" defect means >75% of a segment. The revised PIOPED criteria suggest that summations of defect size arithmetic equivalents can be used, so that two defects that each are 50% of a segment can be counted as equivalent to a large defect.

4. Widespread ventilatory abnormalities. Widespread ventilatory abnormalities usually would be interpreted as intermediate (or indeterminate) probability for PE. Pulmonary infarction may show matched V/P abnormalities and matched chest x-ray infiltrate, and an intermediate probability interpretation would result.

5. Right to left shunts. When lung perfusion scan particles (20–50 μm) are injected intravenously in patients with large right to left shunts, there is concern about embolization of shunted particles, particularly to the brain. Shunting occurs in proportion to percent of cardiac output that goes to the organ. To minimize embolization, the number of particles injected can be reduced for patients with right to left shunts, particularly small children.

II. ACUTECT VENOUS THROMBUS SCAN

The clinical diagnosis of DVT often is unreliable without objective testing. Most patients with clinical symptoms suggesting possible DVT do not have DVT. Of

2

those with DVT, 80% have proximal venous disease (above the popliteal), and 20% have DVT limited to the calves. Proximal disease is associated with PE in 50% of cases. Proximal extension of calf vein thrombosis occurs in 30% of those cases. As many as 23% of PEs have been estimated to derive from calf venous thrombi. Diagnostic approaches for DVT have relied on the clinical presentation, risk factors and symptoms, supplemented with noninvasive tests, primarily Doppler ultrasound. Limitations of the Doppler ultrasound are that it does not distinguish between acute and chronic DVT and does not perform well in diagnosing calf thrombi. A new nuclear medicine study, using AcuTect, images active thrombi and is particularly sensitive for detecting acute thrombi in calves.

AcuTect is ^{99m}Tc-labeled to a low molecular weight synthetic peptide that binds to receptors on the surface of activated platelets. AcuTect is injected intravenously; it is not immunogenic and not associated with risk of viral contamination. Anticoagulants will not interfere with imaging acute venous thrombosis with this agent.

Imaging of the pelvis, thighs and calves is performed 30 min and 4 hr after injection (Fig. 2). There is no special patient preparation. The patient needs to be able to lie flat on the imaging table for about 30–45 min. Diet and medication routines can be continued as usual.

III. RADIONUCLIDE VENOGRAPHY

Radionuclide venography using ^{99m}Tc-MAA can be performed in conjunction with routine perfusion lung scanning. The deep venous system of the lower extremities is visualized by sequential scintillation camera images after injection of a radiopharmaceutical into dorsal pedal veins with tourniquets tied proximally to occlude superficial veins. DVT is indicated by nonfilling of all or a portion of the deep venous system, by filling of abnormal collateral vessels or by the delayed clearance of the particulate tracer. Ultrasound is much easier to perform, and this test is used rarely.

CLINICAL QUESTIONS

1. Does my patient have a pulmonary embolus?

The clinical signs and symptoms for PE can be so elusive and the consequences of unrecognized PE so serious that if the possibility of PE occurs to the clinician as he/she examines a patient, a V/P scan should probably be obtained.

The V/P lung scan is interpreted as high, intermediate, low or very low probability of PE. High probability V/P scan is strong evidence for instituting appropriate therapy. Even in the face of an estimated low clinical probability, there is still an 83% chance of an underlying pulmonary embolus (Table 1), and most clinicians would consider this sufficiently high odds to treat without an angiogram. Low probability V/P scan is strong evidence against PE, but in the face of a high clinical pretest probability estimate, additional tests are warranted.

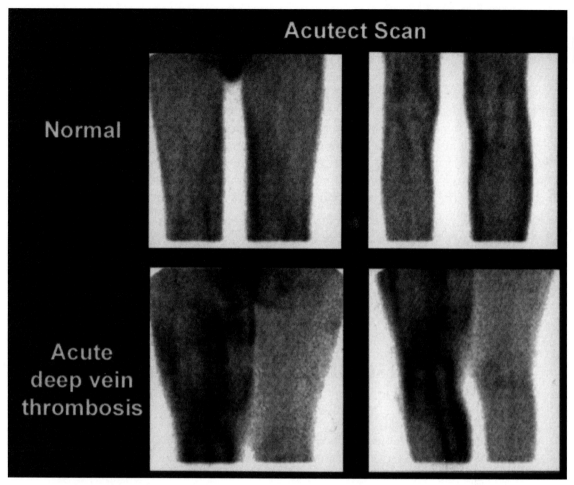

Figure 2. AcuTect venous thrombosis imaging. Lower extremity images of a normal patient are shown (above). Markedly abnormal images (below) show a swollen left lower extremity with increased technetium-labeled AcuTect deposition in the femoral, popliteal and posterior tibial distributions, indicating acute venous thrombosis.

2. What tests other than the V/P scan are available to diagnose PE?

Laboratory tests. Electrocardiogram, blood chemistry, arterial partial pressure of carbon dioxide (pCO_2) and arterial partial pressure of oxygen (pO_2) are not sufficiently sensitive or specific to diagnose PE. Similarly, the chest x-ray is not sensitive for PE, and when findings are present, they are often nonspecific. A blood marker of coagulation, D-dimer assay (DDA), measures fibrin degradation products in blood. The test is quite sensitive (95% in one study) for PE, but of low specificity (31%). Therefore a negative D-dimer result using the enzyme-linked immunosorbent assay (ELISA) method would weigh heavily against PE and could be used to help the clinician exclude the need for a V/P lung scan in cases in which a pretest probability is low. However, the American College of Chest Physicians consensus committee on PE recently concluded that until D-dimer testing is standardized and more widely validated in prospective outcome studies, widespread use of D-dimer measurement is not recommended.

Imaging tests. Pulmonary angiography is the gold standard for diagnosing PE. It provides an image that shows the emboli as filling defects in the contrast-enhanced blood within the pulmonary vasculature. Pulmonary perfusion imaging and pulmonary angiography agree closely in detecting pulmonary emboli, although both tests miss some emboli. Selective pulmonary angiography is more sensitive than perfusion lung imaging for detecting small, peripheral emboli and emboli that partially obstruct pulmonary vessels. But lack of good interobserver agreement in reading small emboli on the pulmonary angiogram somewhat diminishes that advantage. The pulmonary angiogram is expensive and has morbidity associated with injection contrast material and the highly invasive nature of the test.

Contrast-enhanced CT (spiral or electron-beam) can be performed as a rapid scan technique, which combined with intravenous contrast media, permits visualization of the central pulmonary artery and its proximal branches during a single breath-hold of 20 sec or less (electron-beam technique permits 1- to 2-sec imaging). Before spiral CT technology, prolonged scanning times resulted in respiratory and cardiac motion artifacts and poor definition of pulmonary vasculature. Sensitivity of 86% and specificity of 92% has been reported for central vessel PE and lower sensitivity, 63%, and specificity, 89%, for smaller vessel PE compared with pulmonary angiography. Assessments show that it may still be too early to tell if and how spiral CT will fit in the clinical workup of patients suspected of having PE. Recommendations have focused on patients with indeterminate V/P lung scan results or those with extensive chest x-ray infiltrates who are likely to have indeterminate V/P scans (Fig. 3). However, negative CT does not exclude PE because thromboemboli in subsegmental pulmonary arteries are not detected by CT.

Because of intravenous administration of iodinated contrast material and the associated mortality of 1 in 40,000 and morbidity reactions of 1 in 4,000, spiral CT and pulmonary angiography are less desirable alternatives than radionuclide V/P lung scan, which has almost no associated morbidity. Cost is variable, but usually lower for lung scans (see Chapter 29, Comparative Costs of Diagnostic Procedures). Cost of pulmonary angiography is far higher, as is risk to the patient. Some investigators have recommended that the contrast-enhanced CT study may prove to be a less costly alternative to pulmonary angiography and, occasionally, an alternative to radionuclide lung scan and pulmonary angiography (e.g., patients who cannot perform the ventilation test). Magnetic resonance imaging (MRI) is also at an investigational assessment stage in the workup of patients with suspected PE.

3. What is the role of the pretest probability estimate of PE?

The clinician can estimate the pretest probability for PE based on risk factors and clinical symptoms. Risk factors for PE and DVT include conditions that lead

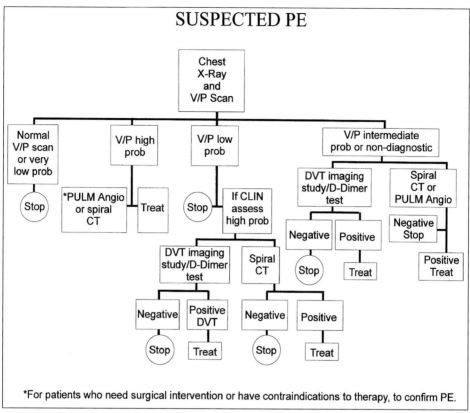

Figure 3. Schematic workup for suspected PE, starting with chest x-ray and V/P scan. Patients whose readings are high probability for PE go directly to treatment for PE, or for spiral CT or pulmonary angiography if therapy is high risk for the patient. For patients whose V/P scans are low probability for PE, the workup would be terminated, unless clinical pretest assessment is high probablity, in which case DVT Doppler and D-Dimer, or spiral CT would follow. For intermediate probability cases, DVT Doppler, D-Dimer or spiral CT, or pulmonary angiogram are warranted.

to venous stasis and intimal injury, e.g., pelvic and lower extremity trauma and surgery, burns, pregnancy, postpartum state, estrogens, prolonged general anesthesia, prior DVT, mass or fibrosis impinging on venous drainage, congestive heart failure, prolonged immobility, obesity, cancer and advanced age. The most common clinical presenting signs and symptoms of patients with PE are dyspnea or tachypnea (96%), which are nonspecific signs and occur in a variety of other non–PE conditions. The classically quoted triad of PE—dyspnea, pleurisy and hemoptysis—occurs in only a small percentage of patients with PE. Hemoptysis is probably present only if pulmonary infarction has occurred, and fewer than 10% of PEs result in clinically evident pulmonary infarction.

As illustrated in Table 1, and demonstrated by the PIOPED multicenter study using pulmonary angiography as the gold standard, estimates of pretest likelihood of PE based on the clinician's assessment are useful in maximizing the accuracy of the lung scan probability interpretation.

- Of patients with the combination of high clinical probability and high probability V/P scan, 95% had PE.

2

- Of patients with the combination of low clinical probability and high probability V/P scan, 83% had PE.
- Of patients with high clinical probability and low probability V/P scan, 43% had PE.

Further refinement of the low probability scan has led to the very low probability category which is associated with PE in <5–10% of cases with the identified scan findings.

4. How does the clinician proceed if the patient has an intermediate probability scan result?

Faced with an inconclusive V/P scan, the next step can be a contrast-enhanced spiral CT scan or a pulmonary angiogram. Algorithms for approaching the workup are suggested in Figure 3. Most physicians would probably agree that the upfront costs of additional diagnostic tests to diagnose PE when an inconclusive V/P scan result is obtained are outweighed by the benefits of basing anticoagulant therapy on a well-founded diagnosis. The incidence of nondiagnostic V/P scans range from about 10% to 50%, depending largely on the patient population sampled. At many hospitals only 10% of V/P scans are interpreted as intermediate probability for PE, whereas 90% are low or high probability. In the PIOPED population, 38% were intermediate probability. Patients with chronic obstructive pulmonary disease are more likely to have intermediate probability for PE, or nondiagnostic scans. But, the almost nonexistent morbidity and relatively low cost compared with pulmonary angiography make the V/P scan the most desirable first line test for PE, after the chest x-ray, which may identify pathology and is needed to correlate with the V/P scan.

Risk of inconclusive PE diagnosis and anticoagulation therapy risks. The risk of death from anticoagulation without a definite diagnosis is low (0.1%). But morbidity from anticoagulant therapies is higher (major bleeding in 5% and heparin-induced thrombocytopenia in 1%). Furthermore, the patient is committed to multiple months of anticoagulation, with considerable cost and inconvenience, as well as the morbidity risks described above. There is also a medicolegal risk to the physician in the event of morbidity from anticoagulation therapy despite an uncertain diagnosis. Therefore, some physicians order duplex ultrasound to diagnose DVT before starting anticoagulation therapy when the V/P scan is inconclusive or when it is delayed for 10–12 hr until morning. Anticoagulation therapy certainly is warranted for DVT, and 70% of patients with PE have positive ultrasound studies for DVT.

Most physicians experienced in diagnosis and therapy of patients with PE prefer to focus the diagnostic workup for PE on the chest, i.e., start with the chest x-ray and V/P lung scan. If an indeterminate probability for PE is found, lower extremity venous imaging may be performed to assist in assessing the likelihood of PE, in hopes of circumventing pulmonary angiography. If compression

Doppler ultrasound, for example, is positive, appropriate anticoagulation therapy is instituted, but if negative, pulmonary angiography or spiral CT still may be needed because the absence of a diagnosis of DVT does not exclude PE.

5. If the chest x-ray shows an infiltrate or effusion, can the V/P scan diagnose PE?

It is reasonable to perform the V/P scan in patients with an infiltrate or effusion; if the effusion is large, it is advisable to remove fluid before the scan, if possible, to assess the underlying lung. If the perfusion scan is relatively normal or low probability, despite focal lung opacification from fluid, the patient is spared more extensive testing. An infiltrate on chest x-ray can be a pulmonary infarct, pneumonia or a host of other pathologies. V/P scan with matched defect(s) leads to an intermediate probability for PE interpretation unless there are other mismatched defects with no accompanying density on chest x-ray. The triple-match, for which the infiltrate on x-ray and the V/P defect are equal in size, is interpreted as intermediate probability for lower lung zone lesions or very low probability for triple-matched defects in upper or middle lung fields. An effusion on chest x-ray usually will correspond to a matched V/P defect. Some data suggest that a small pleural effusion has a higher liklihood of PE than a large pleural effusion, although this interpretation is debated.

6. Should a patient being treated for PE have a follow-up scan? If so, when?

A corollary question, which sometimes arises, particularly if the patient has had a diagnosis of PE in the past, is can the V/P scan distinguish between acute and unresolved (chronic) PE? The V/P scan may not distinguish old from new PE without a prior study. Accurate interpretation of a new V/P scan in a patient with known prior PE requires comparison to a baseline V/P scan acquired after treatment of the prior PE.

The perfusion may normalize after anticoagulation therapy, but long-standing perfusion defects can remain, mimicking acute PE on a V/P scan. A baseline scan after anticoagulation is important in case the patient becomes symptomatic in the future and requires a new diagnostic V/P scan. Persistence of an unresolved defect, particularly if mismatched, will be difficult to sort out if a baseline scan is not available for comparison. The post-therapy lung scan can be obtained at the time of discharge from the hospital or at 3–6 wk as an outpatient.

7. What are the risks of PE, anticoagulation and a V/P scan during pregnancy?

During pregnancy, the incidence of PE and DVT are elevated. Mortality of untreated PE in pregnancy is 12.8%, whereas it is only 0.7% with therapy. Thus, the risk associated with untreated, undiagnosed PE in pregnancy is extremely high. However, the risk related to unnecessary anticoagulation therapy is also high. By contrast, the small risk to a fetus of radiation exposure (see below) from diagnostic testing for PE in the mother is far outweighed by the risks of not diagnosing PE. A diagnosis of PE during pregnancy carries with it prolonged heparin therapy during pregnancy, potential need for prophylaxis if future pregnancies occur, concern about oral contraception and, later in life, concern about estrogen replacement therapy. Thus, a reasonably definitive diagnosis of PE must be pursued, starting with the V/P scan.

Radiation to the fetus from a radionuclide lung V/P study, in a nutshell, is a nonissue if the suspicion for PE exists. Although calculated fetal exposures from a diagnostic lung V/P scan are low, it is advisable to minimize the administered doses.

Many nuclear medicine physicians and radiologists obtain written informed consent from the pregnant patient before performing a lung scan or any necessary procedure involving radiation. In the report, it is advisable for the radiologist or nuclear physician to document the discussions with the patient about the risks and benefits of the test (see V/P Lung Scan Patient Information).

8. If a postpartum patient has a V/P scan, can she continue to breastfeed?

The postpartum patient who is nursing an infant is advised to discontinue nursing for 24 hr. Because the radiation is concentrated in the patient's chest, holding the infant against the chest to nurse should be avoided for several hours. More importantly, a small amount of technetium from the ^{99m}Tc-MAA complex may be excreted in the breast milk. However, because of the 6-hr physical half-life of technetium combined with biologic elimination, after 24 hr the amount of radioactivity excreted in the breast milk will be negligible. If there is any doubt, the best proof would be to count 1.0 ml of expressed milk, which should be close to background ($< 3 \times$ background) before resuming breastfeeding.

9. How much lung function will my patient lose if he/she has a partial lung resection?

Normal individuals have split lung functions of 52% right lung and 48% left lung. If global lung function as measured by pulmonary function indices is compromised substantially, the quantitative radionuclide lung V/P scan can assist in the critical surgical decision of how much lung can be removed while preserving remaining pulmonary function. The loss of lung function resulting from excision of a lobe or lung can thus be predicted in advance of the surgery.

10. Should a V/P scan be obtained to diagnose and quantitate right to left cardiac shunts?

Right to left shunts can be accurately quantitated by a perfusion lung scan that is modified to be a whole-body scan. When a right to left shunt is present, the first capillary bed to which intravenously injected shunted particles come is that of any organ system: brain, liver, kidneys, myocardium, etc., in proportion to the percent of cardiac output blood delivered to that organ system. Thus, by imaging the whole body and measuring the lung counts compared with whole-body counts, the shunted blood (right to left) can be quantitated:

Percent right/left shunt =
(whole-body counts − lung counts) ÷ whole-body counts.

Calculation of differential pulmonary blood flow, i.e., percentage of pulmonary artery blood going to each lung, is commonly used in the pediatric population in the assessment of severity of pulmonary artery stenosis, particularly before and after balloon dilation or stent placement.

11. Does my patient have DVT?

Venous imaging can be performed by several techniques. The traditional gold standard is contrast radiographic venography. This test is based on visualizing filling defects in well opacified venous channels to detect DVT. The major disadvantage of the radiographic contrast venogram is (a) pain, particularly if there is any extravasation of the contrast; (b) iatrogenic thrombosis induction (incidence about 10%); (c) problems of potential reaction to contrast material, which carries a mortality rate of 1:40,000; and (d) potential renal toxicity.

Noninvasive venous imaging using ultrasound (venous duplex scanning) has reasonably high accuracy with sensitivity and specificity of 90% or better and is the current preferred modality. Compression ultrasonography assesses compressibility of the femoral and popliteal veins, i.e., noncompressibility is diagnostic of DVT. The limitations of ultrasound include the following: (a) unreliable accuracy in calf DVT; (b) inability to differentiate acute from chronic recurrent DVT; and (c) highly operator-dependent nature.

Magnetic resonance venography has reported sensitivities of 90–100% and specificities of 93–100%; thus, it may be an excellent noninvasive approach for DVT. Because of cost considerations, it can follow the less expensive ultrasound if nondiagnostic or may be the first-line noninvasive test for some patients at particularly high risk for DVT. Another advantage of magnetic resonance venography is that it appears to be more sensitive than ultrasound in the pelvis and calf. However, it is not yet widely available and is more difficult to obtain than ultrasound on an emergency basis.

Impedance plethysmography is an indirect indicator of blood flow that is sensitive for proximal (above the knees) DVT in symptomatic patients. Impedence plethysmography is not sensitive in the calves, and it may miss nonocclusive proximal thrombi.

The newest imaging test for acute DVT diagnosis uses AcuTect (Fig. 2), a low molecular weight synthetic peptide labeled with technetiun. This test is sensitive in the calf, giving an advantage over Doppler ultrasound for below-knee thrombosis. Statistical analyses from clinical trials indicate that AcuTect's sensitivity to detect acute calf thrombi is 90.6% (specificity 83.9%), using contrast venography as the gold standard. Acute thrombosis imaging will play a role in patients with indeterminate or nondiagnostic ultrasound and in patients with chronic venous disease who have symptoms of recurrent acute thrombosis. The diagnosis of DVT is sometimes used to aid in estimating a higher or lower likelihood of PE when the V/P scan is intermediate probability. Radionuclide venography (see section III, above), compared with contrast venography, has limitations including nonvisualization of the full extent of the thrombus, failure to detect nonocclusive and small thrombi and false-positive results when collateral vessels are visualized but no active thrombosis is noted by contrast venography.

For patients with suspected PE and DVT in whom ultrasound of the lower extremities is performed first and anticoagulation therapy is planned, the V/P scan should be performed as well. Besides documenting PE, the V/P scan can be used to document recurrence of PE by comparison with a subsequent V/P scan if the patient experiences symptoms of recurrence while on anticoagulant therapy. This indicates treatment failure, requiring alternative treatment measures.

WORTH MENTIONING

1. Fibrinogen uptake test

This test measures active deposition of fibrinogen. It is no longer available, because the radiopharmaceutical, ^{125}I-labeled fibrinogen, is not commercially produced in the United States.

2. Impedance plethysmography

Impedance plethysmography is based on the electrical conduction of blood, such that the amount of blood in an extremity is inversely related to the impedance to the electrical conduction. An inflated cuff is used to impede venous drainage. When the cuff is released, there is a rapid fall in volume, but when obstruction is present, this fall is less pronounced and less rapid; in 86–94% of patients with DVT by renography proximal thrombi are detected by impedance plethysmography, but only 30% sensitivity is seen for thrombi in the calf.

PATIENT INFORMATION

I. VENTILATION/PERFUSION LUNG SCAN
A. Test/Procedure

The lung perfusion and ventilation scan gives your doctor pictures of the blood flow patterns and the ventilation (movement of air in your bronchial airway) in your lungs. These scans are used to detect blood clots blocking the blood flow in your lungs. They also tell your doctor which parts of your lungs are functioning well and which parts are not. This test uses small amounts of radioactive materials to show blood flow in the lungs and air movement in the airway.

The ventilation and perfusion procedures take about 30–60 min. The perfusion lung scan is done by injecting a small amount of a radioactive material into a vein and then taking pictures. The ventilation lung scan is done by having you breathe in a small amount of a radioactive gas or aerosol and then taking pictures of your lungs.

B. Preparation

Diet. There is no special preparation for these studies. You can eat and drink fluids as usual.

Medications. There are no medication restrictions for this test. Depending on the findings and whether you need anticoagulation or other therapy, it may be advisable to repeat the lung scan at some time after therapy has been instituted or just before its completion to document the changes that have occurred in response to the therapy and to have this new baseline lung scan to compare with any scan needed in the future if this problem should recur.

C. Radiation risks

The amount of radiation used is small and similar to that given by other diagnostic x-ray tests. The radiation exposure to your whole body from this test is about 50% of the dose the average person living in the United States receives each year from cosmic rays and naturally occurring background radiation sources. The radiation dose is about 3% of the yearly dose considered safe for doctors and technologists who work with radiation. You can be around other people and use a bathroom normally without risk to others.

D. Pregnancy

If you are pregnant or think you might be pregnant, or if you are a nursing mother, please tell your physician so that this can be discussed with the nuclear medicine physician.

II. ACUTECT VENOUS THROMBOSIS SCAN

A. Test/Procedure

The AcuTect scan helps your doctor determine if you have had a recently formed blood clot in a vein, usually in your legs. After an intravenous injection in a vein unrelated to the suspected problem area, pictures will be obtained at 30 min and 4 hr after the injection.

B. Preparation

There is no special preparation and no medication restriction for this test.

2

C. Radiation risks

The amount of radiation used is small and similar to that given by other diagnostic x-ray tests. The radiation exposure to your whole body from this test is about 23% of the dose the average person living in the United States receives each year from cosmic rays and naturally occurring background radiation sources. The radiation dose is about 1.5% of the yearly dose considered safe for doctors and technologists who work with radiation. You can be around other people and use a bathroom normally without risk to others

D. Pregnancy

If you are pregnant or think you might be pregnant, or if you are a nursing mother, please tell your physician so that this can be discussed with the nuclear medicine physician.

References

1. Stein PD, Gottschalk A. Critical review of ventilation/perfusion lung scans in acute pulmonary embolism. *Prog Cardiovasc Dis* 1994;37:13–24.
2. The PIOPED Investigators. Value of the ventilation/perfusion scan in acute pulmonary embolism diagnosis (PIOPED). *JAMA* 1990;263:2753–2759.
3. Biello DR, Mattar AG, McKnight RC, Siegel BA. Ventilation-perfusion studies in suspected pulmonary embolism. *AJR Am J Roentgenol* 1979;133:1033–1037.
4. Webber MM, Gomes AS, Roe D, et al. Comparison of Biello, McNeil and PIOPED criteria for the diagnosis of pulmonary emboli on lung scans. *AJR Am J Roentgenol* 1990;154:975–981.
5. Gottschalk A, Juni JE, Sostman D, et al. Ventilation-perfusion scintigraphy in the PIOPED study, part I: data collection and tabulation. *J Nucl Med* 1993;34:1109–1118.
6. Sostman HD, Coleman RE, Delong DM, Newman GE, Paine S. Evaluation of revised criteria for ventilation-perfusion scintigraphy in patients with suspected pulmonary embolism. *Radiology* 1994;193:103–107.
7. Fennerty T. The diagnosis of pulmonary embolism. *BMJ* 1997;314:425–429.
8. Servatjoo P. Deep venous thrombosis: the dilemma of diagnosis. *J Am Podiatr Med Assoc* 1997;87:224–232.
9. Goodman LR, Curtin JJ, Mewissen MW, et al. Detection of pulmonary embolism in patients with unresolved clinical and scintigraphic diagnosis: helical CT versus angiography. *AJR Am J Roentgenol* 1995;164:1369–1374.
10. Stein PD, Hull RD, Pineo GF. The role of newer diagnostic techniques in the diagnosis of pulmonary embolism. *Curr Opin Pulm Med* 1999;5:212–215.
11. Ralph D. Pulmonary embolism: the implications of prospective investigation of PE diagnosis. *Radiol Clin North Am* 1994;32:679–687.

3
The Genitourinary System

Radionuclide renal scintigraphy provides important functional data to assist in the diagnosis and management of patients with a variety of suspected genitourinary problems. Not all renal scans, however, are the same; there is a choice of five different renal radiopharmaceuticals and several imaging protocols. To make sure the patient receives the optimal radiopharmaceutical and the most appropriate test procedure, it is essential to clearly specify the clinical question when referring a patient for renal scintigraphy.

SCANS AND PRIMARY CLINICAL INDICATIONS

3

CLINICAL QUESTIONS

Obstruction

Renovascular hypertension

Kidney function

Bladder outlet obstruction

Renal transplant

Testicular torsion

SCANS

I. BASIC RENOGRAM
A. Background

The basic renogram is the backbone of the more advanced procedures, such as the diuresis and ACE-inhibition renograms. The basic renogram includes a series of images of the kidney as the tracer is removed from the blood, transits the kidney and enters the bladder (Fig. 1). Renogram curves quantitating the tracer movement through each kidney are typically generated; these curves complement the images and are used in the interpretation of the study. At a minimum, the basic renogram also should provide a measurement of relative renal function. In some institutions, a measurement of total renal function and additional quantitative data are provided to facilitate interpretation of the study. The integration of the clinical presentation with the images and physiologic data derived from the scan often can provide important diagnostic and prognostic information for patients with known or suspected renal disease. The more advanced procedures (diuresis and ACE-inhibition renograms) are modifications of the basic renogram to answer specific questions.

3

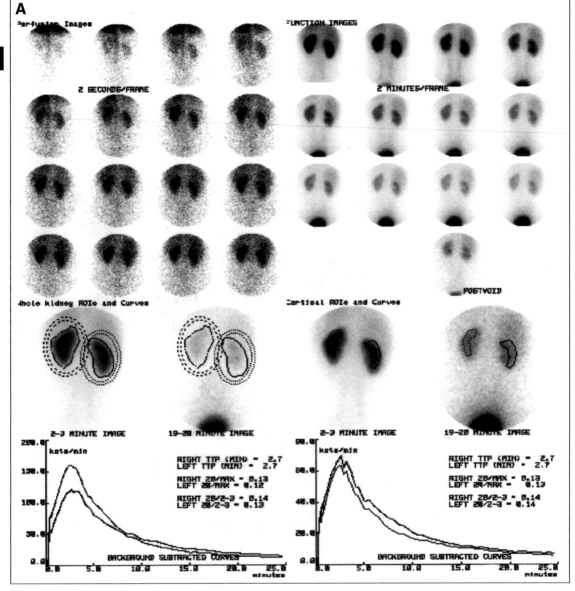

Figure 1A. Normal renal scan. The patient received an intravenous injection of 10.3 mCi (381 MBq) of ^{99m}Tc-MAG3. The images were acquired with the patient's back facing the camera. The left kidney is on the reader's left. Upper left panel. Sixteen sequential 2-sec dynamic flow images are presented showing the initial bolus of activity traveling down the abdominal aorta into both kidneys. Upper right panel. Twelve sequential 2-min images showing the rapid MAG3 uptake by the kidneys at 2 min. Ureters can be faintly visualized, and the bladder first appears on the 2–4 min image. A postvoid image also is shown at the bottom of this panel. Lower left panel. The regions of interest used to correct for background and used to generate the renogram curves are displayed on the 2- to 3-min image and on the 19- to 20-min image. The curves peak by 5 min and show rapid washout of the tracer from the kidneys. The time to peak height for both kidneys is 2.7 min. The 20 min/maximum and 20 min/2–3 min activity ratios also are displayed and are normal. Lower right panel. The regions of interest used to generate the cortical renogram curves are displayed. The cortical quantitative data also are displayed. Because the patient was well hydrated and there was no significant retention of the tracer in the collecting system, the quantitative data for the cortical and whole-kidney renogram curves are essentially identical.

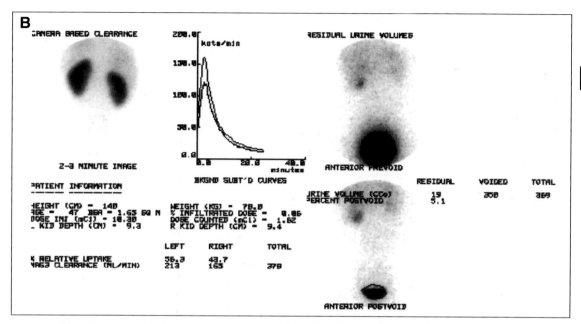

Figure 1B. Left panel. This panel displays quality-control data, including the patient's height, weight, dose injected and infiltrated dose. There was no significant infiltration—0.06% of the injected dose. The panel also shows the relative uptake—56.3% in the left kidney and 43.7% in the right kidney—as well as the individual and total MAG3 clearance using a camera-based technique. The MAG3 clearance was 378 ml/min, which is normal. Right panel. The panel displays the prevoid and postvoid bladder images used to calculate residual volume. The patient voided 350 ml of urine and had a residual urine volume of 5% or 19 ml.

B. Radiopharmaceuticals

1. Technetium-99m-mercaptoacetyltriglycine (MAG3). MAG3 is the most commonly used renal radiopharmaceutical in the United States. After intravenous administration, about 40–50% of the MAG3 in the blood is extracted by the proximal tubules with each pass through the kidneys; the proximal tubules then secrete the MAG3 into the tubular lumen. MAG3 has a much higher extraction fraction than DTPA (see below); consequently, it is a better diagnostic agent than ^{99m}Tc-DTPA, particularly in neonates, in patients with impaired function and in patients with suspected obstruction. The MAG3 clearance is highly correlated with the effective renal plasma flow (ERPF), and the MAG3 clearance can be used as an independent measure of renal function.

2. Technetium-99m-diethyenetriaminepentaacetic acid (DTPA). DTPA is the second most commonly used renal radiopharmaceutical in the United States primarily because it is the least expensive. Technetium-99m-DTPA is filtered by the glomerulus and may be used to measure the glomerular filtration rate (GFR). The extraction fraction of ^{99m}Tc-DTPA is approximately 20%, about half that of MAG3.

3. Iodine-131-orthoiodohippurate (OIH). OIH is extracted primarily by the proximal tubules although a small component is filtered. The extraction fraction of

OIH is 80% in normal individuals, and the OIH clearance often is called the ERPF. The typical adult dose is 300 μCi (11.1 MBq) but ^{131}I-OIH is used rarely in the United States because of suboptimal imaging characteristics of ^{131}I and its beta emission. The beta emission from ^{131}I can lead to a relatively high radiation dose to the kidney and thyroid, particularly if a patient has obstruction or impaired renal function.

C. How the study is performed

The patient lies in the supine position and the usual adult dose of 1–10 mCi (37–370 MBq) of MAG3 or DTPA is injected into a peripheral vein. Images are acquired dynamically for 20–30 min; post-void views may be obtained at the conclusion of the study. The technologist must then process the study on the computer to generate the renogram curve and various qualitative and quantitative indices.

Renal clearance measurements. Advances in nuclear medicine methodologies provide the opportunity to assess renal function (GFR, ERPF and MAG3 clearance) using either plasma sample clearances or camera-based methods. Plasma sample clearances involve blood sampling. Camera-based techniques do not require blood or urine samples to measure GFR, ERPF or a MAG3 clearance, but these measurements are not considered to be as accurate as plasma sample techniques and require specialized software (See F2 below, availability of clearance measurements under Potential Problems).

D. Patient preparation

The patient should be well hydrated when he/she comes to the nuclear medicine department for a basic renogram; there are no medication or dietary restrictions. (For diuresis or ACE-inhibition renography, there are diet and medication restrictions [see Patient Preparation for Diuresis and ACE-Inhibition Renograms, IID and IIID, respectively].)

E. Understanding the report

The report sent to the referring physician may include a description of the renogram curve and various quantitative indices of uptake and excretion. These data are integrated with the clinical presentation and other imaging data to provide the final impression.

The renogram curve is the time activity curve of the tracer as it transits the kidney; this curve is displayed routinely along with sequential timed images of the kidneys. In some institutions, two sets of renogram curves are generated: (a) a renogram curve from a region of interest (ROI) over the whole kidney and (b) a renogram curve from an ROI over the renal cortex (Fig. 1). As renal function deteriorates, the renogram curve often will flatten, reflecting delayed uptake and delayed washout.

3

The relative uptake of the radiopharmaceutical provides a measure of relative renal function and should be described in the report because it is an important clinical parameter. The report also may refer to the following indices:

1. T_{max} is the time to peak height of the renogram curve. MAG3, DTPA and OIH renograms normally peak by 5 min after injection and reach half peak height by about 15 min after injection; however, physiologic retention of the tracer in the renal calyces or pelvis can alter the shape of the renogram curve and lead to prolonged values for the time to peak, 20 min/max ratio and half-life ($T_{1/2}$).

2. The *20 min/max activity ratio* is the ratio of the activity at 20 min to the maximum (peak) activity and provides an index of the transit time and parenchymal function. With the tubular agents, it is an especially useful index in the detection of renovascular hypertension.

3. $T_{1/2}$ refers to the time it takes for the activity in the kidney to fall to 50% of its maximum value. This measurement is most useful after diuretic administration in patients with suspected obstruction (see below).

4. The *20 min/2–3 min ratio* relates the rate of washout (activity at 20 min) to the renal function (activity at 2–3 min); it is used in monitoring renal transplants and may prove to be useful in patients with suspected obstruction. Renogram curves generated from cortical ROIs (ROIs placed over the renal parenchyma that avoid the collecting system) and the indices generated from the cortical renogram curves may provide a clearer index of parenchymal function (Fig. 1).

F. Potential problems

1. *Hydration.* Occasionally there is nonspecific retention in the renal pelvis or calyces that distorts the whole kidney curve, whereas the cortical or parenchymal renogram curve is normal. Mild dehydration, for example, can cause calyceal or pelvic retention. This potential problem can be minimized by instructing the patient to be well hydrated when he/she comes for the study.

2. *Availability of clearance measurements.* Plasma sample clearances are not available in most nuclear medicine departments in the United States. Plasma sample clearance methods require meticulous attention to detail and are subject to error if performed infrequently or by inexperienced personnel. Validated camera-based clearance measurements require specialized software and are not available in many institutions. Camera-based clearances are not as accurate as properly performed plasma sample clearances, but they appear to be equally reproducible. Often a precise measurement of renal function is not as important as being able to reliably determine if the renal function is improving, remaining the same or deteriorating.

3

3. Availability of correlative imaging studies. Interpretation of the renal scan may be less useful if the interpreting physician does not have access to any correlative imaging studies of the kidney that may have been obtained.

II. DIURESIS RENOGRAM
A. Background
Obstruction usually results in a loss of function by the affected kidney unless it is an acute process. The purpose of intervention is to preserve renal function. Diuresis renography is a noninvasive test and the only study that can evaluate renal function and urodynamics in a single test. Urine outflow obstruction may be suspected based on clinical findings, the incidental detection of a dilated renal collecting system, or the previous diagnosis of obstruction in a patient referred for follow-up. Obstruction to urinary outflow may lead to obstructive uropathy (dilation of the calyces, pelvis or ureters) and obstructive nephropathy (damage to the kidney itself). Diuresis radionuclide renography is the noninvasive equivalent of a Whitaker test. The Whitaker test (pressure perfusion flow study) is an invasive nonphysiologic study that requires a percutaneous nephrostomy; the diagnosis of obstruction is based on an abnormal rise in pressure after perfusion of fluid directly into the dilatated system. Because of its invasive nature, the use of the Whitaker test tends to be reserved for special situations. Diuretic renography is based on a high endogenous urine flow rate stimulated by the administration of furosemide. Instead of a rise in pressure, the diagnosis of obstruction is based on an abnormally slow washout of the tracer from a dilatated collecting system. Furthermore, diuresis renography is widely available.

B. Radiopharmaceuticals
MAG3 is preferred over DTPA for diuresis renography (See IB above, Radiopharmaceuticals). The use of MAG3 results in fewer false-positive or indeterminate studies than DTPA, particularly in neonates or in patients with impaired function. Although it is not the optimal agent, DTPA is sometimes used because it is less expensive than MAG3.

C. How the study is performed
The study usually consists of a basic renogram followed by the intravenous administration of furosemide and another 20–30 min of imaging. Typically, the scan takes no longer than 1 hr to complete. In equivocal cases, some investigators recommend repeating the study with the "F − 15 renogram," in which the furosemide is administered 15 min before the injection of the tracer such that the patient is in a state of maximum diuresis at the time of MAG3 or DTPA administration. In selected cases, an equivocal study will become clearly normal or abnormal. Although furosemide will not affect the relative function measurements, many clinicians prefer to visualize the baseline urodynamics and do not make the "F − 15 renogram" the routine procedure.

D. Patient preparation

The patient should be well hydrated as for the basic renogram. Some physicians withhold diuretics for 24 hr before the study to minimize the chance of the patient arriving for the study dehydrated (see Patient Information for Radionuclide Renography).

E. Understanding the report

The report contains the same information as the basic renogram report. In addition, the report comments on the washout of the tracer after furosemide administration, may provide the $T_{1/2}$ measurement and states whether the kidney is obstructed or nonobstructed or if the study is indeterminate (see Potential Problems, below).

Interpretation of the test. Interpretation of the test is based on the rate of washout of the tracer from the dilatated collecting system. If there is prompt renal uptake of the tracer and prompt washout from the upper urinary tract collecting system, there is no obstruction (Fig. 2). Rapid washout of the tracer may occur before furosemide is administered, and depending on the local protocol, furosemide may not be necessary. The response to furosemide usually begins 2–4 min after injection, but the maximum diuresis usually is not reached until 15 min after injection. Some experts interpret the study based on a visual analysis of the washout curve; others, however, attempt to quantitate the rate of washout by measuring the $T_{1/2}$ (time for the activity in the collecting system to fall to 50% of its original value). Prompt clearance of the tracer from the renal pelvis with a $T_{1/2}$ <10 min is a normal response and excludes obstruction, and some authors will accept a $T_{1/2}$ <15 min as normal. Values between 15 and 20 min are often considered to be indeterminate, and a $T_{1/2}$ >20 min is considered suspicious for obstruction (see F1, below).

F. Potential problems

1. $T_{1/2}$. The $T_{1/2}$ not only depends on the presence or absence of obstruction but also on the level of function of the kidney in question, the placement of the ROI around the whole kidney or just around the dilatated collecting system, the radiopharmaceutical used in the study, the delay between administering the tracer and administering furosemide, the method of hydration, the presence or absence of a bladder catheter, the dose of furosemide and the interval used to make the measurement. For the reasons just outlined, measurement of the $T_{1/2}$ has not been standardized, and an isolated $T_{1/2}$ value should not be the sole criterion for determining the presence or absence of obstruction; the $T_{1/2}$ must be interpreted in the context of the whole set of images, curves and data analysis.

2. Equivocal or false-positive studies. Equivocal or false-positive studies may result from the following:

    1) The failure of the kidney under investigation to respond to furosemide. Urine flow rates decrease as renal function decreases,

3

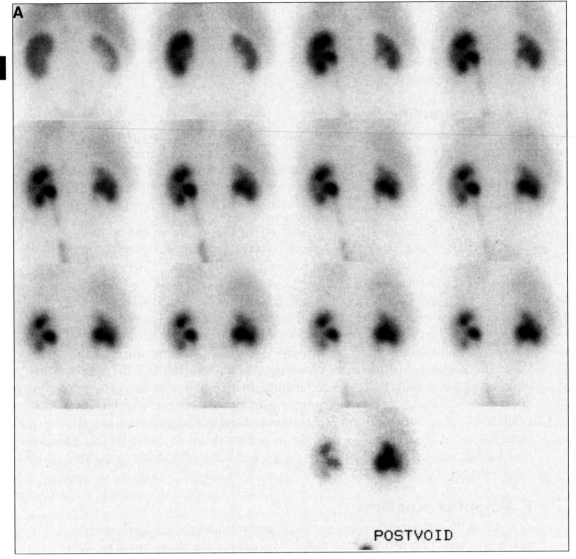

Figure 2A. A patient presented with a dilatated renal pelvis and possible obstruction of the right kidney. Sequential 2-min images show prompt uptake in both kidneys with marked retention in the right renal pelvis. There was no significant drainage from the right pelvis when the patient voided.

but urine flow rates as high as 4 ml/min have been reported from kidneys with creatinine clearances 15–20% of normal. This flow rate often makes it possible to obtain a diagnostic test even in patients with poor renal function, particularly if the renal pelvis is not massively enlarged.

2) *Slow washout of the tracer due to a grossly dilatated collecting system.* A greater problem than reduced function is a grossly dilatated collecting system. For any given rate of urine flow, the rate of tracer

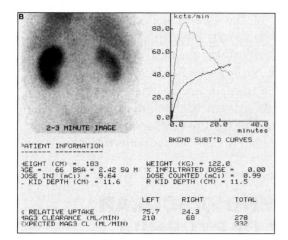

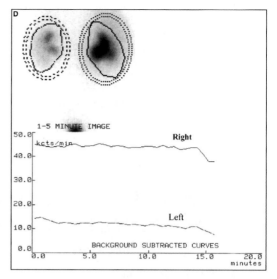

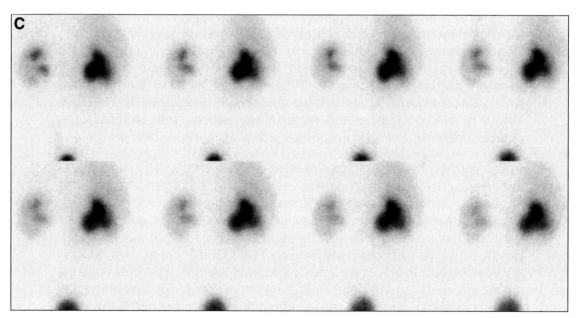

Figure 2B–D. (B) This figure displays the 2- to 3-min image, whole-kidney renogram curves and quality-control and functional data. The renogram curve of the left kidney peaks by 5 min and shows a normal washout pattern. The renogram curve of the right kidney is continuously rising and is abnormal. The left kidney contributes approximately 76% of the total renal function, whereas the right kidney contributes 24%. The total MAG3 clearance is 278 ml/min, which is normal. (C) Because of the persistance of MAG3 activity in the right renal pelvis, the patient received 40 mg of furosemide and additional 2-min images were obtained. There is no significant washout of tracer from the right kidney; the tracer has already largely washed out of the left kidney. (D) Regions of interest were assigned over each kidney, and background regions were automatically assigned. Both curves are relatively flat with a $T_{1/2} > 20$ min. The scan pattern, functional data, washout curves and $T_{1/2}$ show obstruction of the right kidney. The prolonged $T_{1/2}$ of the left kidney reflects the fact that the tracer was largely eliminated from the kidney before the furosemide portion of the study was begun.

3

washout decreases as the size of the dilated collecting system increases; consequently, a dilatated renal collecting system may result in a prolonged $T_{1/2}$, even in the absence of obstruction.

3) *Slow washout of the tracer due to a distended bladder.* A distended bladder may slow washout of the tracer from the renal collecting system. Many institutions have the patient void before furosemide administration. Patients usually are upright to void, and gravity can facilitate drainage from a dilatated but nonobstructed collecting system.

III. ACE INHIBITION (RENOVASCULAR HYPERTENSION OR CAPTOPRIL) RENOGRAM

A. Background

Renovascular hypertension is estimated to affect <3% of the unselected hypertensive population and up to 30% of patients referred to a subspecialty center for problematic hypertension. Renovascular hypertension is defined as an elevated blood pressure caused by renal hypoperfusion, usually due to anatomic renal artery stenosis and activation of the renin-angiotensin system. Advances in percutaneous renal angioplasty, renal artery stenting and surgical techniques have renewed interest in developing better tests for identifying patients with potentially correctable hypertension or renal dysfunction secondary to renovascular disease.

1. Renovascular hypertension versus renal artery stenosis. It is important to distinguish between renovascular hypertension and the presence of anatomic renal artery stenosis. Renal artery stenosis may be a consequence of hypertension rather than its cause and is common even in normotensive individuals over age 50. Renal artery stenosis may be an incidental finding in a hypertensive patient. Revascularization is expensive, is not without risk and may not result in any improvement in blood pressure in as many as 30–40% of patients undergoing the procedure. An ACE-inhibition renogram interpreted as high probability for renovascular hypertension carries a high predictive value (90%) that renal artery stenosis is present and that the hypertension will be ameliorated or cured by revascularization.

2. Mechanism of an abnormal scan after ACE inhibition. Renovascular hypertension is dependent on renin secretion from the juxtaglomerular apparatus of the underperfused, stenotic kidney. Renin converts angiotensinogen to angiotensin I, which is in turn converted to angiotensin II by ACE. Angiotensin II causes preferential vasoconstriction of the postglomerular (efferent) arteriole. Vasoconstriction of the efferent arteriole increases resistance to flow and can maintain the transglomerular pressure gradient and, thereby, maintain GFR even in the presence of a reduced perfusion pressure. Within the stenotic kidney, ACE inhibition reduces the angiotensin II dependent constriction of the postglomerular arteriole, decreases the resistance to flow and thereby lowers the transcapillary pressure gradient maintaining GFR. The resulting decrease in glomerular filtration of the stenotic kidney can be detected noninvasively with ACE-inhibition renography by either a change in relative function or retention of the tracer in the renal tubules due to decreased GFR and decreased flow of the filtrate through the tubules (Fig. 3).

B. Radiopharmaceuticals

Technetium-99m-MAG3 is preferred in azotemic patients. In patients with normal function, MAG3 and DTPA are equally acceptable. (See IB, Basic Renogram Pharmaceuticals, above).

C. How the study is performed

ACE-inhibition renography may be performed using oral captopril or intravenous enalaprilat (Vasotec) as the ACE inhibitor. A normal renogram that becomes abnormal in the left or right kidney after ACE inhibition is highly specific for renovascular hypertension. Two diagnostic approaches can be taken; the choice depends on local factors.

1. Basic renogram followed by an ACE inhibitor (oral captopril or intravenous enalaprilat) and a repeat renogram. This option provides the most definitive information but it requires two renograms and requires the patient to spend 2–3 hr in the nuclear medicine department.

2. The baseline renogram is omitted, and the patient receives the ACE inhibitor followed by a renogram. If the ACE-inhibition renogram is normal, the study is low probability for renovascular hypertension, and there is no need for the baseline renogram. If it is abnormal, the patient needs to return another day for the baseline study to maximize specificity; alternatively, high-risk patients with an abnormal study may be referred for angiography. This option provides the same diagnostic information as option 1 above if the study is normal, but it is less specific if the study is abnormal; however, only one renogram is required, and the patient spends only 1–2 hr in the department.

D. Patient preparation

1. Hydration. The patient should be instructed to be well hydrated when he/she arrives for the examination.

2. No food before captopril renography. If oral captopril is to be given, the patient should be instructed not to eat any solids after midnight before the examination. Food may delay gastric emptying and interfere with the absorption of captopril. The instructions should clearly distinguish between avoiding solid food and the importance of drinking water.

3

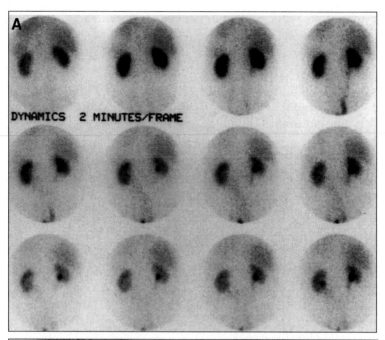

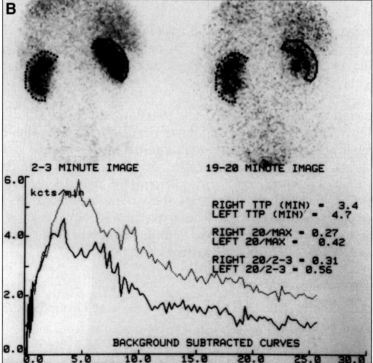

Figure 3. A 78-yr-old man presented with dizziness and was found to have a creatinine of 1.7 mg/dl and blood pressure of 230/120. He underwent baseline scintigraphy with 1.2 mCi of ^{99m}TC-MAG3. (A) Images obtained at 2-min intervals for 24 min show prompt uptake and washout of the tracer. The relative uptake at 2–3 min was 52% in the right kidney and 48% in the left kidney. (B) The cortical renogram curves, however, show that the left kidney had an elevated 20 min/max ratio of 0.42, which is more than three standard deviations above normal.

3

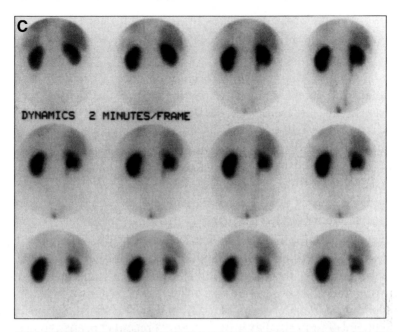

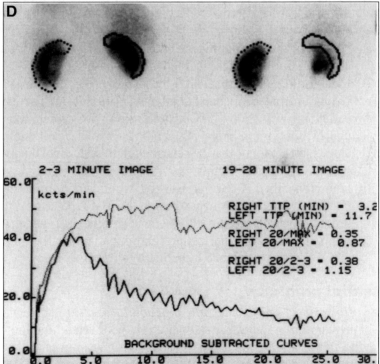

Figure 3 (continued). (C) After completion of the baseline study, the patient was given 50 mg of captopril. Approximately 1.5 hr later, ^{99m}Tc-MAG3 scintigraphy was performed with 9.3 mCi. Sequential 2-min images show cortical retention in the left kidney; however, the right kidney appears normal. (D) The left cortical renogram curve is markedly abnormal with a 20 min/max ratio of 0.87. The 20 min/max activity ratio for the right cortical region of interest has increased slightly from a baseline high normal value of 0.27 to a borderline elevated value of 0.35. Angiography demonstrated bilateral renal artery stenosis. A revascularization procedure was not performed. (Reprinted with permission from Taylor A, Nally JV. Clinical applications of renal scintigraphy. *AJR Am J Roentgenol* 1995;164:31–41.)

3

3. Diuretics. Diuretics should be discontinued for 3 days before the study to avoid dehydration and minimize the risk of hypotension.

4. ACE inhibitors and angiotensin II receptor blockers. Chronic ACE inhibition and angiotensin II receptor blockade may reduce the sensitivity of the test. For optimal sensitivity, these drugs should be discontinued for 4–7 days before the study with the longer half-life drugs discontinued for 7 days. With the exception of diuretics, other antihypertensive medications can be substituted for ACE inhibitors and angiotensin II receptor blockers if the patient requires replacement therapy during the 4–7 days before the ACE-inhibition renogram.

E. Understanding the report

The accuracy of ACE-inhibitor renography in identifying patients with renovascular disease appears to be high, with studies reporting sensitivities and specificities of around 90% in patients with normal renal function. Furthermore, most investigators have observed that a positive test predicts a successful reduction in blood pressure after revascularization, whereas a negative test indicates a low likelihood of renovascular hypertension. A recent consensus panel has recommended that the test be interpreted as high, low or indeterminate probability for renovascular hypertension:

1) High probability. Significant deterioration of the renogram curve after ACE inhibition compared with the baseline study.
2) Indeterminate (intermediate) probability. An abnormal baseline renogram that is unchanged after ACE inhibition. The majority of patients in this group have hypertension with azotemia or a small, poorly functioning kidney. Depending on the level of clinical suspicion, such a patient may be referred for an additional diagnostic test (see Clinical Question 6).
3) Low probability. A normal ACE-inhibition renogram is low probability for renovascular hypertension. Even if renal artery stenosis is present, hypertension in this group of patients is much less likely to improve with revascularization than in patients with a positive test (See Potential Problems, Ischemic Nephropathy, below).

F. Potential problems

1. False-positive or false-intermediate probability studies. These can occur because of dehydration, radiotracer extravasation, poor renal function, obstruction or a distended patient bladder at the start of the scan. A false-positive test also can be obtained if the patient becomes hypotensive during the study.

2. ACE inhibitors or angiotensin II receptor blockers. The sensitivity of the test may be reduced in patients on chronic ACE inhibition. To maximize sensitivity, ACE inhibitors and angiotensin II receptor blockers should be withheld for 3–7 days before the study depending on the half-life of the particular ACE inhibitor. When patients arrive for an ACE-inhibitor study and are found to be on chronic ACE inhibition, most centers elect to proceed with the scan and accept a slightly lowered sensitivity.

3. Ischemic nephropathy. A positive test result in a patient with azotemia or in a patient with a small, poorly functioning kidney indicates a high likelihood that the hypertension will be ameliorated by revascularization. Unlike the population of patients with normal renal function, as many as 50% of patients in this patient population may have an indeterminate or intermediate probability test result (an abnormal baseline study that does not change after ACE inhibition). A false-negative study also is more likely to occur in this patient population, possibly because of the absence of renin-dependent hypertension. Depending on the diagnostic goals, some clinicians will refer patients with ischemic nephropathy and a high pretest probability for renovascular hypertension directly to angiography. Magnetic resonance angiography or Doppler ultrasound are alternatives if there is a need to avoid constrast.

IV. RENAL TRANSPLANT SCINTIGRAPHY
A. Background
Complications of renal transplantation can be divided into parenchymal failure (acute tubular necrosis [ATN], acute and chronic rejection and cyclosporine/tacrolimus toxicity) and mechanical failure (injury to the renal artery or vein, ureteral obstruction and urine leak). A normal scan immediately after transplant excludes mechanical complications. Serial scans during the first 1–3 wk after transplantation can be used to monitor recovery from post-transplantation ATN and may detect early rejection 24–48 hr before biochemical abnormalities occur. Classically, rejection presents as diminished flow with delayed uptake and excretion, and ATN presents with good flow and delayed uptake and excretion, but severe ATN also can present with diminished flow. Indices such as the 20 min/2–3 min ratio and clearance measurements can be useful, but their use and availability varies from center to center.

B. Radiopharmaceuticals
Technectium-99m-MAG3 and DTPA are used to assess transplant function, but MAG3 is preferred in patients with impaired renal function (see Basic Renogram, Radiopharmaceuticals, above).

C. How the study is performed
The typical adult patient receives an intravenous injection of 1–10 mCi (37–370 MBq) of MAG3 or DTPA, and imaging is performed as described in the basic renogram with the camera positioned over the transplant.

D. Patient preparation
The patient should be well hydrated; otherwise, no special preparation is required.

3

E. Understanding the report

Images and renogram curves are evaluated for adequacy of flow, uptake and excretion. The report is similar to that described for the basic renogram (See Basic Renogram, Understanding the Report, above).

F. Potential problems

1. Hydration. See Basic Renogram, Potential Problems, above.

2. Cyclosporine/tacrolimus toxicity. Interpretation takes into account the clinical presentation including the number of days after transplant and knowledge of cyclosporin level. An abnormal scan indicating poor function may exclude infarct, leak and obstruction, but it may not reliably distinguish between rejection and cyclosporin/tacrolimus toxicity. Once renal damage is advanced, it is difficult for any imaging study to distinguish causes.

V. RENAL CORTICAL SCINTIGRAPHY
A. Background

Technetium-99m-dimercaptosuccinic acid (DMSA) and ^{99m}Tc-glucoheptonate (GH) provide excellent visualization of the renal cortex. These agents are used most often to detect pyelonephritis (Fig. 4) and are more sensitive than ultrasound or intravenous urography in detecting pyelonephritis. Cortical scans also can confirm a suspected column of Bertin, measure relative function and identify functioning renal tissue in patients with congenital abnormalities

B. Radiopharmaceuticals

1. Technetium-99m-DMSA. DMSA is an excellent cortical imaging agent. Approximately 40% of the injected dose binds to the renal tubules within 1 hr after injection; the remainder is excreted slowly in the urine over the subsequent 24 hr. DMSA is used when high-resolution anatomic images are required, such as for the detection of pyelonephritis. In patients with poor renal function, delayed images 2–24 hr after injection can substantially improve kidney visualization.

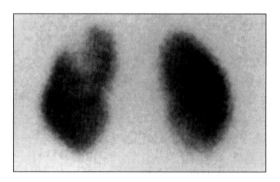

Figure 4. A 3-yr-old child presented with fever, leukocytosis and pyuria. A ^{99m}Tc-DMSA scan shows a focal wedge-shaped abnormality in the upper pole of the left kidney consistent with acute pyelonephritis.

2. Technetium-99m-GH. GH is cleared by GFR and the renal tubules. In patients with normal renal function, most of the dose is excreted rapidly; however, 10–15% of the injected dose remains bound to the renal tubules and high-resolution delayed static images can be obtained. Because of the cortical retention, GH is not recommended in patients with possible obstruction or to detect renovascular hypertension. Furthermore, some GH also may be excreted via the hepatobiliary system with resultant gallbladder visualization.

C. How the study is performed

The usual adult dose of 1–5 mCi (37–185 MBq) of DMSA or 1–10 mCi (37–370 MBq) of GH is injected intravenously. After GH administration, sequential images often are obtained as the tracer enters and transits the kidney; delayed images are obtained 1–4 hr after injection. Delayed images 1–4 hr after injection are obtained after DMSA administration. If a patient has impaired renal function, delaying the images up to 24 hr will provide better cortical detail. Standard images take approximately 30 min, and up to 1 hr is required if SPECT images are obtained.

D. Patient preparation

No special preparation is required.

E. Understanding the report

The relative renal uptake of ^{99m}Tc-DMSA or GH can be quantitated to provide an index of relative renal function. The cortical images are evaluated for homogeneous distribution throughout the renal cortex. Pyelonephritis is recognized by decreased uptake of DMSA or GH in the renal parenchyma (Fig. 4). Normal scintigraphic findings effectively exclude acute pyelonephritis. A column of Bertin can be confirmed when functioning renal cortical tissue corresponds to the mass questioned on ultrasound or CT.

F. Potential problems

Any process that replaces, injures or destroys normal cortical parenchyma will result in an abnormal scan. The configuration of the abnormality may suggest renal cyst, infection, tumor, infarct or scarring, but the study must be used and interpreted in the proper clinical context. Correlation with other imaging modalities is important to confirm the presence of a column of Bertin.

VI. TESTICULAR SCAN
A. Background

Spermatic cord torsion is a medical emergency and prompt surgical exploration is necessary to salvage the involved testis. The cause of acute unilateral testicular swelling and pain is usually torsion of the spermatic cord or acute epididymitis. Other possibilities include torsion of the testicular appendage, orchitis, strangulated hernia or hemorrhage. Radionuclide scrotal imaging can distinguish between acute epididymitis (no surgical intervention) and probable torsion, which requires prompt surgical exploration. Adequate examinations will detect more than 95% of patients with torsion; 80–85% of patients with nontorsion will be correctly identified and spared unnecessary surgery (See Clinical Question 16).

B. Radiopharmaceutical

Technetium-99m-pertechnetate is inexpensive and is commonly used to evaluate blood flow to the testicles.

C. How the study is performed

The study can be performed in 10–15 min. The patient is given a bolus injection of ^{99m}Tc-pertechnetate, and a radionuclide angiogram of testicular perfusion is obtained, followed by additional static images. The typical adult dose of ^{99m}Tc-pertechnetate is 10–20 mCi (370–740 MBq); the pediatric dose is appropriately reduced.

D. Patient preparation

None required.

E. Understanding the report

An area of decreased vascularity corresponding to the involved testis indicates that torsion is likely. If the clinically involved testis is normally perfused or hypervascular, emergency surgery is unnecessary.

F. Potential problems

Correlation of the scan results with the history and physical examination is vital for proper interpretation; this correlation should be done by the physician performing the study. Decreased flow to the affected testicle could be interpreted as increased blood flow to the contralateral testicle if the contralateral testicle were wrongly identified as the testicle at risk.

VII. RADIONUCLIDE CYSTOGRAPHY
A. Background

Vesicoureteral reflux, urinary tract infections and renal scarring can lead to hypertension and end-stage renal disease; however, a large percentage of patients with pyelonephritis do not have reflux. Furthermore, reflux often resolves spontaneously. Management of patients with urinary tract infection and/or reflux tends to be individualized and may vary from center to center. Reflux may be suspected based on an antenatal ultrasound showing ureteral or calyceal dilatation, acute pyelonephritis or documented reflux in a sibling. Conventional voiding cystourethrography (VCUG) with fluoroscopy is usually the first test in males to evaluate the possibility of posterior urethral valves as well as to grade the degree of reflux. Because congenital abnormalities of the bladder and urethra are rare in girls, radionuclide cystography may be used as the initial test. If follow-up studies are required in males or females, the patient should be followed up with radionuclide cystography; the technique is accurate for detecting reflux, and the radiation dose to the gonads is much less than with VCUG. Radionuclide cystography also is used to assess the results of antireflux surgery and in the serial evaluation of reflux in a patient with a neurogenic bladder.

B. Radiopharmaceuticals

Technetium-99m-pertechnetate, DTPA or sulfur colloid usually are infused directly into the bladder via a catheter (See Basic Renogram, Radiopharmaceuticals, above). Technetium-99m sulfur colloid is composed of radioactive particles about 0.5 μm in diameter (See Chapter 6, Infection Imaging). These agents are not absorbed into the blood from the urinary bladder.

C. How the study is performed

1. Direct radionuclide cystography. The bladder is catheterized, and the study is performed by instilling saline containing approximately 1 mCi (37 MBq) of a ^{99m}Tc radiopharmaceutical into the bladder. Imaging is performed continuously during filling of the bladder and subsequent voiding. Reflux can be quantitated by recording data on the computer during the study.

2. Indirect radionuclide cystography. Bladder catheterization is not required. The patient receives an intravenous injection of a ^{99m}Tc radiopharmaceutical. Because of its more rapid clearance, MAG3 is preferred to DTPA. The patient then undergoes evaluation of individual kidney function, urine drainage and reflux with dynamic images obtained during bladder filling, during voiding and after voiding. Indirect radionuclide renography avoids catheterization, but it is not as sensitive as direct radionuclide cystography for detecting reflux.

D. Patient preparation

None is required.

E. Understanding the report

The presence of reflux, as well as the grade, and whether reflux occurs during filling and/or voiding should be reported. The total bladder capacity and bladder capacity at the time of reflux also may be reported. These data can provide guidance regarding patient management and prognosis.

F. Potential problems

As with any pediatric imaging study, meticulous attention to detail in a facility with experience in pediatric imaging is important.

CLINICAL QUESTIONS

3

1. Ultrasound or CT shows a dilated collecting system. Is there ureteral obstruction?

Dilatation of the urinary tract with no apparent cause may be incidentally detected by ultrasound, CT or MRI in a patient with no symptoms of acute obstruction. If the dilated collecting system represents chronic obstruction, an intervention may be required to preserve renal function; if there is simply dilatation of a nonobstructed collecting system, no further work-up is required. Diuresis renography is preferred in the evaluation of the nonacute dilated collecting system because it is noninvasive and it is the only test that can evaluate renal function and urodynamics in a single examination. Diuresis renography allows the clinician to quantitate the physiologic significance of the anatomic abnormality by measuring the relative renal function and the diuretic stimulated washout of the tracer from the dilated system. Furthermore, contrast is avoided and the gonadal radiation dose is reduced substantially, being only 20% of the gonadal dose from intravenous urography.

In 10–15% of diuresis renography studies, the renal scan will be equivocal because washout of the tracer from the collecting system is not rapid enough to exclude obstruction and not slow enough to definitively diagnose obstruction. Indeterminate rates of tracer washout are most likely to occur in kidneys with poor function or massively dilated collecting systems (see Basic Renography, Potential Problems, above). Even if the washout rate is indeterminate, the measurement of relative function provides important clinical information. If a kidney with an equivocal washout rate contributes 50% of a patient's total renal function, there has been no functional compromise and obstruction is less likely. In the chronic setting, it may be appropriate to follow up with serial scans to ensure that function does not deteriorate rather than intervene surgically. If the kidney in question has reduced function, a percutaneous nephrostomy may be performed.

2. A patient with previous obstruction has recurrent symptoms. Has obstruction recurred?

A patient with previous documented and treated obstruction may present with symptoms suggesting recurrent obstruction; ultrasonography often is not helpful in this setting because the urinary tract can be dilated secondary to the previous episode of obstruction. Diuresis renography is the preferred examination (see Clinical Question 1, above).

3. Has surgery successfully relieved a documented obstruction?

A radionuclide scan can document adequate urine flow and relief of obstruction; at the same time, the scan can evaluate the function of the kidney in question

3

and determine (assuming the existence of a preobstruction scan) if there has been any improvement in renal function after the surgical procedure. Furthermore, the scan then serves as a baseline if the patient subsequently becomes symptomatic.

4. Does a patient presenting with flank pain have acute renal colic? If so, can he be managed conservatively?

Knowledge of the size of the obstructing calculus is important because calculi <5 mm generally pass spontaneously; as the size of the calculus increases, spontaneous passage becomes less likely. Intravenous urography (IVU) is often the first procedure performed, but it does involve risk of contrast reaction. Relative contraindications to IVU include renal insufficiency, diabetes, dehydration, allergy to iodinated contrast agents and pregnancy. Renal ultrasound with intrarenal Doppler and a plain x-ray of the abdomen are less accurate than IVU and requires skilled personnel; furthermore, ultrasound cannot differentiate dilatation without obstruction from true obstruction. Noncontrast enhanced spiral CT is rapidly gaining acceptance as an accurate screening method and is becoming the procedure of choice for patients presenting with acute renal colic.

There are acute situations, however, in which renal scintigraphy may be preferred. Many calculi between 3 and 8 mm are followed up conservatively in the hope of spontaneous passage, and patients may be managed on an outpatient basis. In this setting, it may be important to know that renal function is preserved and that delay is unlikely to lead to renal damage. Repeat abdominal x-rays can show that the calculus is moving downward. A baseline renal scan defines the relative function and degree of obstruction. Serial scans can confirm that renal function is preserved and that conservative management is safe. Deteriorating renal function of the affected kidney or increasing obstruction may point to the need for an intervention. The radionuclide renal scan can be used in patients allergic to contrast or with renal insufficiency.

5. Antenatal sonography showed a dilated pelvis or ureter. Is there obstruction or loss of renal function?

The significance of an abnormal antenatal renal sonogram can be readily evaluated by diuresis renal scintigraphy in the newborn (see Clinical Question 1). Because of its higher extraction efficiency, MAG3 is superior to DTPA in this setting.

6. Does a hypertensive patient have renovascular hypertension?

Risk factors for renovascular hypertension include abrupt or severe hypertension, hypertension resistant to medical therapy, abdominal or flank bruits, unexplained azotemia in an elderly hypertensive patient, worsening renal function during therapy with ACE inhibitors, grade 3 or 4 hypertensive retinopathy, a history of heavy smoking, occlusive disease in other vascular beds and onset of hypertension under age 30 or over age 55. To determine the most appropriate test, patients need to be categorized into (a) those with low likelihood of renovascular hypertension, (b) those with moderate to high likelihood of renovascular hypertension and normal renal function and (c) those with moderate to high likelihood of renovascular hypertension and compromised renal function.

Low likelihood of renovascular hypertension. The utility of a test to detect renovascular hypertension depends on the prevalence of the disease in the population studied. If a hypertensive patient has no risk factors, there is a low likelihood of renovascular hypertension and diagnostic tests for renovascular hypertension are not indicated.

Moderate to high likelihood of renovascular hypertension, normal renal function. ACE-inhibitor renography is highly accurate in patients with normal renal function (normal creatinine and the absence of a small, poorly functioning kidney); the sensitivity and specificity of ACE-inhibitor renography for renovascular hypertension in this patient population approach 90%. As an initial approach, angiography in this clinical setting is not cost effective; moreover, the presence of renal artery stenosis does not indicate that revascularization will be beneficial. The strength of ACE-inhibition renography is that it is the only widely available examination that directly examines for the presence of renovascular hypertension.

Moderate to high likelihood of renovascular hypertension, compromised renal function. Patients with impaired renal function often have nondiagnostic ACE-inhibition renograms. A positive ACE-inhibition test result indicates that hypertension is likely to improve after revascularization, but many patients with azotemia or a small, poorly functioning kidney have an intermediate probability or nondiagnostic ACE-inhibition test result (abnormal baseline study that does not change after ACE inhibition). Even if a small, poorly functioning kidney is supplied by a tightly stenotic renal artery, kidney function may not be salvageable, and the kidney may need to be removed or embolized.

In the appropriate clinical setting, an intermediate test result may be sufficient to refer a patient for angiography. Alternatively, patients may be referred for duplex sonography or magnetic resonance angiography. Duplex sonography can be time consuming to perform, and it has achieved reliability only at certain dedicated centers because of difficulties inherent in performing and interpreting the examination.

When there is a high index of suspicion, azotemic patients may be referred directly for angiography. Revascularization is sometimes performed in azotemic patients with renal artery stenosis in an attempt to improve renal function and ameliorate any co-existing hypertension. Intuitively, it seems reasonable to revascularize an azotemic patient to improve renal function, and renal function may be improved, but there are no controlled studies showing that survival after revascularization is superior to available medical therapy.

Prognosis and alternative tests. The renovascular hypertension renogram has important prognostic value in determining which patients will benefit from revascularization. Other imaging examinations only evaluate for the presence of renal artery stenosis. Conventional angiography or digital subtraction angiography are the gold standards for the diagnosis of renal artery stenosis (not necessarily renovascular hypertension), but they are invasive and subject the kidney to a contrast load. Thus, they are of less utility as screening examinations, especially for patients with poor renal function. CT angiography is noninvasive but subjects the kidney to a contrast load. Magnetic resonance angiography is gaining wider appeal because of its noninvasive nature and lack of iodinated contrast. These tests may be more useful in older patients who are most likely to have proximal renal artery stenosis; they are less sensitive for segmental or distal renal artery stenosis. Other tests such as renal vein renin sampling, hypertensive IVU and intravenous digital subtraction angiography are not appropriate as screening procedures, although renal vein renin assays, as well as ACE-inhibitor renography, can be used to evaluate the significance of a renal artery stenosis.

Summary. ACE-inhibition renography provides a logical diagnostic approach to the patient with one or more risk factors for renovascular hypertension, normal renal function and no known unilateral kidney disease. A normal ACE-inhibition renogram obviates further work-up. An abnormal study should lead to referral for angiography and revascularization. If a small, poorly functioning kidney is identified, angiography, CT angiography, magnetic resonance angiography or duplex sonography, depending on local experience and expertise, would be a reasonable next step. The evaluation of the patient with azotemia or a patient known to have a small, poorly functioning kidney is more problematic. ACE-inhibitor renography is a noninvasive procedure, and a positive test result should lead to angiography and revascularization if technically feasible. A disadvantage of ACE-inhibitor renography in this patient population is that as many as half of the test results may be intermediate probability; false-negative test results also can occur in this patient population. The advantages and disadvantages of other diagnostic approaches have been described, and test selection should be based on how the test result will influence patient management.

7–9. What percent does each kidney contribute to total function? What is the global (total) renal function? Is the global (total) renal function stable compared with the most recent measurement?

Relative renal function. The renal scan excels in determining relative function; the measurement can be made using the standard renogram or a cortical scan.

Total renal function. Quantitation of total renal function is often critical in patient management, particularly if there is underlying azotemia, the patient is taking nephrotoxic drugs, or the surgical question is total versus partial nephrectomy. In

3

many patients, a precise measurement of renal function is not as important as being able to reliably determine if the total renal function is increasing, remaining the same or deteriorating. The most common measurements of renal function are the serum creatinine and the creatinine clearance. Often these determinations are sufficient, but both are global indices and provide no information regarding regional or individual function. More than 50% of the renal function may be lost before the serum creatinine rises to an abnormal value. A formal creatinine clearance measurement using blood samples and 24 hr urine collection is cumbersome and often unreliable. Advances in nuclear medicine methodology allow the GFR, ERPF and MAG3 clearance to be measured using either plasma sample clearances or camera-based methods. Available data indicate that radionuclide clearances have less variability than the creatinine clearance and are superior to the creatinine clearance in monitoring changes in renal function; however, radionuclide clearance measurements are not available in many institutions.

10. A patient presents with acute renal failure. What is the cause?

There are various causes of renal failure, and the clinical presentation will dictate the diagnostic approach. Acute failure initially is evaluated best with ultrasound (renal size, atrophy, dilatated collecting system), but if there is a question of obstruction or underlying asymmetrical renal disease, a renal scan can provide important ancillary information. The scan can detect or exclude obstruction and quantitate the relative renal function; furthermore, good renal uptake of the radiopharmaceutical indicates the presence of functioning renal tissue and represents a favorable prognostic sign.

11 and 12. Is there bladder outlet obstruction or bladder dysfunction? What is the postvoid bladder residual?

The postvoid bladder residual can be measured by catheterization; however, ultrasound and radionuclide scintigraphy provide a simple and noninvasive means to answer this question. Residual urine volume can be determined as part of the routine radionuclide renal scan, saving the cost of an additional procedure. The measurement requires a prevoid and postvoid image of the bladder and measurement of the voided urine volume. The main source of error is tracer retained in a dilatated pelvis or ureter that drains into the bladder after voiding. In many nuclear medicine departments, this measurement is not routine and will need to be requested.

13–15. Is the transplant functioning normally? Is there a leak? Is there an obstruction? What is the cause of a poorly functioning renal transplant or rising creatinine?

The radionuclide renal scan can evaluate flow to the transplant, detect infarcts and leaks and distinguish between obstruction and a dilated but nonobstructed collecting system. The ACE-inhibition renogram is useful for detecting reno-vascular hypertension due to transplant artery stenosis. Duplex sonography can evaluate flow. Sonography can detect extrarenal fluid collections and determine if the renal pelvis is dilated. Sonography cannot distinguish between obstruction and a nonobstructed dilated collecting system. Neither test can reliably distinguish between rejection and cyclosporine/tacrolimus toxicity. Interpretation of the renogram requires integration of the test results with the clinical presentation including a knowledge of the antirejection therapy, the number of days that have elapsed since transplantation and the function of the transplant during this period. A scan showing a poorly functioning cadaveric transplant 1 day after surgery typically represents ATN; sequential scans showing a deterioration in function usually represent rejection, although cyclosporine/tacrolimus toxicity can have a similar presentation (See Renal Transplant Scintigraphy, Backgound, above). Institutions vary considerably in regard to how these examinations are used and at what point biopsy is performed.

16. Does the patient presenting with acute scrotal pain have testicular torsion?

The diagnosis of testicular torsion must be made as rapidly as possible because testicular viability decreases to about 80% within the first 5 hr and falls to about 20% after 10–12 hr. Radionuclide scrotal scintigraphy and scrotal sonography with color flow Doppler (duplex imaging) are acceptable diagnostic approaches to distinguish testicular torsion from nonsurgical causes of scrotal pain, such as epididymitis or epididymo-orchitis. The choice depends largely on clinical expertise, cost and availability of the two tests. In patients with suspected torsion, surgery should never be delayed because of a delay in obtaining a test.

17. Is there is a congenital renal abnormality? How well is the kidney in question functioning?

Congenital abnormalities often are detected by sonography in utero. The basic renogram is often important in determining the physiologic significance of a dilated collecting system detected in utero or after birth (See Clinical Question 4, above). In addition to evaluating the presence or absence of obstruction, the scan can determine if both kidneys are functioning, if only a portion of a kidney is functioning or if there is functioning renal tissue in an unusual location such as a horseshoe or pelvic kidney.

18. Does a child presenting with an acute urinary tract infection have acute pyelonephritis?

Pyelonephritis is a serious illness in the pediatric population; renal scarring from recurring infection remains an important cause of end-stage renal disease and hypertension. Clinical and experimental studies have demonstrated that scarring can be prevented or diminished by early diagnosis and aggressive therapy. It is important to emphasize that in infants and young children, pyelonephritis is not always accompanied by high fever, an elevated sedimentation rate and leukocytosis. A normal voiding cystourethrogram does not exclude acute pyelonephritis, and it is increasingly recognized that sonography and excretory urography cannot be used to exclude acute pyelonephritis in infants and children. Renal cortical (DMSA) scintigraphy is much more sensitive for the detection of pyelonephritis than ultrasonography, and many investigators recommend cortical scintigraphy in the initial evaluation of children with suspected pyelonephritis. MRI and CT with contrast are also sensitive tests for the detection of pyelonephritis, but MRI is expensive, and there is the possibility of an allergic reaction to iodinated contrast given during the CT scan.

Will the diagnosis of acute pyelonephritis alter patient management? The diagnostic algorithm depends on what the clinician will do with the information. Some institutions treat pediatric patients with suspected pyelonephritis empirically and only pursue diagnostic studies if the patient does not respond. In other institutions, patients with pyelonephritis receive more aggressive therapy or follow-up in the hope of reducing the risk of scarring and recurrent infection and thereby avoiding the subsequent development of hypertension and renal failure. In these institutions, it is important to distinguish between a lower urinary tract infection and pyelonephritis because the diagnosis of pyelonephritis changes patient management. An episode of acute pyelonephritis in males often leads to VCUG to check for reflux and posterior uretheral valves. In girls, congenital abnormalities are rare but VCUG or radionuclide cystography may be obtained to check for reflux. Once congenital abnormalities are excluded, radionuclide cystography is preferred to VCUG to monitor reflux because the tests are equally sensitive and radiation dose to the gonads from the radionuclide cystogram is only 1–2% of the gonadal radiation dose from VCUG.

Acute pyelonephritis in adults. Acute pyelonephritis generally causes flank pain and fever and frequently is accompanied by signs and symptoms such as urgency, frequency and dysuria. Uncomplicated urinary tract infection is relatively benign, rarely leads to progressive renal failure and usually is diagnosed and treated without the need for imaging studies. The diagnosis is based on the clinical features and results of urinalysis and urine cultures. For these reasons, a cortical scan is not considered necessary in the adult population. For suspected complications such as perinephric abscess, CT is much more valuable.

19–21. Does the patient have ureteral reflux? Is reflux present in an asymptomatic sibling of a child with reflux? Has previously documented ureteral reflux resolved or diminished?

In a male with suspected ureteral reflux, an iodinated contrast examination such as VCUG should be performed initially to evaluate the urethra and reflux. If reflux is established, radionuclide cystography is the ideal follow-up procedure.

Radionuclide cystography is just as sensitive as VCUG in detecting reflux, and the radiation dose to the patient is substantially less (See Question 12, above).

Renal scans can also be important in monitoring individual renal function during conservative management of ureteral reflux. Deterioration of renal function in a refluxing kidney is an indication for ureteral reimplantation.

22. Is a questionable mass on an intravenous urogram a column of Bertin?

Excellent anatomic images of the kidneys can be obtained using renal cortical scintigraphy in patients with allergies to contrast media or in those with a relative contraindication to contrast media administration. Hypernephromas have not been reported to concentrate any renal radiopharmaceutical. Most other renal masses, whether cyst, neoplasm or abscess, fail to concentrate radiopharmaceuticals used for renal imaging. They appear as areas of decreased activity, indistinguishable from one another. A renal column of Bertin is composed of normal cortical tissue, but it can appear as a questionable mass on ultrasound or IVU. The presence of normal cortical tissue can be confirmed by a cortical scan, which shows concentration of the radiopharmaceutical corresponding to the questionable area.

23–25. Is there a urine leak? Is the kidney functioning normally? Is a traumatized kidney recovering its function?

A CT scan is usually the first diagnostic imaging procedure obtained in a patient with suspected abdominal trauma; CT with contrast also can detect a urinary leak. A radionuclide renal scan can determine the effect of trauma on renal function, monitor functional recovery and identify a urine leak.

WORTH MENTIONING

1. Exercise renography

Preliminary studies suggest that many patients with essential hypertension will have abnormal exercise renograms. Exercise renography is performed with the patient exercising at a submaximal level in a sitting position on a stationary bicycle. The test is not widely used because, at present, the significance or clinical utility of the finding has not been determined.

2. Aspirin renography

Preliminary studies suggest that aspirin renography also may be useful in detecting renovascular hypertension. Aspirin blocks the breakdown of bradykinin, which modulates blood flow to the medulla. The role of aspirin renography in conjunction with or versus ACE-inhibition renography has not been determined.

3

3. Angiotensin II receptor blocker renography

Preliminary studies suggest the angiotensin II receptor blockers also may be useful in detecting renovascular hypertension. The role of angiotensin II receptor blocker renography in conjunction with or versus ACE-inhibition renography has not been determined.

4. Suspected infected renal cyst

The largest cyst is not necessarily an infected cyst. When a patient has multiple cysts, a cortical scan to localize the cysts combined with a gallium or labeled white cell scan to determine which cyst is infected can facilitate an appropriate drainage procedure.

5. Renal function and retroperitoneal fibrosis

Ureteral obstruction due to retroperitoneal fibrosis can be detected and followed up by radionuclide renography. This approach can be particularly important when the patient receives nonsurgical therapy such as steroids for retroperitoneal fibrosis.

PATIENT INFORMATION

I. RADIONUCLIDE RENOGRAM
A. Test/Procedure

Your physician has referred you for a kidney scan. This procedure is tailored to fit your individual needs, depending on the clinical question. In most cases, you will lie on a flat table, a large camera will be moved beneath the table and a very small amount of a radioactive tracer will be injected into an arm vein. You will remain on the table for 20–30 min while specialized pictures are being made as the radioactive tracer is removed from the blood by the kidneys and drains into the bladder. If there is suspected obstruction of the kidney, a drug to increase your urine flow may be injected and imaging of the kidneys may continue for another 20 min. If you are referred because of high blood pressure possibly caused by a narrowing of the renal artery, two 20–30 min imaging sessions of the kidney sometimes are performed in the same day.

B. Preparation

Diet. There are no food restrictions unless you are referred for suspected narrowing of the renal artery as the cause of high blood pressure. In this specialized case, you may be given a drug (captopril) in the nuclear medicine department. Food in the stomach may delay stomach emptying or interfere with the absorption of the captopril; for these reasons, you should not eat after midnight before the study, but you should be well-hydrated and continue to drink fluids; water, juice and soft drinks are acceptable. At a minimum, drink at least two large glasses of water when you get out of bed and two more just before coming to the nuclear medicine department. If you have a question, you may want to call the nuclear medicine department to find out if you will be given captopril.

Medications. Check with your doctor before stopping any medications. If you are having the test to determine if narrowing of the artery to the kidney is the cause of your high blood pressure, you may be asked to discontinue certain drugs including diuretics and drugs called ACE inhibitors or angiotensin II blockers.

C. Radiation and other risks

The radiation exposure is minimal and is comparable to that of many other diagnostic x-ray tests. In patients with normal kidney function, more than 95% of the radiation leaves the body by 4 hr. The effective radiation dose to your whole body is less than half of the radiation dose a person living in the United States receives each year from cosmic rays and naturally occurring background radiation. The radiation dose is less than 5% of the yearly radiation dose considered safe for doctors and technologists who work with radiation. You can be around other people and use a bathroom without risk to others.

D. Pregnancy

If you are pregnant or think you may be pregnant, please inform your doctor so that this can be discussed with the nuclear medicine physician before your test.

References

1. Rosenbaum JL. Evaluation of clearance studies in chronic kidney disease. *J Chron Dis* 1970;22:507–514.
2. Brown SCW, O'Reilly PH. Glomerular filtration rate measurement: a neglected test in urological practice. *Br J Urol* 1995;75:296–300.
3. Blaufox MD, Aurell M, Bubeck B, et al. Report of the radionuclides in nephrourology committee on renal clearance. *J Nucl Med* 1996;37:1883–1890.
4. Kass EJ, Fink-Bennett D, Cacciarelli AA, Balon H, Pavlock S. The sensitivity of renal scintigraphy and sonography in detecting nonobstructive acute pyelonephritis. *J Urol* 1992;148:606–608.
5. Rushton HG. The evaluation of acute pyelonephritis and renal scarring with technetium 99m-dimercaptosuccinic acid renal scintigraphy: evolving concepts and future directions. *Pediatr Nephrol* 1997;11:108–120.
6. Conway JJ, Cohn RA. Evolving role of nuclear medicine for the diagnosis and management of urinary tract infection. *J Pediatr* 1994;124:87–90.
7. Rushton HG, Majd M. Dimercaptosuccinic acid renal scintigraphy for the evaluation of pyelonephritis and scarring: a review of experimental and clinical studies. *J Urol* 1992;148:1726–1732.
8. Mittal BR, Kumar P, Arora P, et al. Role of captopril renography in the diagnosis of renovascular hypertension. *Am J Kidney Dis* 1996;28:209–213.
9. Holley KE, Hunt JC, Brown AL Jr, et al. Renal artery stenosis: a clinical-pathologic study in normotensive and hypertensive patients. *Am J Med* 1964;37:14–22.
10. Taylor A, Nally J, Aurell M, et al. Consensus report on ACE inhibitor renography for detecting renovascular hypertension. *J Nucl Med* 1996;37:1876–1882.

11. Blaufox MD, Middleton ML, Bongiovanni J, et al. Cost efficacy of the diagnosis and therapy of renovascular hypertension. *J Nucl Med* 1996;37:171–177.
12. O'Reilly P, Aurell M, Britton K, Kletter K, Rosenthal L, Testa T. Consensus on diuresis renography for investigating the dilatated upper urinary tract. *J Nucl Med* 1996;27:1862–1876.
13. Taylor A. Radionuclide renography: a personal approach. *Semin Nucl Med* 1999;29:102–127.
14. Taylor A, Nally JV. Clinical applications of renal scintigraphy. *AJR Am J Roentgenol* 1995;164:31–41.

4
The Spleen and Hepatobiliary System

Ultrasound, MRI and CT are basically anatomic imaging modalities. Nuclear imaging adds another dimension, that of physiology, in the evaluation of the hepatobiliary system and the spleen. Common procedures include the hepatobiliary (iminodiacetic acid [IDA]) scan, the hemangioma (tagged red blood cell [RBC]) scan and the liver/spleen (radiocolloid) scan. The type of nuclear scan that may be useful depends on the specific clinical question to be answered.

SCANS AND PRIMARY CLINICAL INDICATIONS

I. Hepatobiliary (IDA) scan or cholescintigraphy
Page 79

- To diagnose suspected acute cholecystitis
- To investigate possible biliary obstruction
- To detect biliary leak
- To differentiate biliary atresia from neonatal hepatitis
- To diagnose biliary dyskinesia
- To confirm the presence of a choledochal cyst

II. Hemangioma (tagged RBC) scan
Page 82

- To determine if a liver mass is a hemangioma

III. Liver/Spleen (radiocolloid) scan
Page 84

- To determine if a liver mass is focal nodular hyperplasia

- To confirm the presence of a splenule

- To investigate hepatosplenomegaly and hepatic function

CLINICAL QUESTIONS

4

Gallbladder

Jaundice

Hepatic mass

Spleen and liver size and function

Postoperative

PATIENT INFORMATION

SCANS

I. HEPATOBILIARY (IDA) SCAN OR CHOLESCINTIGRAPHY

4

A. Background

The IDA scan is used most commonly to evaluate the patency of the cystic duct in suspected acute cholecystitis. Other applications include potential biliary obstruction, leaks and atresia, as well as other clinical questions involving biliary dynamics. The scan is not useful to determine the presence or absence of gallstones or common duct stones. It often is called a HIDA scan after one of the first, but no longer used, imaging agents.

B. Radiopharmaceuticals

Technetium-99m-IDA agents (mebrofenin [Choletec] or disofenin [Hepatolite]) are bilirubin analogues with similar uptake and secretion (but not conjugation) into the biliary system. They allow visualization of the bilirubin pathway in the hepatobiliary system, including filling of the gallbladder, and passage through the common bile duct into the duodenum and small bowel.

C. How the study is performed

IDA is injected intravenously (1.5–5 mCi [50–200 MBq] adult dose) and serial images of the abdomen typically are acquired for 1 hr. If duodenum and gallbladder are visualized by this time, the study can be terminated. If the gallbladder is not visualized by 1 hr, this abnormal finding may represent acute or chronic cholecystitis. Failure to visualize the gallbladder on 2–4 hr delayed images increases specificity for acute cholecystitis. With severe hepatic dysfunction, 24-hr delayed views may be required.

Alternatively, many centers use morphine sulfate (0.04–0.1 mg/kg intravenously over 2–3 min) in evaluation of cystic duct obstruction to limit the examination to a total of 60–90 min with high specificity. Morphine causes constriction of the sphincter of Oddi, restricting further passage of bile into the duodenum and redirecting bile flow into the gallbladder with a patent cystic duct.

Cholecystokinin (CCK), which contracts the gallbladder, is given occasionally (0.01–0.02 μg/kg intravenously over at least 3–5 min) to increase diagnostic specificity for acute cholecystitis with prolonged fasting and to determine if there is complete or near-complete obstruction of the common bile duct. It also can be used to establish the gallbladder ejection fraction (percentage of the gallbladder contents that empty with contraction).

D. Patient preparation

The patient should not eat for 4–6 hr (water and non-narcotic medications are permitted) before the examination. Because prolonged fasting may cause false-positive results, if the patient has not eaten for more than 24 hr, CCK pretreatment may be used. An open intravenous line is preferred if morphine or CCK is required. A recent barium examination may obscure activity by blocking photons emitted from the IDA tracer.

Narcotics such as morphine or Demerol that contract the sphincter of Oddi should be withheld for 4–12 hr, if possible, because they alter bile-flow dynamics. The nuclear medicine physician should be aware of a morphine allergy in a patient because morphine is sometimes given during the examination as above. The presence of pancreatitis is also a relative contraindication to morphine.

E. Understanding the report

Typically, hepatic extraction of radiopharmaceutical from the blood is assessed, as well as timely secretion into the intrahepatic biliary system with bile flow into the gallbladder and duodenum. The images can be displayed in a movie format to facilitate viewing and interpretation. The radiopharmaceutical should be evident in the gallbladder and duodenum by 1 hr (Fig. 1).

Various patterns can indicate certain pathologic processes. Nonvisualization of the gallbladder by 4 hr (or approximately 30 min after morphine is given), with visualization of the duodenum, indicates obstruction of the cystic duct (acute cholecystitis) (Fig. 2). Lack of gallbladder visualization, with increased uptake of radiotracer partially surrounding the gallbladder fossa, is called the rim sign and may indicate complicated cholecystitis, such as perforation.

Chronic cholecystitis is suggested if the gallbladder isn't visible by 1 hr, but is visible by 4 hr or after morphine augmentation. Chronic cholecystitis also may be suggested if radiotracer passes into the duodenum before the gallbladder is visualized. In either case, the cystic duct will be reported as patent.

A high-grade obstruction is suspected somewhere in the course of the common hepatic or bile duct if there is good hepatic extraction but no visualization of the intrahepatic biliary system, gallbladder, common duct and duodenum. This intrahepatic cholestasis pattern may be due to retrograde pressure from obstruction or may have other causes including certain drugs such as Dilantin

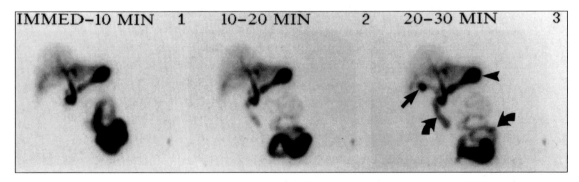

Figure 1. Compressed images from the first 30 min of an IDA examination demonstrate hepatic uptake and excretion with visualization of the gallbladder (straight arrow) and small bowel (curved arrows). Note enterogastric reflux that may be symptomatic in some patients (arrowhead). Also, chronic cholecystitis may be present because radiotracer appeared in duodenum before it passed into the gallbladder.

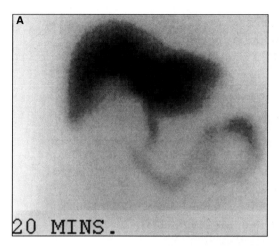

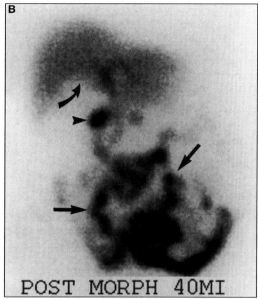

Figure 2. IDA images at 20 min before morphine sulfate (A) and at 40 min after morphine administration (B). The presence of cystic duct obstruction is demonstrated in (B) by small bowel visualization (straight arrows) with nonvisualization of the gallbladder in the gallbladder fossa (curved arrow). A prominent duodenum (arrowhead) may be mistaken for a gallbladder.

(phenytoin), oral contraceptives or phenothiazines. If the biliary system is not visualized, it is not possible to evaluate patency of the cystic duct or to determine the presence or absence of acute cholecystitis. Occasionally, with partial or early obstruction, radiotracer can be visualized to the level of obstruction.

The term delayed biliary to bowel transit may be used in the report if radiotracer takes >1 hr to pass into the duodenum. Delayed transit increases suspicion for partial common bile duct (CBD) obstruction but can be found as a normal variant in up to 20% of the population. If the gallbladder can be seen, but the distal biliary system cannot, CCK may be given to contract the gallbladder and force radionuclide into the duodenum to determine patency.

Modern IDA agents often can provide diagnostic studies even in patients with elevated bilirubin, but it may not be possible to obtain a diagnostic scan in a severely jaundiced patient with poor hepatic extraction. Both long-standing obstruction and primary parenchymal disease can appear similar. The nuclear medicine physician may want to bring the patient back at 24 hr to track the resultant slow progress of radiotracer through the biliary system.

CCK may be given to contract the gallbladder to generate a time activity curve and calculate an ejection fraction of gallbladder emptying. A low ejection fraction (<35%) may indicate gallbladder dysfunction under the appropriate clinical conditions. Too rapid administration of CCK may lead to gallbladder spasm and a falsely low ejection fraction. It is preferable to infuse CCK over 30–45 min.

F. Potential problems

1. Recent meal. It is critical that the patient be fasting except for water and nonnarcotic medications for 4–6 hr. A recent meal may cause gallbladder contraction and result in nonvisualization of the gallbladder, simulating acute chole-cystitis. The nuclear medicine physician should be informed of the time of the last meal or the presence of prolonged fasting (see below).

2. Prolonged fasting and other false-positives. Fasting for >24 hr may cause the gallbladder to distend with viscous bile; as a result, the IDA tracer will not flow into the gallbladder but pass directly down the CBD into the duodenum, simulating acute cholecystitis. In this case, the nuclear medicine physician may elect to pretreat the patient with CCK, contracting the gallbladder, preparing it to receive the radiopharmaceutical. (Unlike a recent meal, which will cause con-tinuous release of CCK and gallbladder contraction during the course of the examination, intravenous CCK will only cause temporary contraction.) Also, severe intercurrent illness, severe hepatocellular disease, chronic cholecystitis and hyperalimentation may cause a false-positive result.

3. Cholecystectomy. A previous cholecystectomy is an occasional cause for a false-positive result. Knowledge of the patient's surgical history is important.

4. Choledocholithiasis. A normal IDA scan does not exclude choledocholithia-sis or partial biliary obstruction. It simply evaluates bile flow.

II. HEMANGIOMA (TAGGED RBC) SCAN
A. Background

The prevalence of hemangiomas in the liver is 5–10%. Even in a patient with primary cancer, a solitary liver mass will more likely represent a benign heman-gioma than a metastasis. Even multiple lesions may represent hemangiomas. Determining which are hemangiomas and which are suspicious for neoplasia will help direct biopsy. Tagged RBC scanning is highly accurate with a speci-ficity of 90–100% and a sensitivity of 65–100% depending on equipment and size and location of the lesion (Fig. 3).

B. Radiopharmaceuticals

Technetium-99m radiolabeled autologous RBCs allow visualization of blood pool structures such as hemangiomas and vasculature.

C. How the study is performed

The patient's RBCs are first radiolabeled with technetium (20–25 mCi [750–925 MBq] adult dose), details about which are provided in Chapter 1, Cardiovascular Diseases, Radiopharmaceuticals. This may take from 30 min to 2 hr if the cells have to be sent to an outside radiopharmacy.

After reinjection of the tagged RBCs, immediate images may be obtained; these can take up to 30 min to acquire. Delayed images 1–3 hr later are always

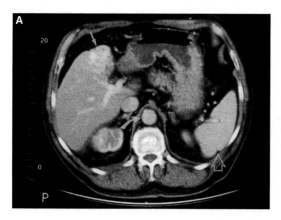
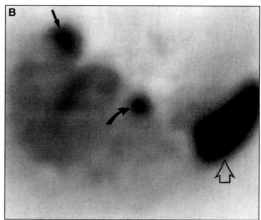

Figure 3. A 73-yr-old man with a bladder mass. Hypervascular liver mass on CT scan (straight white arrow in A) demonstrates intense delayed activity characteristic for hemangioma on the corresponding axial slice from the blood pool scan (straight black arrow in B). The spleen (open white arrow in A, open black arrow in B) and the aorta (curved white arrow in A, curved black arrow in B) also are imaged on both studies.

performed. The use of SPECT is important for the visualization of small lesions (<2–3 cm) and multiple lesions.

D. Patient Preparation

No special preparation is required. The patient does not have to fast. Any patient with poor intravenous access should be discussed with the nuclear medicine physician.

E. Understanding the report

A diagnosis of hemangioma can be made if there is a persistent hot focus compared with surrounding liver. This represents pooling of RBCs in the hemangioma. Its location should correlate with other imaging studies.

F. Potential Problems

1. Lack of correlation. Correlation with other imaging modalities is important, especially if multiple lesions are in question. If pertinent outside studies exist (e.g., the CT scan in which a mass is noted), make them available. Otherwise, a hemangioma may be discovered but could be incidental to the lesion in question.

2. False-Positives. There are rare cases of hepatoma, hemangiosarcoma or hypervascular metastases demonstrating false-positive findings. Comparison of immediate to delayed uptake increases specificity to nearly 100%. Also, knowing what the lesion looks like on other modalities helps increase confidence of a specific diagnosis.

III. LIVER/SPLEEN (RADIOCOLLOID) SCAN

A. Background

The liver/spleen scan is used uncommonly. The liver/spleen scan historically was used to exclude masses, most of which present as photopenic or cold defects (with a reported sensitivity of 80–85%). This role has been supplanted by CT, ultrasound and MRI, which have excellent sensitivity and specificity, as well as better anatomic definition. As outlined below in Clinical Questions 7, 9 and 11–15, there are some instances in which this scan is still useful.

B. Radiopharmaceuticals

Technetium-99m-sulfur colloid consists of 0.1- to 0.5-μm particles that are injected intravenously and are small enough to pass through the pulmonary capillary bed. They are phagocytized by the reticuloendothelial system (RES) and normally distribute in liver Kupffer cells (85%), macrophages of the spleen (10%) and bone marrow (5%). Processes that displace or destroy normal liver or spleen also will replace the Kupffer cells that take up these particles, resulting in an area of decreased radioactivity within the liver (a "cold" defect).

C. How the study is performed

Sulfur colloid (4–6 mCi [150–220 MBq] adult dose) is injected intravenously. The abdomen is then imaged 10–20 min later for 15–30 min or up to 1 hr for SPECT.

D. Patient preparation

No special preparation is required. The patient does not have to fast.

E. Understanding the report

The size and shape of the liver and spleen are noted. The liver and spleen are assessed for homogeneity of uptake and for focal cold or hot abnormalities. The relative uptake of radiocolloid in the liver, spleen and bone marrow gives an indication of colloid shift. Increasing hepatic dysfunction or replacement causes a greater relative shift of particulate uptake from the liver to the spleen and bone marrow.

F. Potential problems

Hepatocellular disease. Severe hepatic dysfunction with portal hypertension produced by cirrhosis or other diseases may result in poor uptake, which would limit evaluation for focal masses.

CLINICAL QUESTIONS

1. Right upper quadrant pain: Acute cholecystitis?

4

Twenty million people in the United States have gallstone disease, but many remain asymptomatic. Sixty percent of patients with acute epigastric or right upper quadrant pain have cholelithiasis, yet most of the time, acute cholecystitis is not present. For the typical case of acute cholecystitis in which a gallstone is causing obstruction of the cystic duct, there is no better test than a properly performed IDA scan (97% sensitivity and 90–95% specificity). Although ultrasound is best to determine if gallstones are present, its specificity is only about 78% in diagnosing cystic duct obstruction. Cholescintigraphy is the only examination that directly determines the patency of the cystic duct in a noninvasive manner. Ultrasound and CT only detect the secondary nonspecific changes that occur from acute cholecystitis.

General guidelines

- For a patient with known gallstones or in whom there is high clinical suspicion of acute cholecystitis: Hepatobiliary IDA scintigraphy is the preferred examination.
- For the patient in whom the presence of gallstones or the clinical question and history are not clear (shotgun approach): Ultrasound, or possibly CT, is preferred. An IDA scan may be indicated if gallstones are confirmed, but classic and specific findings of acute cholecystitis are not present. This may help avoid unnecessary emergent surgery.

2. Intensive care unit patient with unexplained fever: Acute acalculous cholecystitis?

In this special situation, ultrasound should be done first because it is easily performed in the intensivce care unit and is relatively inexpensive. If normal, the evaluation can then be focused elsewhere. If suspicious, the IDA scan should be done.

These patients have often been fasting for >24 hr. A dilatated, sludge-filled, somewhat thickened gallbladder on ultrasound is a common and nonspecific finding in this population. Most do not have acalculous cholecystitis. To make matters worse, because IDA may not be able to enter the distended, sludge-filled but otherwise healthy gallbladder, false-positive scans can occur. Pretreatment with CCK, or possibly morphine during the examination, may be used by the nuclear medicine physician to improve accuracy.

Although specificity may be decreased, the sensitivity of IDA scanning in this situation is still 90%. If the gallbladder fills, acalculous cholecystitis is excluded with 90% confidence, and a percutaneous or operative cholecystectomy can be avoided. (Acalculous cholecystitis can be excluded with near 100% certainty if intravenous CCK administration stimulates significant contraction.) In addition, for problem situations with a positive IDA scan, it may be worthwhile considering a radiolabeled white blood cell scan or a 4-hr gallium scan.

3. Right upper quadrant pain: Chronic calculus cholecystitis?

Most patients with chronic cholecystitis will have a normal IDA scan. Furthermore, almost all patients with gallstones demonstrate some pathologic evidence of chronic cholecystitis. Cholescintigraphy can demonstrate patency of the cystic duct. Although chronic cholecystitis can be inferred from delayed visualization of the gallbladder, neither IDA nor other imaging modalities are specific for chronic cholecystitis beyond establishing the presence of stones.

4. Chronic biliary symptoms and normal gallbladder ultrasound: Biliary dyskinesia?

There are entities known as chronic acalculous cholecystitis, gallbladder dyskinesia, and sphincter of Oddi dysfunction that are increasingly recognized as a source of treatable abdominal pain. IDA scanning can serve as a useful tool to determine abnormal biliary dynamics, however it should not be used as a blind screening examination, but only after other causes of abdominal pain have been excluded. Usually this test involves giving CCK to determine if normal gallbladder contraction, ejection fraction and bile flow are present. Also, the presence of enterogastric reflux as a cause of unexplained abdominal pain may be detected on IDA scanning.

5. Jaundice: Biliary obstruction?

IDA scanning is not a good first-line test in the evaluation of jaundice because only complete or near-complete obstruction can be detected with high sensitivity and specificity. Yet, there are many situations in which IDA scanning proves useful, especially if more invasive procedures, such as diagnostic endoscopic retrograde cholangiopancreatography (ERCP), are not an immediate or safe choice.

IDA can demonstrate obstruction in the first 24–72 hr before the biliary system has a chance to dilate. In a patient with acute elevation of bilirubin, this study can identify high-grade obstruction requiring emergent ERCP or percutaneous biliary intervention. Intermittent or partial obstruction may be missed on IDA scan, as well as ultrasound. ERCP is required in this situation. (Some centers may attempt CT or MRI first.) Thus, one shouldn't depend on the IDA scan to exclude obstruction completely. But knowing that there isn't a complete or near-complete obstruction can defer emergent ERCP.

This examination is also most helpful in the first week of jaundice to differentiate elevated liver function tests due to obstruction from other nonobstructive causes. In the presence of long-standing elevated bilirubin and liver failure, the IDA scan becomes harder to interpret and less specific in diagnosing obstruction.

After obstruction causing biliary dilation has resolved, the CBD may not return to a normal size. IDA scanning can be useful to separate obstructive biliary dilation from nonobstructive causes.

6. Newborn with jaundice: Biliary atresia versus neonatal hepatitis?

In the evaluation of the newborn with elevated bilirubin, IDA scanning is considered the primary test in differentiating biliary atresia from other causes of neonatal jaundice, such as hepatitis. It is more accurate when carried out after phenobarbital pretreatment, and 24-hr imaging often is needed to visualize radiotracer in the bowel, which excludes biliary atresia.

7. Potential hepatic mass?

As noted above, other imaging modalities have supplanted the radiocolloid scan in the search for hepatic masses. Yet there are some instances in which this scan may be useful such as in the markedly obese patient. If the patient has surpassed the weight limit of the CT or MRI table, he/she is probably past the weight limit of the nuclear gamma camera table, although the nuclear scan can be done standing or on a stretcher with some machines. In addition, if the patient is too large for ultrasound to penetrate well, there will likely be increased attenuation of the photons from the radiocolloid, degrading the quality of the scan. Even so, attenuated planar images of the liver can be of diagnostic quality and are worth a try.

8. Hepatic mass on CT or ultrasound: Hemangioma?

Ultrasound may demonstrate findings suggestive of hemangioma, but it is not definitive. A classic ultrasound appearance of homogeneous increased echogenicity with follow-up to document stability may be adequate for a patient with an incidentally discovered mass and no history of primary cancer, but it is not as desirable an option in a patient undergoing staging for primary neoplasia.

A hemangioma has highly specific characteristics on an intravenous contrast-enhanced CT (i.e., nodular centripetal fill-in with contrast), but they are often not met in a screening examination. Small and multiple lesions can be difficult to characterize. If a lesion is found on ultrasound or CT that is likely to be a hemangioma, but for which definitive proof is required short of biopsy, what is the next logical step?

Certainly a repeat focused CT can be performed, exposing the patient to more iodinated contrast. Alternatively, tagged-RBC scanning and MRI have high sensitivity and specificity if properly performed. With SPECT and correlation with other imaging modalities in which the lesion was first noted, a positive RBC scan is virtually diagnostic of hemangioma. The use of SPECT will identify 1- to 2-cm lesions with high sensitivity, and ones as small as 0.5–1 cm with less sensitivity. Depending on which MRI protocols are used, there can be overlap

4

of the appearance of hemangiomas and malignant lesions. It often is easier to be definitive on a positive nuclear hemangioma scan than it is on MRI.

This is a suggested algorithm: For a lesion >2 cm, or for multiple lesions, RBC scanning is an excellent choice. For lesions 1–2 cm, RBC scanning may be preferred depending on location of the lesion in the liver. If a 1- to 2-cm lesion is deep-seated or near portal vessels, MRI is more accurate. For a lesion <1 cm, MRI is the better choice, although it still may be difficult to make a definitive diagnosis. Multiple modalities may be required. The uncommon fibrosed or thrombosed hemangioma will be difficult to diagnose with any modality short of biopsy. It is best to discuss the issues with the nuclear medicine physician before ordering the tests.

9. Hepatic mass on CT or ultrasound: FNH?

The appearance of FNH and malignant liver lesions can overlap on CT, ultrasound and MRI. Homogeneity, isointensity on T1 and T2 sequences and a hyperintense central scar are characteristic appearances of FNH on MRI, yet this classic triad is present in <10% of cases. Thus, nuclear imaging can add important ancillary information if a biopsy is not desired.

Fifty percent to 60% of FNHs demonstrate normal or slightly increased uptake on radiocolloid scan. Ten percent have intense uptake, and the remaining 20–30% have decreased or no uptake. Therefore, if the lesion in question shows intense uptake, it is pathognomonic for FNH. Small lesions (<1–2 cm) may be difficult to detect depending on imaging equipment. If there is normal or slightly increased radiocolloid uptake, it is still probably FNH. (Some adenomas can have this degree of uptake.) If one combines this appearance on radiocolloid scan with findings suggestive of FNH on other modalities, such as central scar, a confident diagnosis can be made. Hepatoma, metastases, most adenomas or benign lesions such as cysts and hemangiomas will not have colloid uptake and appear as cold defects.

10. Right upper quadrant mass: Choledochal cyst?

IDA will fill a cyst which communicates with the biliary tree, and an IDA scan is an ideal method to confirm this entity.

11. Abnormal physical examination: Is hepatomegaly or splenomegaly present?

The liver/spleen (radiocolloid) scan can determine if hepatomegaly or splenomegaly is present. The classic use of this examination is for the patient with chronic obstructive pulmonary disease in whom the liver may be normal size but is pushed inferiorly by hyperinflated lungs, simulating hepatomegaly on physical examination. Although ultrasound and CT are not as convenient for imaging overall hepatic and splenic size due to limited fields of view, they are used most often for evaluating hepatosplenomegaly because of higher sensitivity and specificity than the liver/spleen scan in the detection of masses.

12. Can I get an image of my patient's impaired liver function to encourage lifestyle change?

As hepatic dysfunction deteriorates, there is a shift of particles away from the liver to the spleen and bone marrow. This can be followed visually on radiocolloid scanning, but is somewhat nonspecific because there are other causes of colloid shift, such as certain anemias. Although plasma liver function tests such as albumin, prothrombin time and bilirubin are inexpensive and easy to perform, a physiologic/anatomic picture of hepatic dysfunction may prove useful to help the patient and family understand the disease or even to encourage a lifestyle change. After alcohol is ceased, the scan may return to normal if liver function improves.

13. Splenule versus neoplasia?

Although radiocolloid scanning also can be used to judge spleen size and search for abnormalities, it is much more useful in evaluating a mass in the abdomen that could be an accessory or residual spleen versus neoplasia. This problem may occur after a splenectomy in a patient with lymphoma. By demonstrating a mass to be splenic tissue, biopsy can be avoided. Neoplasia or lymph nodes will not take up radiocolloid. Correlation with other imaging modalities and SPECT capability are helpful for a more specific diagnosis.

A different nuclear imaging examination, the heat-denatured RBC scan, is sensitive for splenic tissue but is not as readily available (see Worth Mentioning #2, below). Radiolabeled leukocyte scanning also can be used to visualize the spleen.

14. Functional asplenia/polysplenia?

The radiocolloid scan also is useful in the evaluation of the asplenia/polysplenia syndromes and in the determination of functional asplenia due to infarct.

15. Splenic trauma?

CT is the procedure of choice for this question. In the unlikely event that it is not available, radiocolloid imaging can be used to evaluate for splenic trauma, but its sensitivity is low.

16. Postoperative problem solving: Bile leak?

With the advent of laparascopic cholecystectomy there has been an increase in the incidence of bile leaks. Bile leaks can also occur after liver transplants and biliary diversion surgery. ERCP remains the gold standard for determining the presence of bile leaks and answering detailed anatomic questions, but it is invasive. In addition, the endoscopist may not be able to cannulate the CBD. IDA scanning is approximately 85% accurate in demonstrating if a leak is present and is an excellent, noninvasive, first-line test.

17. Postoperative problem solving: Afferent loop obstruction status post Billroth II anastomosis?

The afferent loop is difficult to fill on upper gastrointestinal series. An IDA scan can fill the loop via the biliary system and demonstrate emptying; it also can be used to help determine what surgery has been performed, if there is any doubt.

18. Postoperative problem solving: Patency after biliary diversion procedure?

This examination is an ideal, noninvasive method to ensure not only mechanical but physiologic patency after biliary diversion and liver transplant surgery.

WORTH MENTIONING

1. Hepatic arterial chemotherapy pump

Although usually confined to specialty centers, imaging with ^{99m}Tc-macroaggregated albumin (MAA) injected through the hepatic arterial port is used to determine if the pump catheter is in the proper location for infusion of chemotherapy to liver lesions. It may be performed in conjunction with the radiocolloid scan. The relatively large MAA particles are trapped by the first capillary bed they encounter, and their use can ensure that the chemotherapeutic agent is not being delivered to vital organs such as the stomach or spleen.

2. Heat-denatured RBC scan

This study is used for highly sensitive imaging of only splenic tissue but is not commonly offered. The patient's blood is withdrawn and the RBCs are heat denatured, then radiolabelled with ^{99m}Tc. The RBCs are reinjected and imaging is carried out 30–120 min later. The report will describe the technique used as well as the number, size and location of functioning splenic tissue.

3. RBC (splenic) sequestration study

This is a nonimaging nuclear medicine study performed with RBCs labeled with ^{51}Cr, which tracks their removal from the circulation by the spleen. The study may extend over 2–3 wk, is technically demanding and is not widely offered.

4. Potential hepatoma or hepatic abscess

In the evaluation of potential hepatoma, a gallium scan may be useful because hepatoma is gallium avid. Radiolabeled white blood cells also can be used to evaluate a mass that may be a liver abscess.

4

5. MRI contrast agents

Some newly developed contrast agents are taken up by RES cells in the liver, but early reports suggest that they might not exactly mimic radiocolloid uptake in FNH.

6. Technetium-99m-galactosyl-neoglycoalbumin

This is a new radiotracer that specifically binds to hepatocytes and holds promise in diagnosing FNH.

PATIENT INFORMATION

I. HEPATOBILIARY (IDA) SCAN
A. Test/Procedure

Your doctor has ordered a hepatobiliary (IDA) scan to determine if you have a problem with your gallbladder or bile duct system.

A small amount of radioactive material called a tracer will be injected into your vein. This tracer normally is taken up by your liver, which then passes it into your gallbladder and bowel.

You will be positioned next to a special machine called a gamma camera, which doesn't produce radiation but detects radiation that is coming from the injected tracer in your body. A series of pictures of your abdomen will then be taken, typically for 1 hr. You may have to come back for delayed images up to 4 hr later and, uncommonly, at 24 hrs.

Before or during the examination you may be given certain medications to help with the study. One is called CCK and makes your gallbladder contract. It is given slowly, but it may cause some queasiness, nausea or other abdominal discomfort. If this happens, please inform the doctor or technologist. No serious side effects have been reported for this use of CCK. Another medication that may be used is morphine sulfate, a common pain killer, which also can help direct the tracer into your gallbladder. It is given in a small and safe dose. If you have an allergy to either of these medications, please inform your doctor.

B. Preparation

You should fast (water is permitted) for 4–6 hr before the test. Most medications will not interfere with the study. Some types of pain killers may cause a problem and should be stopped for 4–12 hr before the test. If you are taking pain killers, please discuss this with your doctor. Also, if you have fasted for >24 hr, inform your doctor because it may affect the way the study is performed and interpreted. If you have had surgery on your gallbladder, please tell this to your doctor and the nuclear medicine personnel.

4

C. Radiation and other risks

The amount of radiation used is small and similar to that given by other diagnostic x-ray tests. The effective adult radiation dose to your whole body from this test is about the dose the average person living in the United States receives in 6 mo to 1.5 yr from cosmic rays and naturally occurring background radiation sources. The radiation dose is about 5–10% of the yearly dose considered safe for doctors and technologists who work with radiation. You can be around other people and use a bathroom normally without risk to others.

D. Pregnancy

If you are pregnant or think you could be pregnant, inform your doctor so that this can be discussed with the nuclear medicine physician.

II. HEMANGIOMA (TAGGED RBC) SCAN

A. Test/Procedure

Your doctor has ordered a hemangioma (tagged RBC) scan to determine if the suspected growth in your liver is a benign collection of blood vessels called a hemangioma.

Your RBCs will be labeled with a small amount of radioactive material called a tracer either by a series of injections or by withdrawing a small amount of blood from your vein and then reinjecting it with the tracer attached to the RBCs.

You will be positioned next to a special machine called a gamma camera, which doesn't produce radiation but detects radiation that is coming from the injected tracer in your body. A series of pictures of your abdomen will then be taken 1–3 hr later that take 30–60 min to complete. Images also may be obtained immediately after the injection.

B. Preparation

There is no special preparation. Eating, drinking and taking medications do not interfere with this examination.

C. Radiation and other risks

The amount of radiation used is small and similar to that given by other diagnostic x-ray tests. The effective adult radiation dose to your whole body from this test is about the same dose as the average person living in the United States receives in 2–2.5 yr from cosmic rays and naturally occurring background radiation sources. The radiation dose is about 10–15% of the yearly dose considered safe for doctors and technologists who work with radiation. You can be around other people and use a bathroom normally without risk to others.

D. Pregnancy

If you are pregnant or think you could be pregnant, inform your doctor so that this can be discussed with the nuclear medicine physician.

III. LIVER/SPLEEN (RADIOCOLLOID) SCAN

A. Test/Procedure

Your doctor has ordered a liver/spleen scan to examine your liver and/or spleen for abnormalities.

4

A small amount of radioactive material called a tracer will be injected into your vein. You will be positioned next to a special machine called a gamma camera, which doesn't produce radiation but detects radiation that is coming from the injected tracer in your body. A series of pictures of your abdomen will then be taken, typically for 30–60 min.

B. Preparation

There is no special preparation. Eating, drinking and taking medications do not interfere with this examination.

C. Radiation and other risks

The amount of radiation used is small and similar to that given by other diagnostic x-ray tests. The effective adult radiation dose to your whole body from this test is about the dose the average person living in the United States receives in 8 mo to a year from cosmic rays and naturally occurring background radiation sources. The radiation dose is about 5% of the yearly dose considered safe for doctors and technologists who work with radiation. You can be around other people and use a bathroom normally without risk to others.

D. Pregnancy

If you are pregnant or think you could be pregnant, inform your doctor so that this can be discussed with the nuclear medicine physician.

References

1. Davis LP, McCarroll K. Correlative imaging of the liver and hepatobiliary system. *Semin Nucl Med* 1994;24:208–218.
2. Rubin RA, Lichtenstein GR. Hepatic scintigraphy in the evaluation of solitary solid liver masses. *J Nucl Med* 1993;34:697–705.
3. Middleton ML. Scintigraphic evaluation of hepatic mass lesions: emphasis on hemangioma detection. *Semin Nucl Med* 1996;26:4–15.
4. Ziessman HA. Cholecystokinin cholescintigraphy: victim of its own success? *J Nucl Med* 1999;40:2038–2042.
5. Shea JA, Berlin JA, Escarce JJ, et al. Revised estimates of diagnostic test sensitivity and specificity in suspected biliary tract disease. *Arch Intern Med* 1994;154:2573–2581.
6. Rosenberg DJ, Brugge WR, Alavi A. Bile leak following an elective laparoscopic cholecystectomy: the role of hepatobiliary imaging in the diagnosis and management of bile leaks. *J Nucl Med* 1991;32:1777–1781.
7. Krishnamurthy S, Krishnamurthy GT. Biliary dyskinesia: role of the sphincter of Oddi, gallbladder and cholecystokinin. *J Nucl Med* 1997;38:1824–1830.

8. Lillemoe KD. Chronic acalculous cholecystitis: are we diagnosing a disease or a myth? *Radiology* 1997;204:13–14.
9. Howman-Giles R, Uren R, Bernard E, Dorney S. Hepatobiliary scintigraphy in infancy. *J Nucl Med* 1998;39:311–319.

4

5
The Gastrointestinal System

Nuclear imaging of the gastrointestinal (GI) system is most commonly used to localize acute lower tract hemorrhage and to evaluate gastric emptying. A number of other studies are performed less frequently but may be valuable in specific clinical settings. It is best to inquire about the available protocols, not during the heat of an acute workup, but in a general dialogue with the nuclear medicine physician. This chapter also includes brief descriptions of nuclear medicine studies that do not use imaging such as the Schilling test and Helicobacter pylori *screening.*

SCANS AND PRIMARY CLINICAL INDICATIONS

5

CLINICAL QUESTIONS

GI bleeding

GI motility/aspiration

Postsurgery/pernicious anemia/*H pylori*

PATIENT INFORMATION

SCANS

I. GI BLEEDING SCAN

A. Background

GI bleeding scans can be used to visualize bleeding at almost any site in the body but are used most commonly to localize suspected bleeding distal to the ligament of Treitz (lower GI tract). The GI bleeding scan can be performed using ^{99m}Tc-radiolabeled red blood cells (RBCs), or ^{99m}Tc-sulfur colloid.

B. Radiopharmaceuticals

Technetium-99m-radiolabeled autologous RBCs are prepared by attaching or "tagging" a radiotracer to the patient's own RBCs. This tagging is completed in one of three ways, details for which are provided in Chapter 1, Cardiovascular Diseases, Radiopharmaceuticals. This may take from 30 min up to 2 hr if the cells have to be sent to an outside radiopharmacy. Because the attached radiotracer emits gamma rays that can be detected by a gamma camera, blood in the patient's vascular spaces, as well as blood extravasated into the GI tract, can be imaged.

Technetium-99m-sulfur colloid is injected intravenously but doesn't attach to RBCs. Tagged RBCs remain in the vascular space unless there is bleeding, but ^{99m}Tc-sulfur colloid is rapidly cleared from the circulation by the reticuloendothelial system (RES) with a $T_{1/2}$ elimination time of 2–4 min. The radiotracer emits gamma rays that are detected by the gamma camera allowing visualization of the vascular space and possible blood extravasation during the study.

C. How the study is performed

1. RBC imaging. The patient's blood must first be radiolabeled with ^{99m}Tc-pertechnetate (20–30 mCi [750–1100 MBq] adult dose). After the tagging, a rapid angiogram sequence is acquired for 1 min, followed by a series of images for typically 1–2 hr. This is done in the supine position. The patient may then be routinely reimaged up to 24 hr after injection if no bleeding site is found or if continued blood per rectum is noted. In some departments, the series of images can be viewed as a movie (cine mode), which increases sensitivity of detection.

2. Sulfur colloid. Sulfur colloid (10 mCi [370 MBq] adult dose) may be injected all at once or in fractions. A series of images is then obtained. With a single injection, the study typically lasts approximately 20–30 min because of the rapid clearance of the sulfur colloid from the circulation by the RES. Delayed images are not obtained, but the study can be repeated in its entirety if the patient rebleeds. Cine viewing can also be helpful as described above.

D. Patient preparation

A suspected upper GI source of blood per rectum should be excluded with nasogastric lavage or endoscopy as appropriate. A recent barium study may obscure the site of bleeding by blocking photons from the tagged RBCs or the ^{99m}Tc-sulfur colloid extravasated into the bowel. The patient does not need to fast for the scan. If unusual postsurgical anatomy is present, or if there are known prior barium studies, this should be pointed out to the nuclear medicine physician, as it will help in the interpretation of the bleeding scan.

E. Understanding the report

The *sine qua non* of GI blood extravasation is accumulation of luminal activity that moves with time (Fig. 1). Blood in the GI tract may have anterograde

5

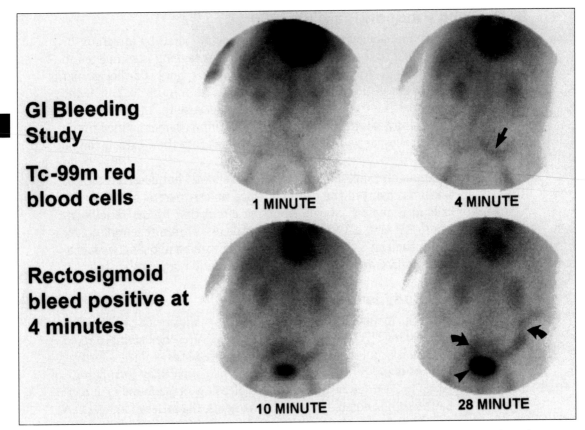

GI Bleeding Study

Tc-99m red blood cells

1 MINUTE

4 MINUTE

Rectosigmoid bleed positive at 4 minutes

10 MINUTE

28 MINUTE

Figure 1. Tagged RBC scan demonstrates rectosigmoid blood extravasation (arrow) that moves with time (curved arrows). Note renal excretion of radiotracer breakdown products distending the bladder and obscuring the pelvis (arrowhead).

and retrograde motion because of the stimulatory effect of heme products on the GI mucosa. The report will describe the examination methodology and will characterize abnormal activity, if present, including the location in the GI tract where the activity was first detected, as well as the time of the scan in which it was visualized. The earlier in the study the activity is seen, the higher the confidence of localization. A scan may be interpreted as negative, positive and localizing, or positive and nonlocalizing. A positive study at 24 hr is likely to be nonlocalizing (see Potential Problem 2, below). Sometimes a stationary blush is reported on the angiographic phase of imaging. This may indicate an area of increased vascularity, such as arteriovenous malformation (AVM), tumor or inflammation.

With tagged RBCs, blood pool structures normally are seen, such as the heart, great vessels, spleen, and less so the liver. The gallbladder may also be seen normally at 24 hr because of heme breakdown products. A sulfur colloid scan will typically demonstrate liver, spleen and bone marrow uptake; blood pool structures are not seen on delayed images.

F. Potential problems

1. Active bleeding. The study will not detect prior bleeding. Only active bleeding (at least 0.05–0.1 ml/min) while the radiotracer is in the vascular space can be imaged. Thus, there will be a smaller window to detect bleeding with the sulfur colloid study because of rapid vascular clearance.

2. Motility. Once extravasated, blood usually moves in anterograde and retrograde motion in the bowel. This can happen within minutes, obfuscating exact localization. This is why rapid dynamic imaging is important to freeze frame initial bleeding. With tagged RBCs, delayed images can be acquired up to 24 hr. Yet, the further out that imaging is performed, the less confident one can be that an exact bleeding location will be identified due to this peristalsis. For example, if a static 24-hr view was performed after an initially negative scan, the entire colon may be filled with activity. Some may perform dynamic cine imaging and computer manipulation at this point in an effort to visualize new bleeding.

3. Quality of the RBC tag. A poor quality RBC tag may result in unattached ^{99m}Tc-pertechnetate (free pertechnetate) which is secreted into the stomach by gastric mucosa cells and may simulate an upper GI bleeding source. Renal excretion of breakdown products also may be problematic.

4. Small bowel. Small bowel bleeding may be difficult to see due to rapid peristalsis if dynamic cine imaging is not done.

II. MECKEL'S DIVERTICULUM SCAN
A. Background

Meckel's is a true diverticulum in distal small bowel found in 1–3% of the population. Most people are asymptomatic. Ectopic gastric mucosa is present in only 10–30% of all Meckel's cases, 60% of symptomatic ones, and 98% of those that bleed. Most symptomatic Meckel's cases are patients less than 2 yr old, and symptoms are rare in those over 40 yr old. Ectopic gastric mucosa elsewhere in the abdomen such as in bowel duplication or, rarely, in small bowel proper also may cause symptoms and can be detected with this study.

B. Radiopharmaceuticals

Technetium-99m-pertechnetate localizes in gastric mucosal cells. This is an advantage when searching for ectopic gastric mucosa in a Meckel's diverticulum or elsewhere in the abdomen.

C. How the study is performed

Technetium-99m-pertechnetate (8–12 mCi [300–450 MBq] adult dose; 50–220 μCi/kg [2–8 MBq/kg] pediatric dose) is injected intravenously, and a series of dynamic and static supine images are obtained. The examination lasts approximately 30–60 min.

A number of techniques may be used in an effort to increase sensitivity and specificity. H2 blockers (cimetidine, ranitidine) can be given orally for 2 days before the examination (or intravenously 1 hr before the examination) to increase retention of pertechnetate in gastric mucosa, including ectopic gastric mucosa, as well as to decrease secretion of interfering pertechnetate into the gastric lumen and subsequent passage into small bowel. Glucagon also can be given intravenously 10 min after radiotracer injection to decrease peristalsis of normally secreted gastric pertechnetate into the small bowel and to prevent rapid motion of the Meckel's diverticulum during the examination.

D. Patient Preparation

Patients are required to fast for at least 4–6 hr. A recent barium examination may obscure activity by blocking photons emitted from the radiotracer. As above, pretreatment may be part of the usual protocol. If this study and a bleeding scan are desired, the order and timing should be discussed with the nuclear medicine physician (See Clinical Question 5, below).

E. Understanding the report

The report will include the imaging method, including medications used for the study. The stomach normally secretes ^{99m}Tc-pertechnetate. A confident diagnosis of Meckel's diverticulum can be made when there is almost immediate right lower quadrant activity that appears as intense as stomach (Fig. 2). But a Meckel's diverticulum or other ectopic gastric mucosa may be present anywhere

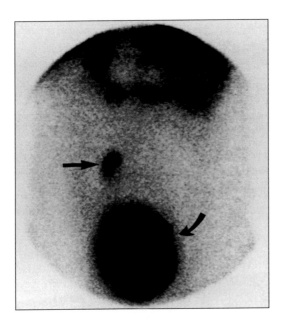

Figure 2. Intense right lower quadrant activity on a Meckel's scan performed on a child confirms the presence of a Meckel's diverticulum (straight arrow). Activity in a distended bladder also can be seen (curved arrow).

within the abdomen, and a small diverticulum may become apparent at a later time than stomach.

F. Potential problems

1. Gastric secretion. Normally secreted gastric pertechnetate that peristalsis distally may interfere with scan interpretation.

2. Other false-positive results. Confounding urinary system activity, GI obstruction, tumor and inflammation can cause false-positive results.

3. False-negative results. False-negative results may be secondary to lack of sufficient ectopic gastric mucosal cells in a Meckel's diverticulum, as well as washout from rapid bleeding.

III. GI MOTILITY STUDIES
A. Background

Nuclear imaging provides tools for in vivo detection and quantitation of various GI motility disturbances. The sophistication to which these are applied depends on the interest of the nuclear medicine physician and involved clinician. Because methodology varies among institutions, normal values should be established by each facility. The key ingredient in a useful examination is consistency, as well as communication between the nuclear medicine physician and ordering clinician. This section will focus on gastric and esophageal studies. Small bowel and colon motility examinations can be performed but are not commonly available.

B. Radiopharmaceuticals

Technetium-99m-sulfur colloid can be incorporated in specific foods for motility investigations. By using food rather than barium, a physiologic evaluation of solid-food gastric emptying can be performed.

Indium-111-DTPA can be used as a marker in the liquid phase of swallowing studies and for evaluating the liquid phase of gastric emptying.

Technetium-99m-DTPA is also used as a liquid radiotracer.

C. How the study is performed

1. Gastric emptying. The gastric emptying study is the most commonly performed of all GI motility examinations. Radiolabeled solid, liquid or combination meals can be used. The most frequent solid meal is ^{99m}Tc-sulfur colloid (0.2–1 mCi [7–37 MBq] adult dose) complexed to eggs or liver pâté as they are being cooked. Other meals such as oatmeal, hamburger, potato, or banana have been used. Patients may be studied supine or standing, using a series of static or continuous dynamic images, for up to 3 hr after ingesting the meal, or until a $T_{1/2}$ emptying time can be calculated. If liquids are used, the same procedure is followed. A dual solid-liquid emptying study can be performed using

^{111}In-DTPA (0.1–0.2 mCi [3–7 MBq] adult dose) for the liquid phase, which has a different photon energy than the ^{99m}Tc-sulfur colloid. Both qualitative and quantitative analysis is completed, and an emptying curve as well as a $T_{1/2}$ emptying time are generated (Fig. 3). In addition, a special study can be carried out for gastric emptying in which the patient is given promotility agents before or during the examination to determine if they affect the emptying curve.

2. Esophagus. The esophagus also can be evaluated for motility and reflux. An abdominal binder may be applied in an adult to increase abdominal pressure to provoke reflux. Delayed images of the lungs also may be obtained to determine if aspiration is occurring.

3. Pediatric motility studies. Motility studies in children can be performed as a continuum, especially using milk or formula. Esophageal, gastric, small bowel and colon transit, as well as aspiration, can be evaluated in one setting. This is more expensive and requires expertise.

D. Patient preparation

In general, patients should fast for 8 hr before the examination. No special diet is required, and there is no bowel preparation. Smoking can affect the examination. A detailed medical and surgical history should be provided to aid in meaningful interpretation and expected normal values.

Some medications such as narcotic analgesics, certain antidepressants, anticholinergics, calcium channel blockers and aluminum-containing antacids can delay gastric emptying and prokinetic agents such as metoclopramide, cisapride, erythromycin and bethanechol accelerate gastric emptying. Often the gastric emptying examination is performed while the patient is taking his or her usual medications. If a baseline study is desired while a certain medication is withheld, careful consideration should be made of the risks and benefits to the patient of withdrawing a particular medication before the examination. These issues should be discussed with the nuclear medicine physician.

Diabetics should bring their insulin with them to titrate with the meal because hyperglycemia can delay gastric emptying. If possible, premenopausal women should be studied on day 1–10 of their menstrual cycle because hormonal variation affects gastric motility.

It is preferable that the patient be prepared for the type of meal that is used. For example, some centers use liver pâté and beef stew that could present a problem for strict vegetarians.

E. Understanding the report

The report will vary depending on what is being imaged and the examination methodology. The type of food ingested, imaging technique, interfering medication the patient may be taking, as well as normal ranges for that particular procedure may be described. Characterization of the transit or emptying curve, as well as numerical values, usually are included in the report.

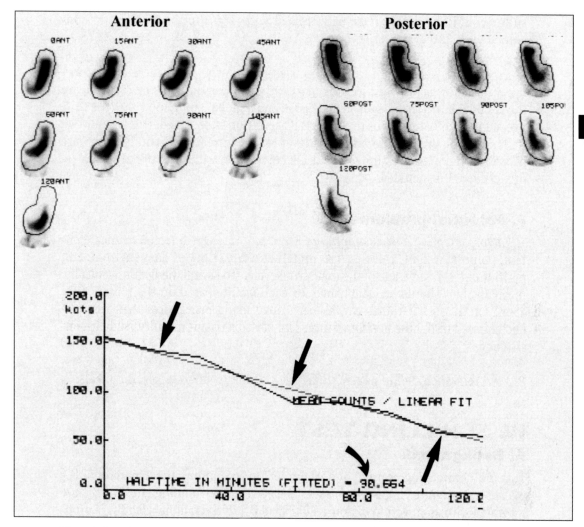

Figure 3. Normal gastric emptying study. Anterior and posterior sequential images of the stomach with regions of interest drawn around them. (Time in minutes is at upper right of each stomach image.) The curve (straight arrows) describes the gastric emptying and the $T_{1/2}$ value (curved arrow) quantifies it.

1. Gastric emptying. For gastric studies, the rate of emptying can be approximated by a monoexponential emptying curve for liquids and a linear emptying pattern for solids. The shape of the curve and the time it takes for one half the meal to leave the stomach ($T_{1/2}$) usually are reported. It is important to realize that normal values vary depending on the protocol used for the study, but a typical $T_{1/2}$ for liquids is between 10 and 20 min, and solid meals normally demonstrate 40–50% emptying by 90 min. These values have wide standard deviations. (Normal solid $T_{1/2}$ values at Emory University are 77.9 ± 32 min for men; 92.4 ± 15 min for premenopausal women and 77 ± 32 min for postmenopausal women. These normal values are based on published studies using a standard meal consisting of [99mTc-]

sulfur colloid bound to liver pâté, mixed with 150 g of beef stew and consumed with 150 g of orange juice.)

2. Esophageal transit and reflux. Transit time for the esophageal bolus (normally 6–15 sec) is provided in the report. Other values that may be reported are the residual in the esophagus at a set time and a global emptying time (the time needed to eliminate 90% of the bolus). If aspiration is observed, this is reported. Reflux may be graded; the anatomic level reached, frequency and duration are described. If a pressure binder was used, correlation with pressure at which reflux occurred is included.

F. Potential problems

1. Factors affecting gastric emptying. Emptying rates are affected by meal content, volume, weight, calories, fat, protein, acidity, time of day, environment, positioning, gender, stage of the menstrual cycle, stress and medications. Ideally, normal values should be established for each facility based on their study variables; alternatively, studies can be performed using procedures that are well-documented in the medical literature. The key to a useful motility study is consistency.

2. Meal tolerance. Some patients may not be able to tolerate specific meals.

IV. SCHILLING TEST

A. Background

This is a nonimaging examination useful for understanding the dynamics of B_{12} malabsorption. After ingestion of radiolabeled B_{12}, liver binding sites for B_{12} are saturated with an injection of nonradiolabeled B_{12}. If the radiolabeled B_{12} is properly absorbed across the gut, it will have no place to bind, and it will then be excreted in the urine. Thus, the urine excretion is proportional to absorption.

B. Radiopharmaceuticals

Cobalt-57 and ^{58}Co are complexed in trace amounts to vitamin B_{12} to determine percent urinary excretion.

C. How the study is performed

1. Stage I. The patient ingests a ^{57}Co labeled B_{12} capsule (0.5 μCi [18.5 KBq] adult dose) and is then injected with 1000 μg of nonradiolabeled cyanocobalamin (B_{12}) intramuscularly 1–2 hr later. (For convenience, certain facilities inject the nonradiolabeled B_{12} at the time of radiolabeled B_{12} ingestion.) The patient typically collects urine for 24 hr and returns it to the nuclear medicine department, where the percent of the ingested dose in the urine is measured.

2. Stage II. If the excretion is abnormally low, a second stage Schilling test can be performed in which the patient is given ^{57}Co B$_{12}$ with intrinsic factor, and the percent excreted is then measured as before.

3. Stage III. A third stage scan also can be carried out when poor gut absorption of B$_{12}$ may be due to bacterial overgrowth; ^{57}Co B$_{12}$ is then given following a course of oral antibiotics.

Stages I and II of the Schilling test also can be performed as a single step in which ^{57}Co B$_{12}$ bound to intrinsic factor is ingested with a second capsule of ^{58}Co. These two radionuclides have different energies that can be counted separately in the urine, and excretion with or without intrinsic factor can be calculated simultaneously.

D. Patient Preparation

Exogenous B$_{12}$ is withheld for 24 hr before the examination. The patient should fast (water is permitted) for 8–12 hr before the Schilling test, which is typically done in the morning. A light breakfast may be eaten after ingestion of the ^{57}Co-labeled B$_{12}$ capsule, and normal lunch and dinner meals may be taken thereafter. (Some centers withhold exogenous B$_{12}$ for 3 days before the study and maintain the patient's fasting status for 2 hr after the radiolabeled B$_{12}$ capsule ingestion.) The patient must be able to collect urine for 24 hr and return it to the department the next day. A recent radionuclide examination of any kind may contaminate the urine. Obtain blood for B$_{12}$ and folate serum measurements before the examination, because the injected flushing B$_{12}$ dose can affect serum B$_{12}$ and folate values.

E. Understanding the report

Urinary excretion <10% is considered abnormal. This may be due to a lack of intrinsic factor (pernicious anemia) or inability to absorb B$_{12}$ through the gut. If there is normal urine excretion when B$_{12}$ is given with intrinsic factor (stage II Schilling test), pernicious anemia can be diagnosed. If urinary excretion remains low despite administration of intrinsic factor, malabsorption due to such problems as short gut syndrome, sprue, regional enteritis or bacterial overgrowth from a blind loop or diverticulosis are suspected. Malabsorption due to bacterial overgrowth can be confirmed if urinary excretion normalizes during a stage III Schilling test.

F. Potential problems

1. Incomplete urine collection. If the patient fails to collect all the 24 hr urine, the measured B$_{12}$ in the urine will be falsely low. Some centers measure urine creatinine and urine volume as a control.

2. Renal failure. If the patient has renal failure, a 48-hr urine collection is usually required.

3. False-negative examination. Uncommonly, some patients may be able to absorb the crystalline B_{12} used with the standard Schilling test, yet have malabsorption of food-bound B_{12}. If a false-negative examination is suspected, the Schilling test can be repeated with radiolabeled B_{12} bound to egg yolk.

V. *H PYLORI* (UREASE) BREATH TEST

Detecting the presence of *H pylori* in the stomach does not always require invasive endoscopy. This nonimaging radioactive test uses a trace amount of ^{14}C urea (1 μCi [37 KBq] adult dose) ingested by the patient in capsule form. If *H pylori* is present, it will split the urea and release the ^{14}C as radiolabeled carbon dioxide, which is absorbed across the gut into the bloodstream and exhaled by the patient into a collection device.

False-negative results may be caused by prior therapy with antibiotics or bismuth (Pepto-Bismol), and patients should be told to withhold them, if possible, for 30 days before the examination. Sucralfate (Carafate) and proton pump inhibitors such as omeprazole (Prilosec) and lansoprazole (Prevacid) should be stopped, if possible, 2 wk before the examination because they also may cause false-negative results. Some patients may not tolerate this preparation. Please consult with the physician performing the study if withholding the above medications for the examination will not be possible. Alternative medications such as H2 blockers may be substituted. Patients should fast for 6 hr before the test. False-positive results may occur secondary to achlorhydria or the presence of other urea-splitting bacteria.

CLINICAL QUESTIONS

1. Acute blood per rectum: What is the source of lower GI bleeding?

Eighty percent of acute GI bleeding in adults originates in the upper tract, and 20% originates distal to the ligament of Treitz. Most lower GI bleeding is caused by colonic diverticula or angiodysplasia. In the pediatric population, Meckel's diverticulum is the most common cause of lower GI bleeding. Clinical findings are frequently not reliable in differentiating upper from lower GI bleeding. In addition, GI bleeding is often intermittent, confounding attempts at localization.

The evaluation of GI bleeding should be a multidisciplinary team effort. The workup of this entity is often institution specific, depending on the strengths of nuclear imaging, angiography and endoscopy, as well as physician preference. With an organized approach, and early involvement of the surgical team, there is a high likelihood of identifying the source of GI bleeding.

There is controversy over the role of nuclear imaging in acute lower GI bleeding. The goal of any approach is to avoid emergent subtotal colectomy in favor of limited colon resection. How best can this be accomplished?

Barium studies have almost no place in the evaluation of acute GI bleeding.

Colonoscopy in the acute setting is seldom revealing in unprepared bowel. In addition, the rate of perforation and other complications increases because of obscuring blood. Often, bleeding can be seen, but the exact location goes undetermined. Colon preparation is usually impractical in the acute situation. Proctosigmoidoscopy, on the other hand, while seldom definitive, is simple and has low morbidity. If a rectal source of bleeding is identified, such as hemorrhoids, an expensive workup can be avoided.

Angiography is considered the principal initial modality by some investigators. It has a relatively low morbidity, and therapy can be performed at the same setting, such as using intra-arterial vasopressin, coils or Gelfoam to stop bleeding. Yet angiography is only 10–20% as sensitive for the evaluation of GI bleeding as is nuclear imaging. Angiography can image bleeding at rates of 0.5–1 ml/min or greater; the GI bleeding scan will image bleeding at rates as low as 0.05–0.1 ml/min. Also, angiography will detect bleeding only if extravasation is occurring during the injection of contrast. Nuclear imaging may detect bleeding that can occur intermittently over a prolonged period of time after injection of the radiopharmaceutical. In addition, angiography is more costly than nuclear imaging and carries a small risk of morbidity and mortality.

Nuclear imaging is inexpensive, safe and effective. While angiography is being arranged, a nuclear test often can be completed. In fact, some angiographers insist on a positive nuclear imaging study before angiography is undertaken because of the increased sensitivity of the bleeding scan and its ability to help guide the angiographic procedure. Each nuclear imaging method has advantages and disadvantages, although tagged RBCs are more commonly used. With tagged RBCs, patients can be followed up for longer periods of time, and intermittent bleeding can be detected. Sulfur colloid scanning is easier to perform and theoretically more sensitive in detecting even slower bleeding because of rapid elimination of the radiotracer from the blood pool; however, ^{99m}Tc-sulfur colloid has two drawbacks: first, intense activity in the liver and spleen may mask transverse colon extravasation; second, because of the rapid clearance of sulfur colloid from the circulation, it can only detect bleeding that occurs within approximately 15 min of injection. (Repeat injections can be performed if bleeding recurs.) Usually a department will choose one protocol based on cost, throughput and patient population, as well as needs of the clinical services. The most successful localization of the bleeding site is accomplished with high-quality RBC labeling, when rapid sequential images are acquired in cine mode and image acquisition is repeated frequently over several hours or for the longest continuous time practical.

Most bleeding is moderate or intermittent. Nuclear imaging, especially the RBC-labeled study, is an excellent first-line examination. If no bleeding is identified with an RBC study even on delayed images, studies indicate these patients do well with conservative therapy and outpatient endoscopic/barium evaluation. If the bleeding site is confidently identified on nuclear imaging, the patient can go on to angiography for an attempt at noninvasive therapy or temporizing measures before localized surgery is performed. It is not uncommon for the nuclear scan to be positive and localizing but angiography to be negative.

Acute GI bleeding flowchart

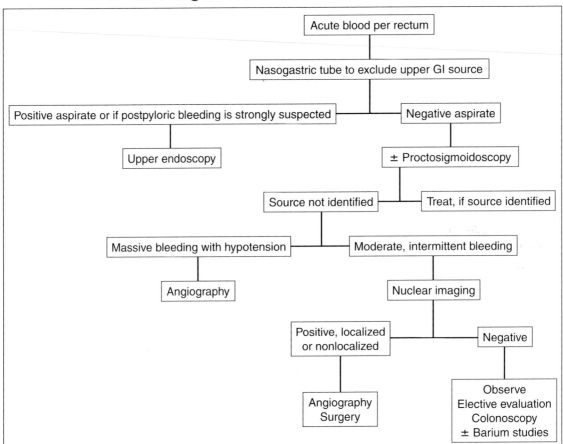

2. GI bleeding: Upper GI tract source?

The investigation of suspected upper GI bleeding is best done with endoscopy, through which treatment can also be performed, such as sclerotherapy.

3. GI bleeding with negative upper GI and colon evaluation: Small bowel source?

In the setting of acute GI bleeding when no source is identified, dynamic cine imaging with ^{99m}Tc-radiolabeled RBCs or sulfur colloid may identify a small bowel source of hemorrhage. In the chronic setting, a detailed barium small bowel series or small bowel endoscopy may be required.

4. Positive stool hemoccult test: Chronic low-grade GI bleeding?

Nuclear imaging is rarely useful in the evaluation of chronic low-grade GI bleeding because the bleeding is too slow and intermittent; endoscopic techniques and barium studies are preferable.

5. Toddler with lower GI bleeding: Meckel's diverticulum?

5

Meckel's scanning is highly sensitive and specific in children but less so in adults because of confounding abdominal disease and lower prevalence of Meckel's diverticulum. An initial GI bleeding scan using tagged RBCs may interfere for days to weeks with later extraction of ^{99m}Tc-pertechnetate by gastric mucosa during a Meckel's scan. Also, normal gastric excretion of ^{99m}Tc-pertechnetate from a Meckel's scan can confound interpretation of a GI bleeding scan performed less than 24 hr later. In general, if active GI bleeding is occurring, a GI bleeding scan is recommended for most accurate localization. Once bleeding has stopped, it is more appropriate to commence the workup with a Meckel's scan. These are often complicated issues that should be discussed in advance with the nuclear medicine physician.

6. Diabetic with bloating: Gastroparesis?

Gastric stasis can be caused by many acute and chronic conditions, as well as medications. Promotility agents are available that hold some promise in therapy. The nuclear gastric emptying study is the gold standard in the evaluation of gastric emptying. It is physiologic, simple to perform, accurate, quantifiable and noninvasive. It is especially useful in detecting diabetic related gastroparesis, the most common cause of slowed gastric emptying. It also can be used in evaluation of drug interventions. In general, solid-phase emptying is more sensitive to early disturbances than liquid phase.

Sixty percent of patients with gastroesophageal reflux have delayed gastric emptying for solids, which is why many surgeons order this examination before antireflux surgical procedures are performed. It should be kept in mind that the initial workup of dyspepsia should include barium studies and/or endoscopy because nuclear imaging cannot determine an anatomic cause of delayed emptying. A tumor or ulcer may be present.

An upper GI series with barium is neither an accurate nor physiologic method to assess gastric emptying. Other tests such as double sampling gastric aspiration, ultrasound, MRI, electrical impedance and tracer methods are not widely available and have many disadvantages such as cost, invasiveness and inconsistency. A standard workup may consist of a history and physical examination, laboratory work, barium upper GI or endoscopy to exclude an anatomic lesion and then a gastric emptying study. If gastroparesis is present, therapy with promotility drugs may be beneficial. The response can be quantitated by a repeat gastric emptying study.

5

7. Heartburn: Gastroesophageal reflux?

In the evaluation of reflux disease, patients often are diagnosed and treated empirically. If some type of examination is needed, the intraesophageal pH probe is considered the gold standard. Upper GI examination and endoscopy are neither sensitive nor specific in the evaluation for reflux but can be used to document reflux esophagitis. The nuclear imaging examination is relegated to a supporting or problem-solving role.

If patients do not respond to empiric therapy, an upper GI series or endoscopy should be performed. If this is not revealing, a pH probe study is the next logical choice. If equivocal, further evaluation with nuclear imaging may then be required. If a patient has significant gastroesophageal reflux, it is desirable to screen for Barrett's disease, which carries an increased risk for adenocarcinoma. A gastric emptying study performed at the same time as the reflux study can yield important diagnostic information. Nuclear imaging is most helpful in children who may not tolerate a pH probe.

8. Dysphagia: Esophageal motility problem?

Endoscopy or barium esophagraphy should always be performed first to exclude anatomic pathology and allow correlation with the nuclear examination. Fluoroscopy of the swallowing bolus can also yield some important information, but it is not quantifiable. Manometry is considered the gold standard in studying esophageal motility. Yet, the majority of those studied will have either normal results or nonspecific abnormalities. Nuclear scanning allows quantification and serves an important complementary role. Up to 50% of symptomatic patients with normal manometry or endoscopy will have an abnormality on nuclear scanning.

The nuclear study is a more physiologic examination than manometry and better tolerated by children. It is most useful to evaluate the response to therapy, to assess progression of disease or to confirm normality when other tests are negative. It involves little radiation and can be repeated. It is also useful for those who cannot tolerate manometry or who have indeterminate results.

9. Child with multiple pneumonia episodes: Aspiration?

The swallowing examination can be important in diagnosing and documenting aspiration. If aspiration is not immediately observed, delayed imaging may demonstrate radiotracer activity in the lungs due to aspiration after the initial swallow. Lack of activity on delayed images does not exclude aspiration because the aspirate may have been cleared from the lungs by coughing, or sufficient radiotracer may not have been present in the stomach when reflux and aspiration finally occurred.

10. Is the gastric emptying scan useful for the postsurgical syndromes?

The dumping syndrome often is diagnosed clinically. The interpretation of postsurgical patterns on the gastric emptying scan is not well defined but can be useful to help confirm dumping. Upper GI and endoscopy should be performed first. Expected findings depend on the type of surgery performed.

11. Question pernicious anemia?

The nonimaging Schilling test is considered the gold standard in confirming this entity as well as other causes of B_{12} deficiency. Because the Schilling test can be cumbersome because of the requirement for 24-hr urine collection, some clinicians advocate identifying pernicious anemia through the use of serologic studies. The presence of autoantibodies to intrinsic factor and parietal cells, decreased serum pepsinogen I and hypergastrinemia may be used alone or in combination to diagnose pernicious anemia in the presence of low serum cobalamin levels. The clinical accuracy of these serum tests has not been well defined in relation to the Schilling test; if the serology is not conclusive, a Schilling test should be performed.

12. Gastric or duodenal ulcer: *H pylori?*

Endoscopy with biopsy is considered the gold standard in the diagnosis of *H pylori*, but it is expensive and invasive. The nonimaging ^{14}C urease breath test can be used for diagnosis and follow-up. There is also a nonradioactive counterpart of this breath test that uses ^{13}C labeling. An antibody test is available that documents past infections, but does not tell if active infection is present. The antibody test may be useful in initial diagnosis of selected patients but is not recommended for post-therapy follow-up. Which test or tests are used is contingent on local practice patterns, experience and availability.

WORTH MENTIONING

1. Ectopic gastric mucosa

The Meckel's scan can be used to find other ectopic gastric mucosa such as in suspected GI duplications, retained gastric antrum after surgery and suspected Barrett's esophagus.

2. Protein losing enteropathy

This can be evaluated by injecting ^{99m}Tc-human serum albumin or ^{111}In-chloride, which binds to transferrin intravenously. The abdomen is then imaged to determine if this leaks from blood into bowel. This test is not widely available.

3. Salivary scintigraphy

Salivary scintigraphy using ^{99m}Tc-pertechnetate can be useful to distinguish between xerostomia secondary to Sjögren's syndrome and physiologic dry mouth, as well as to assess the patency of the salivary duct after citric acid stimulation.

It should be noted that the contrast sialogram is considered the gold standard, and CT or MRI should be obtained to examine the anatomy.

4. Tear duct study

The patency of the lacrimal duct can be evaluated with the nuclear tear duct study, which involves placing a drop of radionuclide in the eye.

5. Small bowel and colon motility scintigraphy

Small bowel and colon motility studies are finding increasing use in some centers for the diagnosis and management of patients with suspected transit abnormalities, and these studies may become more widespread in the future.

PATIENT INFORMATION

I. GI BLEEDING SCAN

A. Test/Procedure

Your doctor has ordered a GI bleeding scan to try to find the site of your GI bleeding.

The study will be performed in one of two ways. A small amount of radioactive material called a tracer will be injected into your vein. Alternatively, your RBCs will be labeled with a small amount of radioactive tracer, either by a series of injections or by withdrawing a small amount of blood from your vein and then reinjecting it with the tracer attached to the RBCs.

You will be positioned next to a special machine called a gamma camera, which doesn't produce radiation but detects radiation that is coming from the injected tracer in your body. A series of pictures of your abdomen will then be taken, typically from 20 min to 2 hr. If the area of bleeding is not seen, you may be returned to the nuclear medicine department for additional imaging.

B. Preparation

Eating, drinking or taking medications do not interfere with this examination, but your doctor may have ordered that you fast in case surgery is needed for your GI bleed. Please check with your doctor or nurse. Also, please inform the nuclear imaging staff if you have had surgery on your bowel. This information will help in the interpretation of your study.

C. Radiation and other risks

The amount of radiation used is small and similar to that given by other diagnostic x-ray tests. The effective adult radiation dose to your whole body from this test is about the same dose as the average person living in the United States receives in 2–3 yr from cosmic rays and naturally occurring background radiation sources. The radiation dose is about 10–20% of the yearly dose considered safe for doctors and technologists who work with radiation. You can be around other people and use a bathroom normally without risk to others.

D. Pregnancy

If you are pregnant or think you could be pregnant, inform your doctor so that this can be discussed with the nuclear medicine physician.

II. MECKEL'S DIVERTICULUM SCAN

A. Test/Procedure

Your doctor has ordered a Meckel's scan to determine if you have a small area in your bowel that contains stomach tissue that may be responsible for your GI bleeding.

A small amount of radioactive material called a tracer will be injected into your vein. You will be positioned next to a special machine called a gamma camera, which doesn't produce radiation but detects radiation that is coming from the injected tracer in your body. A series of pictures of your abdomen will then be taken, typically from 30 to 60 min. In an effort to maximize the success of the study, you may be given oral medication to take at a certain time before the examination or given an injection of medicine before the study.

B. Preparation

You should not eat anything for 4–6 hr before the examination. Also, please inform the nuclear imaging staff if you have had surgery on your bowel. This information will help in the interpretation of your study.

C. Radiation and other risks

The amount of radiation used is small and similar to that given by other diagnostic x-ray tests. The effective adult radiation dose to your whole body from this test is about the dose the average person living in the United States receives in 1–2 yr from cosmic rays and naturally occurring background radiation sources. The radiation dose is about 10% of the yearly dose considered safe for doctors and technologists who work with radiation. You can be around other people and use a bathroom normally without risk to others.

D. Pregnancy

If you are pregnant or think you could be pregnant, inform your doctor so that this can be discussed with the nuclear medicine physician.

III. GI MOTILITY STUDIES

A. Test/Procedure

Your doctor has ordered a GI motility (gastric emptying) scan to determine if you have a problem with movement of food through your stomach. Your esophagus or bowel may be examined also.

5

You will be asked to eat a meal or drink liquid that contains a small amount of radioactive tracer. The meal will consist of _____. You will be positioned next to a special machine called a gamma camera that doesn't produce radiation but detects radiation that is coming from the radioactive meal in your body. A series of pictures of your abdomen will then be taken for up to 2–3 hr. If you are to be examined for esophageal reflux, a special binder may be applied around your abdomen and inflated with air. You also may be asked to return the next day to obtain pictures of your lungs if your doctor is worried about aspiration of food into your lungs.

B. Preparation

You should not eat or drink anything for 8 hr before the study, and you should refrain from smoking. If you are a diabetic, please bring your insulin in preparation to adjust with the meal. Certain medications may interfere with the study. Please discuss your medications with your doctor to determine if any should be withheld. Also, please inform the nuclear imaging staff if you have had surgery on your stomach. This information will help interpret your study.

C. Radiation and other risks

The amount of radiation used is small and similar to that given by other diagnostic x-ray tests. The effective adult radiation dose to your whole body from this test is less than the dose the average person living in the United States receives in 1 yr from cosmic rays and naturally occurring background radiation sources. The radiation dose is <5% of the yearly dose considered safe for doctors and technologists who work with radiation. You can be around other people and use a bathroom normally without risk to others.

D. Pregnancy

If you are pregnant or think you could be pregnant, inform your doctor so that this can be discussed with the nuclear medicine physician.

IV. SCHILLING TEST

A. Test/Procedure

Your doctor has ordered a Schilling test to determine the cause of your vitamin B_{12} deficiency.

You will be given one or two capsules to take orally that contain a tiny amount of radioactive labeled B_{12}. Approximately 1–2 hr later you will be given an intramuscular injection of nonradioactive B_{12}. You will be asked to collect all your urine for 24 hr in the provided container and return it the next day to the nuclear medicine department. (If you have kidney problems, you may be asked to collect urine for 48 hr.) If you have not collected all your urine, please inform the nuclear medicine staff, as this will affect the interpretation of the test.

B. Preparation

You should not eat or drink anything for 8–12 hr before the study except for water. Please withhold any vitamin preparations containing B_{12} for 3 days before the examination. You may take your other medications.

5

C. Radiation and other risks

The amount of radiation used is small and similar to that given by other diagnostic x-ray tests. The effective adult radiation dose to your whole body from this test <5% of the dose the average person living in the United States receives each year from cosmic rays and naturally occurring background radiation sources. The radiation dose is <1% of the yearly dose considered safe for doctors and technologists who work with radiation. You can be around other people and use a bathroom normally without risk to others.

D. Pregnancy

If you are pregnant or think you could be pregnant, inform your doctor so that this can be discussed with the nuclear medicine physician.

References

1. DeMarkles MP, Murphy JR. Acute lower gastrointestinal bleeding. *Med Clin North Am* 1993;77:1085–1100.
2. Maurer AH. Gastrointestinal bleeding and cine-scintigraphy. *Semin Nucl Med* 1996;26:43–50.
3. Suzman MS, Talmor M, Jennis R, Binkert B, Barie PS. Accurate localization and surgical management of active lower gastrointestinal hemorrhage with technetium-labeled erythrocyte scintigraphy. *Ann Surg* 1996;224:29–36.
4. Notghi A, Harding LK. The clinical challenge of nuclear medicine in gastroenterology. *Br J Hosp Med* 1995;54:80–86.
5. Maurer AH, Fisher RS. Current applications of scintigraphic methods in gastroenterology. *Baillieres Clin Gastroenterol* 1995;9:71–95.
6. Parkman HP, Miller MA, Fisher RS. Role of nuclear medicine in evaluating patients with suspected gastrointestinal motility disorders. *Semin Nucl Med* 1995;25:289–305.

6
Infection Imaging

Inflammatory and infectious processes can be insidious, occult and easily escape clinical detection, or they can be explosively declarative with alarming clinical presentations. Even after a meticulous history, physical examination, blood cultures and standard radiographs, the site of infection still may be undetected or the presence of infection still may be unconfirmed. Nuclear medicine offers a number of tools to localize and confirm the site of infection.

SCANS AND PRIMARY CLINICAL INDICATIONS

I. ¹¹¹In or ⁹⁹ᵐTc-HMPAO-labeled leukocyte scan

Page 119

- To diagnose infection/abscess in soft tissues anywhere in the body, but particularly in the abdomen/pelvis

- To evaluate extent and severity of inflammatory bowel disease

- To diagnose postoperative abscess in patients with fever, after inconclusive or negative CT scan in patients with high clinical suspicion

- To diagnose infection in a patient with known tumor and fever

- To diagnose vascular graft infection

- To diagnose osteomyelitis in diabetics with nonhealing ulcers

- To diagnose osteomyelitis in patients with inconclusive three-phase bone scan or MRI

II. Gallium scan
- To diagnose and evaluate severity and extent of infection/inflammation in the lungs
- To determine the cause of fever of unknown origin (FUO), usually infection or occult tumor
- To detect osteomyelitis (often combined with a bone scan) in children or adults

III. Three-phase bone scan
- To diagnose osteomyeltis in children and young adults; if inconclusive, follow up with labeled leukocyte or gallium scan
- To evaluate a variety of bone abnormalities (see Chapter 11, The Skeletal System)

IV. 99mTc-LeukoScan (monoclonal antibody)
- See indications for labeled leukocytes

CLINICAL QUESTIONS

Febrile patients

Pulmonary inflammation

Abdominal-pelvic infection

Osteomyelitis

Orthopedic conditions and possible osteomyelitis

PATIENT INFORMATION

6

SCANS

I. ^{111}In OR ^{99m}Tc-HMPAO-LABELED LEUKOCYTE SCAN

A. Background

Indium-111 leukocytes and ^{99m}Tc-exametazime (HMPAO)-labeled leukocytes localize in sites of soft-tissue infection, inflammation, abscesses and osteomyelitis. Labeled leukocyte scans are used most often when an infection is suspected but no localizing signs are present, after negative or equivocal CT or for suspected osteomyelitis.

B. Radiopharmaceuticals

Indium-111 and ^{99m}Tc-HMPAO-labeled leukocytes are the most sensitive and specific radionuclide imaging tools for detecting infection. These agents image the migration of neutrophils to the site of infection or inflammation and have a sensitivity of 85–90% for detecting soft-tissue infection. Technetium-99m-HMPAO has slightly higher propensity to image nonsignificant bowel uptake, which increases with time after administration, and to show physiologic diffuse lung uptake because of slow clearance. The process of labeling leukocytes with ^{111}In or ^{99m}Tc-HMPAO involves separating leukocytes from the patient's venous blood by sedimentation or centrifugation and incubating with ^{111}In-oxine or ^{99m}Tc-HMPAO. The process requires meticulous quality control because blood is handled by technologists and radiopharmacists and reinjected into the patient. Usually, the labeling is performed by a commercial radiopharmacy, although it also can be done in the nuclear medicine department.

C. How the study is performed

After the labeling process, which takes about 1–1.5 hr, 0.5 mCi (18.5 MBq, adult dose) ^{111}In or 5–15 mCi (185–455 MBq, adult dose) ^{99m}Tc-HMPAO autologous labeled cells are reinjected into the patient's peripheral vein. Imaging is performed 18–24 hr later for ^{111}In (or as late as 48 hr, as needed) and 1–4 hr (or up to 8 hr for lung or bone infection) for ^{99m}Tc-HMPAO. SPECT imaging can be added to enhance the conventional imaging.

D. Patient preparation

There is no special preparation for the patient except placement of an intra-venous catheter for withdrawal of 50 ml blood and reinjection of labeled cells. Diet and medication are continued as usual for the patient. The patient needs to be able to tolerate lying still on the imaging table for about 1 hr. If the patient's white blood cell count is <2000 cells/ml, donor cells can be labeled and used.

E. Understanding the report

Labeled leukocytes normally localize in the liver, spleen and bone marrow. Later imaging times may be needed for most effective imaging of bone infection. Diffuse lung uptake and low-level bowel uptake may be observed in normal subjects after ^{99m}Tc-HMPAO leukocyte administration; the bowel uptake increases with time, whereas the lung uptake decreases with time.

The report describes the abnormalities in terms of focally increased or decreased activity (labeled leukocyte localization). The most characteristic finding of a localized focus of infection or inflammation is increased activity, either separate from the normal physiologic pattern of the radiopharmaceutical localization or superimposed on a region of normal physiologic deposition. It is sometimes difficult to separate bony from adjacent soft-tissue accumulations of labeled leukocytes; in other words, infection can be localized but the resolution of the procedure cannot distinguish between soft-tissue infection and osteomyelitis. Likewise, a deficit, an area of abnormally decreased activity called a photopenic or cold defect, also may represent infection, but this finding is not as specific for infection as a hot focus. The photopenia may be due to an abscess which may be very slow to fill-in with the labeled leukocytes, either because of thick encapsulation or poor vascular supply and inefficient penetration of the abscess wall, resulting in a focus of relatively decreased activity. Other sources of photopenia are tumors, prostheses, infarctions, prior radiation and prior surgery.

F. Potential problems

1. False-positive results. Hematomas, bleeding sites and other noninfected inflammatory processes can cause false-positive results. These occur because of the incomplete separation of leukocytes from other cells during the labeling process, resulting in labeling of a mixed population of cells (leukocytes, red blood cells, platelets) with ^{111}In or ^{99m}Tc-HMPAO.

2. Low white counts. Low peripheral white blood cell count (<2000 cells/ml), particularly a neutrophil count of <1000 cells/ml, results in insufficient autologous cells to maintain the high sensitivity of the test for detecting and localizing infections. Labeling and injecting donor cells has been performed, but only in special circumstances. Gallium might provide a better alternative in those circumstances.

3. Liver abscess. Detecting an abscess in or adjacent to the liver and spleen may be challenging because these organs normally show labeled leukocyte activity.

Some abscesses may fill with labeled leukocytes slowly, and further delayed imaging (which can be done with ^{111}In but not as well with ^{99m}Tc) on rare occasions may be helpful.

4. Chronic vertebral osteomyelitis. The sensitivity of labeled leukocytes for detection of chronic vertebral osteomyelitis is approximately 50%. Gallium combined with bone scanning is sensitive but less specific. But, most importantly, nuclear imaging does not provide information about abscess formation and encroachment on the spinal cord as does MRI. Thus, in this condition, MRI is the recommended procedure.

6

5. Distinguishing osteomyelitis from surrounding soft-tissue infection. In the distal extremities it may be difficult to separate a focus of abnormal increased bone uptake (compatible with osteomyelitis) from increased soft-tissue uptake (compatible with cellulitis). Transmission scans that define the skin surface or simultaneous imaging of the bone scan with the indium leukocyte scan are maneuvers that may assist in distinguishing osteomyelitis from cellulitis.

II. GALLIUM SCAN
A. Background
Gallium was the first radionuclide infection imaging agent to be used clinically and as an infection imaging agent; gallium has been particularly effective in imaging chronic processes, as well as acute disease.

B. Radiopharmaceuticals
Gallium-67 is injected intravenously as ^{67}Ga-citrate and immediately binds to circulating transferrin. Gallium-67 transferrin localizes in sites of infection, inflammation and tumors, as well as the liver, spleen, bone marrow, gastrointestinal tract and kidney. Gallium is excreted primarily in the bowel (see Patient Preparation, below) and in the kidney (apparent on images at 24–48 hr).

Acutely inflamed tissue shows the following effects: vasodilation, expansion of the extracellular space and migration of neutrophilic leukocytes. In chronic inflammation, a predominant mononuclear cell infiltration of macrophages, lymphocytes and plasma cells characterizes the cellular migration to the inflamed site.

To a limited extent, gallium normally localizes in bone and is a calcium analog. This leads to nonspecificity for osteomyelitis, similar to that of the bone scan. Gallium also has been found in regions of infection in association with bacterial cellular debris and leukocytes. Thus, similar to labeled leukocytes, gallium localization in infection apparently is facilitated by a migration of white blood cells, but contrary to labeled leukocytes, gallium is not solely dependent upon that phenomenon. This may explain why agranulocytic subjects can have gallium accumulation at sites of bacterial concentration. High levels of lactoferrin in neutrophilic leukocytes and in abscess fluid has been noted as an important factor in gallium accumulation in infection sites. Strong affinities of gallium for binding to lactoferrin and siderophores (low molecular weight compounds that facilitate iron uptake by microorganisms) are probably also important factors in gallium's propensity to concentrate in infections.

C. How the study is performed

After the intravenous injection of 4–6 mCi (8–10 mCi for SPECT imaging [150–220 MBq, adult dose, or 296–370 MBq]), ^{67}Ga-citrate, whole-body or localized imaging may be performed at 24–48 hr or even as early as 4 hr in cases in which early diagnosis is important. If early images are negative, later imaging (24–48 hr) must be obtained. If bowel activity is particularly increased or focal in nature and overlies or interferes with evaluation of the vertebral spine, repeat imaging 24 hr later often is performed to confirm that the activity represents normal bowel excretion. SPECT imaging of any suspected abnormality often is performed to clarify and better delineate the anatomic abnormality. If needed, repeat imaging up to 96 or 120 hr or even as late as 7 days after the administration of the gallium can be done because gallium has a physical half-life of 67 hr.

D. Patient preparation

There is no dietary restriction before the procedure or the imaging.

Gallium injection should be postponed for at least 24 hr after blood transfusions or gadolinium-enhanced MRI scanning, both of which may interfere with normal gallium biodistribution. Gallium normally is excreted primarily into the bowel; if excessive bowel activity is seen on the first images (24, 48 or 72 hr), the patient may be requested to return the next day after an enema or laxative, which will cause the intraluminal activity to move, thereby clarifying the findings on the scan.

E. Understanding the report

The report usually describes the procedure including administration and dose of gallium injected, the imaging technique including SPECT if performed and the findings, including correlations to other imaging (CT, ultrasound, MRI) or to previous nuclear studies.

Evaluation of possible osteomyelitis often requires comparison of gallium images to the bone scan, particularly in regions of prior trauma, degenerative disease and remote infection. The final impression of the report usually concludes with a summary of the significant results and suggestions for further diagnostic steps, if warranted. A level of confidence (i.e., high, moderate, low) in the interpretation is sometimes added.

F. Potential problems

1. Correlation with bone scan. For bone infection, gallium images may be difficult to interpret and may require an accompanying bone scan to (a) better define the anatomy and (b) analyze for discordant abnormal gallium uptake relative to bone scan activity (criterion for diagnosis of bone infection). The bone scan can be performed before, after or simultaneously with the gallium scan. SPECT of both studies may be advantageous to better localize, delineate and assess any abnormalities.

2. Normal excretion paths. Images earlier than 48 hr usually show kidney activity that is normal renal excretion. Therefore, pyelonephritis (particularly if bilateral) may not be definite on early images (<72 hr) and impaired renal function can accentuate that problem. Normal bowel excretion is evident at all times and may complicate the evaluation of suspected soft-tissue abdominal-pelvic infections. Because indium leukocytes do not accumulate significantly in normal bowel (^{99m}Tc-HMPAO tends normally to show very low grade bowel activity), labeled leukocytes are preferred over gallium for evaluating abdominal-pelvic infections.

III. THREE-PHASE BONE SCAN

A. Background

To detect osteomyelitis, the conventional bone scan is modified to distinguish cellulitis from osteomyelitis. Cellulitis is associated with increased blood flow and localized swelling. Consequently, there is increased delivery of the tracer to the site of cellulitis and diffusion into the interstitial space. The rationale for the three phase is to allow the increased soft-tissue activity seen in cellulitis initially to be gradually cleared from the region because of renal excretion of the tracer from the blood. If osteomyelitis is present, the increased radiopharmaceutical delivered by increased blood flow is incorporated into the osteogenic new bone formation incited by the infection and the scan shows increasing activity relative to the soft-tissue background over time. Thus, by continuing to image a bony region for several hours, the three-phase bone scan increases specificity of the scan to approximately 80–85%, an increase of about 15 percentage points over the conventional bone scan.

B. Radiopharmaceutical

Technetium-99m-methylene-diphosphonate (MDP) is the most widely used of the phosphonate bone scan compounds. Its localization depends upon bone blood flow and osteoblastic activity. Because the bone scan is effective in detecting osteogenesis and because bone reacts to any insult (e.g., infection, trauma, etc.) by making new bone, the scan is a sensitive tool for detecting any insult to bone.

Bone blood flow has been identified as perhaps an even more important factor than osteogenesis in determining radiopharmaceutical uptake in bones. It is clear that an absence of blood perfusion to a localized region of bone prevents delivery of the radiopharmaceutical, and a photon deficit, or cold region, may be apparent on the scan. Thus, a balance between impaired, normal or augmented bone blood flow and impaired, normal or augmented osteogenesis results in decreased, normal or increased activity on the bone scan.

C. How the study is performed

The three-phase bone scan consists of the following: (a) a radionuclide angiogram—sequential images every 2 sec, for 30–60 sec, followed by (b) a static blood pool image for 1 min and (c) the conventional 2–3 hr static image or a further delayed image at about 4–5 hr. The fourth phase is a 24-hr static image, which is warranted only occasionally. The entire study is performed after an intravenous injection of the radiopharmaceutical (20–25 mCi ^{99m}Tc-MDP) as the patient lies under the camera. Each imaging sequence takes 10–20 min; the entire study usually takes 3–4 hr.

D. Patient preparation

There is no special patient preparation for this test, except that the patient needs to be well hydrated. The patient is requested to drink a few glasses of water after the radiopharmaceutical injection during the first 2 hr before imaging.

E. Understanding the report

The report describes why the study is being done, the radiopharmaceutical, injection and imaging procedures, the findings and the concluding impression. Radiographic findings that may affect the scan findings often are described to indicate their potential impact on the scan results.

    The three- or four-phase bone scan interpretation depends on visualizing over time increasingly abnormal activity in the infected bone relative to a normal reference region seen on the angiographic or blood-pool phases and the delayed static images. This is best appreciated if technical imaging factors and patient positioning are reproduced well on the sequence of images.

    The sensitivity of the three-phase bone scan for osteomyelitis exceeds 95%, but specificity of the test is reduced because any insult (trauma, infection, vascular injury or metabolic injury) may show focal areas of increased uptake on the bone scan (see Clinical Questions 8 and 9, below). Pattern reading and modifications of the bone scan to include vascularity and perfusion information can aid in optimizing specificity.

F. Potential problems

1. Nonspecificity. The three-phase bone scan is highly specific, as well as sensitive, in children and adults who have had no previous bone trauma or infection but have clean bones, with no bony baggage (prior bone abnormality). For patients (usually adults) with preexisting bone abnormalities, because the three-phase bone scan loses specificity, it may be reasonable to skip the bone scan and proceed directly to a labeled leukocyte scan.

If an inconclusive result is obtained with the three- or four-phase bone scan, the labeled leukocyte scan or gallium scan or labeled antibody scan may be recommended to clarify the findings. The ^{111}In or ^{99m}Tc-HMPAO leukocyte scan is much more specific (as well as quite sensitive) for nonvertebral bone infection in patients with bony baggage.

2. Photopenic cold bone lesions. Photon deficient areas on bone scans can occur in association with osteomyelitis, tumor, avascular necrosis, radiation and surgical interventions including prostheses and hardware insertions. Because the pathophysiology of osteomyelitis involves slowed intramarrow blood flow because of increased intramarrow space pressures associated with inflammation, infarction is also part of the process. Thus, photon deficiency (cold focus) on the bone scan due to infarction is seen early in the process. These photon deficient lesions often become hot lesions on scans performed days later. The spectrum of cold to hot in such bone abnormalities crosses a normal uptake zone, which would lead to a false-negative result.

IV. ^{99m}Tc-LEUKOSCAN (MONOCLONAL ANTIBODY)

This murine whole monoclonal antibody directed against leukocyte cell membrane antigen has the important advantage over labeled leukocytes of not requiring withdrawal and handling of the patient's blood or blood products. LeukoScan is supplied as a kit for labeling with ^{99m}Tc and intravenous injection. Imaging is early (30 min–4 hr). At the time of this writing, LeukoScan had not yet been approved by the United States Food and Drug Administration.

CLINICAL QUESTIONS

1. FUO: should a nuclear imaging study be obtained to identify the cause?

The dominant cause of FUO is infection, followed by tumor. According to the classical definition of FUO, patients present with a 3-wk or longer history of cyclical fever. Generally, these patients do not have localizing signs to direct tomographic imaging techniques such as CT or sonography to a suspected anatomic site. They may not have the usual positive laboratory tests including blood cultures. Thus, total body nuclear scan is particularly practical and desirable. Because gallium concentrates well in certain tumors, including lymphomas, and approximately 20% of patients who present with FUO have occult neoplasm, gallium may be preferred over indium leukocytes. Gallium imaging has had documented high yield in fever of unknown origin (Fig. 1). However, if there is suspected infection in the abdomen, labeled leukocytes might be preferred because of the decreased sensitivity of gallium for detecting abdominal processes because of normal colonic excretion of gallium. Some published data

6

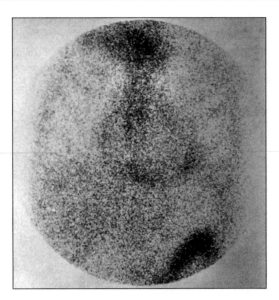

Figure 1. FUO. Gallium scan shows an abnormal rim of gallium activity in the pericardium in this man with FUO. Subsequently, fluid tapped from the pericardial sac cultured *Staphylococcus aureus,* diagnosing infectious pericarditis.

have indicated favorable results of ^{111}In-leukocytes in identifying focal inflammatory lesions in patients with FUO, particularly in patients with known tumor and acquired immunodeficency syndrome (AIDS) (except for suspected pneumocystis because gallium, not labeled leukocytes, is preferred for imaging pneumocystis). For more detailed discussion of infection imaging in AIDS patients, see Chapter 7, AIDS. Thus in FUO, arguments can be made for either technique, but as a general guideline, the arguments for gallium as the first-line total-body imaging technique in these patients appears more compelling.

2. Cancer and FUO: should an imaging study be done? If so, which?

Febrile patients with known tumor present a particular problem because fever may be the result of the tumor or chemotherapy or may be related to an infection or inflammatory lesion. If localizing symptoms are present, CT or ultrasound scans are indicated to evaluate the focus of suspicion. If localizing signs are not present, labeled leukocytes or gallium whole-body imaging in search of a nonsymptomatic focus is warranted. The findings on indium leukocyte and gallium scans in such patients are summarized as follows: Negative indium and positive gallium indicates tumor-chemotherapy fever, whereas ^{111}In identifies infection foci in patients with tumor, regardless of the tumor's affinity for gallium. Thus, ^{111}In or ^{99m}Tc-HMPAO-labeled leukocytes is the imaging procedure of choice in patients with known tumor and fever who may have infection but no localizing signs.

3. Do antibiotics affect the sensitivity of labeled leukocyte or gallium scans?

Antibiotics do not significantly affect the sensitivity of the indium-leukocyte scan, unless the infection has been eradicated. This is probably also true for ^{99m}Tc-HMPAO-labeled leukocytes, but the published data were for indium studies.

4. Worsening chronic interstitial pulmonary disease: Chest x-ray shows no change; can nuclear imaging help?

The extent and severity of gallium uptake in the lungs correlates with abundance of neutrophils in bronchoaveolar lavage samples. Thus, quantitative gallium lung studies in idiopathic pulmonary fibrosis patients have been useful in staging inflammatory activity and in following response to therapy if a baseline study is available.

In contrast, lung uptake with labeled leukocytes is nonspecific. Fewer than 50% of scans with focal uptake of ^{111}In-leukocyte correlate with infectious lesions. Causes of nonspecific ^{111}In-leukocyte uptake in the lungs include congestive heart failure, adult respiratory distress syndrome, atelectasis, aspiration and infarction. Therefore, for pulmonary infection and exacerbation of inflammation, gallium is preferred over indium.

5. Recent abdominal surgery: Patient has fever and normal CT scan. Can a labeled leukocyte scan or a gallium scan help?

Comparative studies of the accuracy of labeled leukocyte scintigraphy and CT for detection of intra-abdominal abscess have shown that both perform with high sensitivity and specificity, particularly when localizing signs are present. If drainage or sampling is warranted, the procedure is best performed under CT guidance. CT permits the identification of surrounding anatomic structures and distortions caused by inflammatory processes or abscesses which may not be apparent on a labeled leukocyte scan. Thus, CT is the first imaging technique used. Labeled leukocyte whole-body imaging may be helpful when CT is problematic to confirm the presence or absence of an abscess or to identify distant foci.

Gallium is not as accurate as labeled leukocytes for the identification of abdominal abscess in postoperative or other patients because the normal bowel excretion of gallium confounds identification of an abscess focus. The sensitivity and specificity of a labeled leukocyte scan for diagnosis of abdominal abscess is 90%, and abscesses at unexpected sites of infection are identified outside the abdomen in 16%. Other abdominal pelvic inflammatory-infectious lesions that will be positive on labeled leukocyte or ^{67}Ga-citrate images include cholecystitis, pyleonephritis, uterine abscess, peritonitis and pancreatitis. Indium-111-labeled leukocytes accumulate in the pancreas only in "severe" cases and can accurately distinguish between pancreatic abscess, a serious complication of acute pancreatitis which requires surgical intervention, and simple pseudocyst.

6. Crohn's disease: Patient with prior partial bowel resection has recurrent symptoms; can nuclear scan assist in guiding therapy?

In patients with inflammatory bowel disease, labeled leukocyte imaging provides a noninvasive method of quantitatively assessing extent and severity of inflammation (Fig. 2). In patients too ill for barium or endoscopy, labeled leukocyte scan can give information on extent of disease that might be useful in guiding need for continuing therapy or perhaps changing therapy. The scan provides an objective measure of inflammatory activity for following response to therapy in occasional circumstances in which objective data are needed. Vascular bowel infarction, pseudomembranous colitis and other inflammatory bowel processes are positive on labeled leukocyte images and may be indistinguishable except perhaps for the distribution of disease sites, i.e., small bowel, large bowel or rectum.

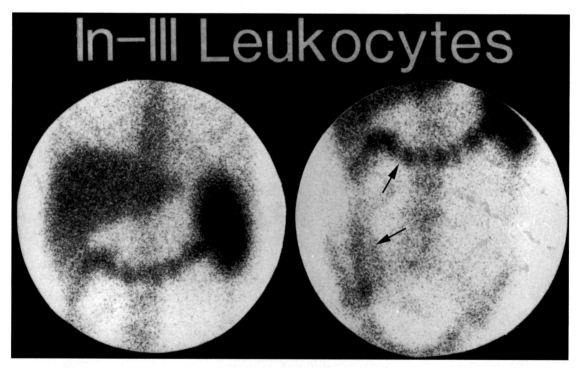

Figure 2. Inflammatory bowel disease. Indium-111 leukocyte image of anterior abdomen and pelvis shows abnormal transverse (arrow), ascending (arrow) and, to a lesser degree, sigmoid colon uptake. The patient has Crohn's disease and is suffering an active inflammatory recurrence involving the regions of bowel that have taken up the labeled leukocytes. Normal labeled leukocyte abdomen scans show no bowel uptake, but only liver, spleen and bone marrow.

Inflammatory bowel disease is probably the only instance when early indium (4-hr) imaging should be performed. Because labeled cells may be sloughed from sites of inflamed mucous in the bowel lumen, a late image (24 hr) may show activity at sites distant from the origin of inflammation because of intralumenal transport of the sloughed labeled cells—retrograde and prograde. Because of its normal excretion into the bowel, gallium is less effective for inflammatory bowel disease.

7. Aortobifemoral vascular graft placed 1 yr ago: Patient has fever and vascular graft infection is suspected; can a nuclear scan help?

Labeled leukocyte imaging is a reliable modality for detecting vascular graft infections. A comparative study of CT imaging and ^{111}In-leukocyte scans in detection of abdominal aortic graft infection gave similar results for the two modalities, with the exception that CT was thought to more accurately depict extension of infection into the retroperitoneum than was apparent from the labeled leukocyte scans. In practice, the CT scan and the ^{111}In-leukocyte study may be complementary in evaluating these patients.

8. A 23 yr old with fever presented to the emergency room with acute hip pain; does he have osteomyelitis?

An x-ray of the hip is done first; if it is negative, the likelihood of osteomyelitis can be effectively evaluated with a three-phase bone scan because it is 95% sensitive and specific in young patients who do not have other bone abnormalities such as prior trauma, degenerative bone changes or arthritis, particularly in the presence of elevated peripheral white blood cell count with left shift and elevated sedimentation rate.

The three-phase bone scan has a reported overall sensitivity of 90–100% and a specificity of 73–87%, which includes patients with complicating preexisting bone conditions, in whom the specificity drops to 33%.

Recent trauma. Inflammation caused by recent (within months) trauma can cause a false-positive three-phase bone scan result. A gallium labeled leukocyte scan might be more specific in such cases. In young adults, children and infants, gallium may be preferred over indium or technetium because it is highly accurate in the absence of complicating bony conditions, less expensive than labeled leukocytes, and somewhat lower in radiation exposure than indium. If traumatic inflammation is suspected, MRI may be recommended to visualize the soft-tissue edema, inflammation or bleeding that may be present but not detected by a bone scan, gallium scan or indium leukocyte scan.

9. Limping toddler with fever; does he have osteomyelitis?

An x-ray should be obtained first. If negative, as it usually is in early osteomyelitis, the three-phase bone scan is the preferred next test, with 95%

sensitivity and 95% specificity. It also is the least expensive imaging test that can be done. Gallium would be the second-line test if the bone scan were inconclusive. Either three-phase bone scan or gallium scan would be expected to have high sensitivity and high specificity for osteomyelitis in a 1-yr-old child without previous trauma or underlying bony abnormality.

Gallium imaging has been used widely in children, particularly if the bone scan is inconclusive or shows a cold defect (see Potential Problems, above). Indium-111 leukocytes are not used widely in children, mainly because of the increased radiation exposure and the need to withdraw blood for labeling.

10. Acute versus chronic osteomyelitis: Which scan is best?

Chronic osteomyelitis is more challenging to evaluate than acute osteomyelitis by any technique: bone scan, labeled leukocytes, gallium or MRI. Gallium is effective, but requires a concomitant bone scan to interpret the gallium result, unless it is negative. A baseline gallium scan is necessary for interpreting response to therapy in chronic bone infection, and gallium performs well as a monitor over time.

The sensitivity of labeled leukocytes to detect osteomyelitis varies with bone location, as well as with the age of the infection. The sensitivity to detect acute osteomyelitis is consistently 90–95% in all skeletal locations. The sensitivity for chronic osteomyelitis varies from 53% in central (marrow containing) locations to 80% in middle (between distal extremities and central locations) to 94% in peripheral bony locations (distal extremities). The specificity for labeled leukocyte imaging is 90% in all cases.

11. Child with sickle cell anemia has right tibial pain and fever. Can nuclear scans distinguish between osteomyelitis and bone infarct?

The differential diagnosis of acute, nontraumatic, painful bones in youngsters with sickle cell anemia is usually osteomyelitis versus bone infarction. In typical sickle cell crises, bone pain is usually infarct. If the presentation is atypical or suggests osteomyelitis, the problem is a particularly challenging diagnostic puzzle. On bone scan, osteomyelitis and bone infarct may be either hot or cold. Gallium scans are more consistently hot in osteomyelitis but also may be hot in acute infarction. The bone marrow scan using ^{99m}Tc-sulfur colloid has been suggested as a potential adjunctive procedure, but it too may show focal cold abnormalities in osteomyelitis and infarction.

One recommended imaging approach to this problem is the combination of bone scan (three-phase) and gallium scan. If the gallium uptake exceeds bone scan uptake, or if there is marked focal bone and gallium scan increased uptake, osteomyelitis is likely. If there is decreased bone and gallium scan uptake, or increased gallium uptake that is less than increased bone scan uptake, then infarct is more likely. All other patterns are indeterminate.

12. Orthopedic surgery 15 mo ago on vertebral spine with increasing pain in recent months; needs assessment for osteomyelitis?

The bone scan is unlikely to be helpful in this setting because of the prior surgical trauma, which will likely result in an abnormal bone scan and be indistinguishable from osteomyelitis. Similarly, gallium scan may be abnormal because of prior bone surgical trauma; the sensitivity of indium leukocyte scans is reduced in chronic vertebral osteomyelitis (50%), although there are reports indicating that ^{99m}Tc-HMPAO-labeled leukocyte scans maintain higher sensitivity in chronic osteomyelitis of the vertebral spine. MRI, however, demonstrates better performance in the spine and has the added important advantage of imaging the surrounding soft tissues so that associated abscess and inflammation are identified, as well as possible disc herniation or threatened encroachment on the spinal cord. Therefore, MRI is recommended as the first-line imaging test in possible vertebral osteomyelitis. If metallic hardware is present in the spine, a ^{99m}Tc-HMPAO scan should be considered.

13. Orthopedic screw and plate surgically placed 1 yr ago for fracture fixation; patient complains of new pain at the site. Does he have bone infection?

The diagnosis of bone infection in the presence of prior orthopedic surgery or other trauma is often difficult because the bone scan (the simplest and least expensive test) has decreased specificity for infection (33%) because of the abnormal findings associated with prior surgical trauma, even though its sensitivity remains 95–100%. If an x-ray shows joint fluid that can be tapped, a needle aspiration may give the answer. But if a noninvasive test is desired, the labeled leukocyte study would be an excellent test. The labeled leukocyte study maintains its high specificity (85%), as well as its sensitivity (85%), in these instances and therefore is a better test. MRI would be at least as good as the labeled leukocyte test, but the presence of the metal hardware precludes MRI. The gallium scan combined with the bone scan also may be effective, although the specificity is not as high as it is for the leukocyte scan. The question of osteomyelitis, as a chronic process with exacerbations, arises in patients with prior orthopedic surgery. In general, sensitivity and specificity of the technetium-gallium combination are variable (25–80%) at sites of prior orthopedic surgery.

Figure 3 shows a labeled leukocyte scan, a colloid bone marrow scan and a new monoclonal antibody product scan (^{99m}Tc-LeukoScan), which targets granulocytes in a patient with a painful knee prosthesis. The images diagnose infection by showing avid increased uptake at the knee and surrounding regions of the labeled leukocytes and the monoclonal antibody. The fact that the bone marrow scan shows lesser increased activity than the other scans confirms that bone marrow uptake alone cannot explain the increased uptake on the other two scans, which normally go to marrow.

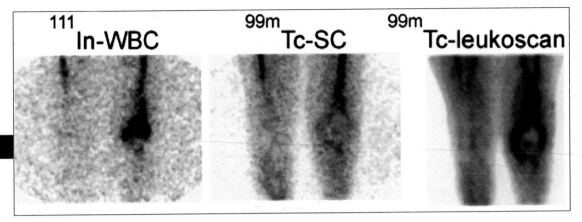

Figure 3. Infected knee prosthesis. Indium-111-labeled white blood cell image shows abnormal increased uptake of the femoral component of the prosthetic knee. This is consistent with infection or inflammation. The marrow scan using ^{99m}Tc-sulfur colloid shows marrow extending into the knee, but much less uptake than the indium leukocytes, confirming that the uptake on the indium scan is much more than can be explained by marrow. The ^{99m}Tc-labeled LeukoScan study also confirms increased uptake extending from the knee proximally, indicating infection. (Photo courtesy of Christopher J. Palestro, MD., Long Island Jewish Medical Center, New Hyde Park, NY)

14. A 60-yr-old patient with diabetes, peripheral vascular disease and nonhealing ulcerations overlying three distal toes. Is there underlying osteomelitits?

Diabetic foot infections account for 20% of all diabetic patient hospital admissions in the United States. Complications of diabetic foot infections lead to almost half of all nontraumatic foot or leg amputations. Thus, appropriate early treatment is often critical to avoid loss of a limb in diabetic patients presenting with foot infections. Diabetics who present with osteomyelitis of the foot require intravenous antibiotics. If the infection is confined to soft tissue, a simple course of short-term antibiotics and good wound care, if ulceration is present, may be all that is needed. Management may consist simply of a trial of antibiotics; if osteomyelitis is considered likely, the diagnosis may be pursued vigorously using plain x-rays, bone scans, leukocyte scans, MRI or bone biopsy. If osteomyelitis is considered unlikely, noninvasive diagnostic imaging is preferred because surgical exploration of a foot can lead to unnecessary damage, particularly in a neuropathic diabetic foot.

The diagnostic problem is more difficult in diabetic patients, in part because of complications of neuroarthropathies, previous bone or tissue infections, previous bone trauma and bone deformities. The labeled leukocyte scan (Fig. 4) is the radionuclide study with the best sensitivity, specificity and cost-effectiveness in patients with prior bone problems (i.e., trauma, degenerative changes, etc.). MRI and labeled leukocytes have approximately the same sensitvity and specificity for detection of osteomyelitis. In diabetic children, or diabetic adults without bony abnormalities, the three-phase bone scan is highly sensitive and specific for suspected osteomyelitis (Fig. 4).

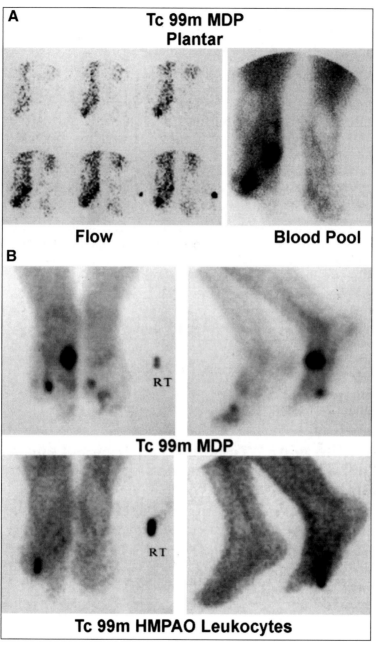

Figure 4. Three-phase bone scan and HMPAO leukocyte scan. (A) Phases 1 and 2 of the three-phase bone scan show a hypervascular response in the left foot, most focally increased to the distal lateral digits on the radionuclide angiogram, which shows sequential images at 2 sec per frame (left panel). The right panel shows increased blood pooling in the same regions noted as hypervascular on the angiographic study: the distal third and fourth digits and a focal medial region over the proximal first metatarsal base-tarsal bones. (B) Phase 3 of the three-phase ^{99m}Tc-MDP bone scan and the leukocyte scan. The delayed images of the bone scan (3 hr, top row) again show persistence of activity in the same regions noted on the early phases (A), consistent with osteomyelitis but not specific in this 60-yr-old man with diabetes, and likely bone degenerative changes. Also evident is that the distal phalanges of the third, fourth and fifth digits are missing (previously amputated), and the abnormal activity is actually in the third digit. The ^{99m}Tc-HMPAO leukocyte images, however, show focal leukocyte migration only to the third digit of the left foot, indicating osteomyelitis. No uptake is seen in the other site of the first metatarsal base-tarsal region, which was seen on the bone scan, confirming absence of bone infection in that region.

MRI may distinguish abscess from osteomyelitis, cellulitis, septic arthritis and tenosynovitis, whereas radionuclide imaging may distinguish between osteomyelitis and cellulitis but does not reliably identify an abscess as separate from cellulitis or osteomyelitis.

CT is not as sensitive for diagnosis of osteomyelitis as MRI or labeled leukocyte imaging. It is, however, effective as a diagnostic aid in the feet of diabetic patients, focusing on plantar compartmental infection. CT can detect extension of superficial diabetic foot infections at an earlier stage and may have a role in amputation-level planning, but no validated data on sensitivity or specificity of CT for these purposes are available.

To summarize, overall, labeled leukocytes and MRI give comparable results; in patients with no underlying bony abnormality, the much less expensive three-phase bone scan gives excellent results, and its high sensitivity and specificity in those with no bony abnormalitiy often allow the diagnosis of osteomyelitis to be made or excluded.

WORTH MENTIONING

1. Malignant external otitis in diabetic patients

Necrotizing external otitis and severe external otitis can be distinguished using a semiquantitative approach of SPECT bone scanning.

2. Other ^{111}In and ^{99m}Tc-labeled monoclonal and polyclonal antibody preparations, antibiotic radiopharmaceuticals and peptides

Several effective antibody products directed against leukocyte antigens are available in Europe but not approved in the United States. These, as well as other radiopharmaceutical compounds (labeled antibiotics), have been shown in European studies to be comparable to ^{111}In leukocytes. The advantage of such agents is that no blood drawing or cell labeling is required. Chemotactic peptides are under investigation.

PATIENT INFORMATION

I. HMPAO LEUKOCYTE SCAN

A. Test/Procedure

Your physician has referred you to the the nuclear medicine department for a technetium white blood cell scan because you may have an infection. The technologist will first withdraw about 3 ounces of blood from a vein (usually in the arm). Your blood will be processed in the laboratory to isolate the white blood cells and label them with a radioactive isotope. Your labeled blood will then be reinjected into your arm vein. A few hr later, pictures will be taken with a special camera to visualize where the radiolabeled blood cells localized in your body. Drawing your blood, labeling it, reinjecting it and taking pictures may take 5–7 hr.

B. Preparation

Diet. There is no particular preparation for this test. You may eat your usual diet.

Medications. You may continue all medications that have been prescribed for you.

C. Radiation and other risks

The only risks to this procedure are those associated with radiation, drawing blood and reinjecting it. These include radiation to your body from the radioisotope and infection, bleeding or hematoma at the vein puncture site. The amount of radiation you get is similar to what you would get from many other diagnostic x-ray tests. The amount of radiation to your whole body is about what people receive from cosmic and naturally occurring background radiation sources for 2 yr. This is equivalent to about 15% of the yearly radiation dose considered safe for doctors and technologists who work with radiation. You can be around others and use a bathroom normally without risk to others.

D. Pregnancy

If you are pregnant or think you could be pregnant, please notify your doctor so that this can be discussed with the nuclear medicine physician.

II. INDIUM LEUKOCYTE SCAN

A. Test/Procedure

Your doctor has ordered a leukocyte scan to assess whether you have an infection. This test is done by withdrawing about 3 ounces of blood from a vein in your arm and tagging your white blood cells with a radioisotope. Your blood is reinjected into your vein, and pictures are taken the next day (18–24 hr later) with a special camera called a scintillation camera. The pictures take about 1 hr.

B. Preparation

Diet. There is no particular preparation for this test. You may eat your usual diet.

Medications. You may continue all medications that have been prescribed for you.

C. Radiation and other risks

The main risks to this procedure are those associated with radiation, drawing blood and reinjecting it. These include radiation to your body from the radioisotope and infection, bleeding or hematoma at the vein puncture site. The amount of radiation you get is similar to what you would get from many other diagnostic x-ray tests. The amount of radiation to your whole body is about what people receive from cosmic and naturally occurring background radiation sources for 7–14 yr. It is equivalent to the amount of radiation considered safe for doctors and technologists who work with radiation to receive during 9 mo to 1 yr.

D. Pregnancy

If you are pregnant or think you could be pregnant, please notify your doctor so that this can be discussed with the nuclear medicine physician.

III. GALLIUM SCAN
A. Test/Procedure

Your physician has referred you to the nuclear medicine department for a gallium scan because you may have an infection. A small amount of radioactive gallium is injected into a vein and then pictures are obtained 48 and/or 72 hr later with a special camera called a scintillation camera. Occasionally pictures are obtained at 4 and/or 24 hr. Each set of pictures may take 45–90 min, depending on the number of pictures needed and the camera being used.

B. Preparation

Diet. There is no particular preparation for this test. You may eat your usual diet.

Medications. You may continue all medications that have been prescribed for you.

C. Radiation and other risks

The risk of this procedure is radiation to your body from the radioisotope. The amount of radiation you get is similar to what you would get from many other diagnostic x-ray tests. The amount of radiation to your whole body is about the amount that people receive from cosmic and naturally occurring background radiation sources for 7 yr. It is equivalent to 50% of the yearly dose considered safe for doctors and technologists who work with radiation.

D. Pregnancy

If you are pregnant or think you could be pregnant, please inform your doctor so that this can be discussed with the nuclear medicine physician.

IV. THREE-PHASE BONE SCAN
A. Test/Procedure
Your doctor has ordered a bone scan to assess whether you have an infection in your bones. A small amount of a radioactive material is injected into a vein. The radioactive tracer preferentially concentrates in infected bone. Pictures usually are taken with a special camera immediately after the injection; additional pictures are taken 2–3 hr later and possibly at 5 or 24 hr. The pictures take about 15–40 min each time, depending on how many pictures are needed.

6

B. Preparation
Diet. There is no special preparation for this test. You may eat as usual. It is recommended that you be well hydrated for the test, i.e., drink lots of fluids (preferably water and juices).

Medications. You should continue taking all medications that have been prescribed for you. If you have had any other recent nuclear medicine test, please inform the nuclear medicine technologist or physician.

C. Radiation and other risks
The risk of this procedure is radiation to your body from the radioisotope. The amount of radiation you get is similar to what you would get from many other diagnostic x-ray tests. The amount of radiation to your whole body is about what people receive from cosmic and naturally occurring background radiation sources for 2–3 yr. It is equivalent to about 10–20% of the yearly dose considered safe for doctors and technologists who work with radiation.

D. Pregnancy
If you are pregnant or think you could be pregnant, please inform your doctor so that this can be discussed with the nuclear medicine physician.

References
1. Schauwecker DS. The scintigraphic diagnosis of osteomyelitis. *AJR Am J Roentgenol* 1992;158:9–18.
2. Datz F. Infection imaging. *Semin Nucl Med* 1994;24:89–91.
3. Corstens FH, van der Meer JW. Nuclear medicine's role in infection and inflammation. *Lancet* 1999;354:765–770.
4. Peters AM. Nuclear medicine imaging in fever of unknown origin. *Q J Nucl Med* 1999; 43:61–73.
5. Palestro CJ. Radionuclide imaging of nonosseous infection. *Q J Nucl Med* 1999;43:46–60.

7
Acquired Immunodeficiency Syndrome

By the end of 1998, nearly 700,000 people had been diagnosed with AIDS in the United States, and more than 33 million people worldwide were living with the disease. Although patients with AIDS often are treated empirically, nuclear imaging can be useful. Specialized scans like thallium-gallium sequential imaging, as well as routine studies such as bone scanning and iminodiacetic acid, have demonstrated value with human immunodeficiency virus (HIV)-infected patients.

SCANS AND PRIMARY CLINICAL INDICATIONS

CLINICAL QUESTIONS

SCANS

I. GALLIUM SCAN

A. Background

Despite certain pitfalls in using a nonspecific tumor and inflammation marker, gallium scanning is invaluable in the hands of a skilled nuclear medicine physician. It is the most widely used nuclear medicine scan to examine AIDS patients. A negative scan in the appropriate setting is highly significant. Patterns of uptake, correlated with other imaging modalities and clinical information, can be highly specific for certain opportunistic infections and help direct workup.

B. Radiopharmaceuticals

Gallium-67-citrate is a nonspecific marker of tumor and inflammation. It acts as an iron analog and is transported in the blood via transferrin. Some tumors have transferrin receptors that avidly bind the gallium and facilitate incorporation into the lysosomes of these active tumor cells. At sites of inflammation, the gallium-transferrin complex leaks into the extracellular space, and gallium preferentially binds to lactoferrin and siderophores, which are released by leukocytes and bacteria. There are also transferrin-independent mechanisms, which make gallium useful in the leukopenic patient.

C. How the study is performed

Gallium is injected intravenously (4–6 mCi [150–220 MBq] adult dose), and images are acquired at 2–3 days (to allow blood pool clearance). Sometimes 4–6 hr images are obtained for early diagnosis of infection or pulmonary disease or to evaluate the abdomen, which is confounded by normal colon clearance at 24 hr. Delayed images may be necessary up to 4–7 days after injection. The imaging may take less than 30 min for planar chest views and up to several hours for a comprehensive examination with whole-body planar views and SPECT. The patient should be prepared for this possibility.

D. Patient preparation

Gallium scanning should be avoided within 24 hr after blood transfusions or gadolinium-enhanced MRI scanning, both of which may interfere with biodistribution. The nuclear medicine physician may prescribe a gentle laxative to assist bowel clearance. The patient may eat, drink and take medications as usual.

E. Understanding the report

Abnormal gallium uptake corresponds to foci of inflammation or certain types of neoplasia. Gallium is distributed normally in the liver, spleen, skeletal system and colon and in varying degrees in salivary and lacrimal glands, nasal region, breast and genitalia. There is faint renal uptake on the 48- to 72-hr images. Mild hilar uptake also may be a normal finding. Minimal lung uptake may be seen up to 48 hr.

Scan interpretation. A normal chest x-ray with diffuse pulmonary gallium uptake, especially if heterogeneous and intense, has a >90% specificity for PCP in the AIDS patient population (Fig. 1). Some may use a quantitative or qualitative reporting scale for degree of uptake, which increases specificity. Other gallium scan patterns suggestive of particular causes include focal lobar uptake—bacterial pneumonia; patchy upper-lobe pulmonary uptake with hilar and nonhilar lymph nodes—mycobacterial disease (or coccidioidomycosis and histoplasmosis in endemic areas); diffuse low-grade pulmonary uptake with renal, adrenal, lacrimal or colonic uptake—cytomegalovirus (CMV); pulmonary and parotid uptake—lymphocytic interstitial pneumonitis; bulky nodal uptake—lymphoma; pulmonary and bone uptake—*Actinomyces/Nocardia;* ileal/cecal and nodal uptake—mycobacteria; proximal small bowel— *Cryptosporidium* (or possibly *Giardia* or *Isospora*). Sarcoid, though not associated with AIDS, demonstrates symmetric hilar and right paratracheal uptake and may be found incidentally in a young patient population.

7

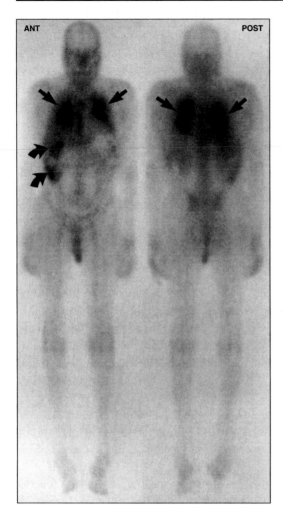

Figure 1. Anterior (ANT) and posterior (POST) views from a gallium scan demonstrate intense bilateral pulmonary uptake (straight arrows) secondary to PCP in this patient infected with HIV. Intense colon uptake in the right upper quadrant on the anterior image (curved arrows) resolved on delayed images and was not a pathologic finding.

There are many other nonspecific patterns. For example, cardiac uptake may be due to pericarditis, myocarditis, endocarditis or neoplasia. Kaposi's sarcoma is not gallium-avid (see below). A negative gallium scan with an abnormal chest x-ray in an AIDS patient suggests Kaposi's sarcoma.

F. Potential Problems

1. Normal distribution. Because gallium has normal distribution in certain organs, diseases affecting them will be less conspicuous. The most frequent such activity confounding interpretation is that of normal bowel excretion. Normal uptake in the pediatric thymus and breast uptake with ongoing lactation are expected findings.

2. Nonspecificity. Infection, inflammation, sarcoid and many cancers can demonstrate abnormal gallium uptake. Although faint renal uptake is seen normally, intense uptake may indicate AIDS-related nephropathy or liver failure but also can be present with acute tubular necrosis (ATN) or CMV. Severe constipation, any bowel inflammation or certain neoplasia can demonstrate abnormal colonic uptake. Increased uptake can occur at sites of recent surgery, fracture, biopsy and intramuscular injections. Findings need to be correlated with the clinical examination and the results of other diagnostic tests.

3. False-negative results and biointerference. Disease therapy may lead to a false-negative result, and treatment of PCP with aerosolized pentamidine can cause atypical upper-lobe pulmonary uptake. Too little gallium accumulation in small foci of disease as well as inadequate blood flow to the area may lead to a false-negative result. In addition, a subset of preterminal AIDS patients have been described in which obvious pulmonary infections are gallium negative. Other potential problems include the alteration of gallium biodistribution caused by recent chemotherapy, radiotherapy, chelation, iron therapy or overload, blood transfusion and gadolinium administration for MRI.

II. THALLIUM SCAN
A. Background
Thallium has primarily been used for myocardial perfusion imaging. Preferential uptake in certain neoplasms, combined with its low avidity for infection, has made it a useful radionuclide in the evaluation of AIDS patients. It is used for brain scanning to help differentiate toxoplasmosis from lymphoma, in conjunction with gallium scanning (see below) to distinguish the many causes of pulmonary disease and as a whole-body scan to survey for Kaposi's sarcoma lesions.

Some centers use sestamibi instead of thallium, which is not as well validated but has better imaging characteristics. Sestamibi can be substituted in chest and musculoskeletal imaging but usually is not used for brain evaluation because of choroid plexus uptake.

B. Radiopharmaceuticals
Thallium-201 is a potassium analog that does not cross the blood-brain barrier unless disrupted. Thallium mainly is concentrated like potassium in viable tumor, to a lesser degree in inflammatory cells and almost negligibly in necrotic tissue. Although early imaging may demonstrate uptake in infection because of passive diffusion, this generally clears on delayed images.

C. How the study is performed
Thallium (3–4 mCi [110–150 MBq] adult dose) is injected intravenously as thallium chloride, and initial images are performed 10–30 min later. The extent of imaging depends on the clinical questions to be answered. A planar survey of the chest will take approximately 15–30 min. SPECT may take up to 1 hr depending on the equipment used. Delayed views at 2–4 hr often are performed.

D. Patient preparation

No special preparation is required for brain scanning. For abdominal imaging, the patient should fast (water is permitted) for 4–8 hr before injection to reduce interference with splanchnic uptake. Thallium uptake is not affected by steroid use.

E. Understanding the report

Normal activity may be present in muscle, myocardium, thyroid, liver, kidney, bowel and bladder. Normal brain should have little or no thallium uptake. Abnormal lesion location and intensity will be described, as well as correlation with other imaging and physical examination, to narrow the differential diagnosis. For example, in the brain, the usual clinical differentiation based on an abnormal CT or MRI scan is between lymphoma and toxoplasmosis. Lymphoma is thallium avid, whereas toxoplasmosis is not. A retentive index of lesion activity to contralateral brain may be calculated. The higher the index, the greater the specificity for lymphoma. Kaposi's sarcoma is thallium avid.

F. Potential problems

1. False-negative results. If a lesion is necrotic, partially treated, near an area of normal uptake or below the resolution of imaging (usually 1 cm), a false-negative scan result may result.

2. False-positive results. There also have been reports of thallium uptake with abscess, certain infections and, rarely, with radiation necrosis. Most of these false-positive occurrences do not demonstrate increased relative intensity on delayed images.

III. THALLIUM-GALLIUM SCAN
A. Background

Thallium is taken up in neoplastic processes such as Kaposi's sarcoma and lymphoma, although generally not in infections. Gallium is avid for infectious etiologies and lymphoma but not for Kaposi's sarcoma. This pattern of differential uptake can be exploited in the combined thallium-gallium scan. Although this scan is mostly used to differentiate pulmonary processes, the same principals can be applied to myositis, pericarditis and even cerebral pathology.

B. Radiopharmaceuticals

Thallium-201-chloride and ^{67}Ga-citrate are the same radiopharmaceuticals used in thallium and gallium scans above.

C. How the study is performed

A thallium scan is first performed. After the delayed views are obtained, gallium is injected and standard gallium views are acquired 1–3 days later. (Some centers perform the thallium scan after gallium scanning if needed.)

D. Patient preparation

Preparation is the same as for the individual scans.

E. Understanding the report

Comparison of differential uptake is the key to diagnosis. A lesion that is thallium-positive and gallium-negative is consistent with Kaposi's sarcoma; one that is thallium-negative and gallium-positive may indicate infection such as PCP or *Mycobacterium tuberculosis* (MTB); and one that is thallium- and gallium-positive points to lymphoma. Moreover, these results can be combined with patterns of anatomic distribution.

F. Potential problems

1. Decreased sensitivity. Although the thallium-positive, gallium-negative pattern has a high specificity for Kaposi's sarcoma, sensitivity has been reported to be decreased in the presence of confounding opportunistic infection if only immediate images were obtained. When 2–4 hr delayed thallium scan views were added, infectious lesions had washout of radiotracer, whereas Kaposi's sarcoma remained intense.

2. Nonspecificity. Although a gallium-positive, thallium-negative pattern with hilar lymph node uptake is highly specific for mycobacterial disease, other infections such as *Cryptococcus* with superimposed lymphadenitis can mimic this appearance.

IV. OTHER SCANS

Any type of nuclear imaging can be used for the HIV-positive patient. Below is a listing of the more useful ones. The reader is referred to specific chapters (in parentheses) that will provide more detail.

1. White-blood-cell scanning (Chapter 6, Infection Imaging)

Patients with AIDS are often neutropenic. Yet this scan can be performed as long as the patient has sufficient neutrophils (>2000). Because this examination involves blood withdrawal and reinjection, scrupulous blood and body fluid precautions must be taken, and a system must be in place to ensure the labeled white blood cells do not get reinjected into a different patient. Because of these concerns, some departments are reluctant to use labeled white blood cells for infection and prefer to use gallium instead. White-blood-cell scanning is generally not as useful for opportunistic infections such as PCP, but it is excellent for bacterial infections.

2. Hepatobiliary scan (Chapter 4, The Spleen and Hepatobiliary System)

This examination can help diagnose AIDS-related chronic cholecystitis and cholangiopathy. Linear defects on initial images that join in a biliary tree pattern with delayed filling and bowel excretion are consistent with cholangiopathy. Delayed gallbladder filling may be seen with chronic cholecystitis.

3. Gastrointestinal bleeding scan (Chapter 5, The Gastrointestinal System)

The radiolabeled red blood cell scan can identify the hypervascular lesions of Kaposi's sarcoma of the bowel.

4. Brain SPECT perfusion imaging (Chapter 8, The Central Nervous System)

This examination can help in the diagnosis of AIDS dementia before findings are apparent on CT or MRI. Classic abnormalities include multifocal cortical or subcortical perfusion defects especially in the frontal, temporal and parietal regions. The basal ganglia also may be involved. A similar pattern also can be present in drug abusers and in AIDS encephalopathy without dementia. In addition, cerebral herpes simplex virus (HSV) infection can present with characteristic increased cerebral uptake. Patients with AIDS also have a higher incidence of cerebrovascular insults that demonstrate larger and more characteristic vascular territory defects than those seen with dementia.

5. Bone scan (Chapter 11, The Skeletal System and Chapter 6, Infection Imaging)

This examination is performed as any other bone scan, either as a three-phase or standard delayed scan, as appropriate. It can help diagnose bacillary angiomatosis and differentiate myositis and cellulitis from osteomyelitis. Gallium and thallium scanning also can be combined with bone scanning to differentiate the many processes affecting bone.

6. Multiple-gated acquisitions (Chapter 1, Cardiovascular Diseases)

Gated radionuclide ventriculography (also known as multiple-gated acquisitions) is useful to track and document AIDS- or drug-related cardiac dysfunction.

CLINICAL QUESTIONS

1. Suspected cerebral disease: Is it toxoplasmosis or lymphoma?

The two most commonly treatable cerebral lesions in patients with AIDS are toxoplasmosis and lymphoma. These conditions usually are identified on CT or MRI but can have an overlapping appearance as ring-enhancing lesions. Stereotactic brain biopsy is considered to be the definitive procedure, but it carries a risk of morbidity and is prone to sampling error. Often patients are treated empirically for toxoplasmosis but concurrent steroids frequently are used to decrease brain edema. This treatment can result in an apparent improvement in lymphoma with antitoxoplasmosis therapy. Furthermore, the failure to establish a diagnosis may delay appropriate therapy. The ^{201}Tl brain scan is a noninvasive study and in this setting is nearly 100% sensitive and 90% specific in diagnosing lymphoma, leading to timely radiation therapy (see Fig. 4 in Chapter 8, Central Nervous System. Central nervous system lymphoma and glioblastoma have a similar degree of uptake on thallium scan.)

2. Suspected cerebral disease: Is it AIDS dementia?

7

Human immunodeficiency virus dementia is common in patients with AIDS. It is thought to be caused by direct HIV brain infection. A CT or MRI should be obtained to exclude infectious and neoplastic lesions. If these are negative, and the clinical diagnosis is in doubt, the brain SPECT perfusion scan is a sensitive indicator of early AIDS-associated dementia. Reversal of changes can be seen with treatment for HIV.

3. What is the source of FUO?

A general algorithm for FUO with no localizing source in a patient with AIDS is the meticulous history and physical examination and collection of blood cultures, relevant serologic tests and a chest x-ray; a gallium scan may be performed if these tests are unrevealing. If there is FUO with localizing symptoms suspicious for acute abdominal infection, CT scan and stool culture are obtained first. If these tests are nondiagnostic, an ^{111}In-leukocyte scan would be an appropriate next examination because of confounding normal bowel excretion in ^{99m}Tc-labeled leukocyte scanning and gallium scans. If lymphoma or mycobacterial infections are likely, gallium is more sensitive than ^{111}In-labeled leukocytes and is preferred. For a suspected acute head and neck infection, CT or MRI are first-line examinations. If they are nondiagnostic, a labeled white-blood-cell scan also would be the appropriate next study, because of confounding normal gallium uptake in the sinuses and salivary glands. More specific discussions are continued below (see Chapter 6, Infection Imaging).

4. Abnormal chest x-ray and diagnostic sputum: Is nuclear imaging of value?

With the advent of effective prophylactic regimens, the incidence of PCP has decreased. Kaposi's sarcoma, lymphoma, bacterial pneumonia and MTB infections are increasingly common. In endemic areas, coccidioidomycosis and histoplasmosis may demonstrate findings similar to MTB. Fungal disease, lymphocytic interstitial pneumonitis, nonspecific interstitial pneumonitis and CMV can affect the lungs.

Chest x-ray and routine sputum smears and cultures, as well as skin testing, lack sensitivity. Yet, chest x-ray should be obtained first because it is inexpensive and noninvasive. If the chest x-ray is positive, induced sputum followed by bronchoalveolar lavage, if necessary, has high sensitivity for PCP, especially with the use of immunofluorescence staining. When the initial chest x-ray is positive followed by diagnostic sputum or lavage, no further imaging is required. With typical clinical and radiographic findings for PCP, some clinicians advocate empiric therapy as a cost-effective alternative to bronchoscopy. Some centers may perform high-resolution CT scanning as a next step instead of bronchoscopy. A "ground-glass" mosaic infiltrate pattern is suggestive of PCP. Bronchial disease that commonly accounts for pulmonary symptoms in the absence of PCP can also be diagnosed by CT.

5. Nondiagnostic chest x-ray and sputum: Is pulmonary disease the cause of illness?

When a patient presents with nonspecific pulmonary symptoms, a normal or near-normal chest x-ray and nondiagnostic sputum, high-resolution CT scanning as described above may be helpful. Gallium scanning is hampered by the 24-hr delay needed for imaging, although some clinicians advocate early imaging at 4–6 hr postinjection. If reliable sputum analysis and bronchoalveolar lavage are not available and high-resolution CT is equivocal or not offered, gallium or thallium scanning or both can play an important role in diagnosis. A negative chest x-ray and negative gallium scan virtually rule out a pulmonary source. Gallium is positive in nearly 100% of PCP cases. A few days of therapy for PCP should not affect gallium uptake. Therefore, treatment can be started before the gallium scan results are available. A normal chest x-ray with diffuse, heterogeneous and intense pulmonary gallium uptake has a greater than 90% specificity for PCP in AIDS. When the gallium scan is combined with the thallium scan, other patterns also can be diagnostic. The specificity of a thallium-positive, gallium-negative pattern for Kaposi's sarcoma is 96%. If a specific diagnosis is not suggested, nuclear imaging can at least direct attention for bronchoscopy or biopsy, especially if abnormal extrapulmonary uptake is identified.

6. Is nuclear imaging helpful in monitoring therapy and recurrence of pulmonary disease?

A chest x-ray can remain positive long after successful therapy, losing its value for the monitoring of therapeutic response. Gallium scanning also can be used to monitor response to treatment and to distinguish active from inactive disease, such as with MTB or PCP. A full course, or at least 2–3 wk of treatment, is required to establish a response on the gallium scan.

7. Nonspecific clinical findings: Is an abdominal process present?

Ultrasound, CT scanning and barium studies often are first-line imaging choices for potential abdominal problems, and the results of nuclear imaging should be carefully correlated with these anatomic modalities. Barium swallow and endoscopy are more useful in the evaluation for potential esophageal lesions. The liver is best examined by ultrasound, CT or MRI combined with needle biopsy of lesions, although nuclear imaging may prove useful for specific questions, especially if biopsy is considered too risky.

A myriad of neoplastic and infectious processes can affect the abdomen, sometimes causing diarrhea. Nuclear scanning plays a more limited role, and diagnostic accuracy has not been as well validated in the abdomen as in the chest. This is confounded by normal bowel excretion of gallium after 24 hr. Nuclear imaging can be helpful in certain situations though, especially if anatomic imaging and stool cultures are unrevealing. Using early (< 24-hr) gallium imaging, a specific diagnosis may be suggested based on the uptake pattern. Fusion of the images with a CT scan can precisely direct biopsy. For example, intense, unchanging colonic gallium activity with a negative stool culture in the appropriate clinical setting may suggest CMV or pseudomembranous colitis. If there is characteristic pulmonary, eye and renal/adrenal uptake, CMV is more likely.

Radiolabeled leukocyte scanning also may be useful in the febrile patient with AIDS in whom an acute abdominal infection is probable. It is considered more sensitive and specific in the abdomen for acute infections but is not sensitive for lymphoma or mycobacterial infections. Labeled leukocyte scanning also involves the handling and reinjection of HIV-infected blood, which makes it a less practical alternative (see Chapter 6, Infection Imaging).

8. Possible abdominal process: Is it AIDS-related cholecystitis or cholangiopathy?

Hepatobiliary scanning can be used to help diagnose various manifestations of AIDS-related cholangiopathy and chronic cholecystitis and help separate them from high-grade biliary obstruction and acute acalculous cholecystitis, respectively. It can identify those patients with delayed biliary drainage into the duodenum who may benefit from endoscopic dilation of the ampulla. Labeled white-blood-cell and gallium scanning also may be helpful in selected cases.

9. Musculoskeletal disease: What is the cause of myositis?

Muscle swelling in patients with AIDS may be due to AIDS-related myositis, Kaposi's sarcoma or lymphoma. Evaluation with MRI, CT, ultrasound and/or biopsy may be useful depending on institutional preference. The thallium or gallium scan also can be used to differentiate these etiologies because myositis is only gallium-avid, Kaposi's sarcoma is only thallium-avid, and lymphoma is gallium- and thallium-avid.

10. Musculoskeletal disease: Is it bone or joint infection or bacillary angiomatosis?

Three-phase bone scanning may help discriminate cellulitis from osteomyelitis in the absence of bone trauma. Gallium scanning also can be used to identify infectious arthritis and monitor response of infections to therapy. Bacillary angiomatosis is gallium-avid, and response to therapy can be monitored by repeat scans; skeletal involvement can be detected by bone scan. White-blood-cell scanning also can be helpful for skin, soft-tissue and skeletal bacterial infections (see Chapter 6, Infection Imaging).

11. Possible cardiac disease: Is it depressed cardiac function or carditis?

AIDS-related cardiomyopathy will demonstrate ventricular dilatation and decreased left-ventricular ejection fraction on multiple gated acquisition scan, although echocardiography can give the same information. Gallium uptake can be demonstrated in pericarditis, myocarditis and lymphoma; it is much less sensitive for endocarditis.

12. Possible renal disease: Is it HIV nephropathy?

Abnormal bilateral gallium renal uptake at 48–72 hr with enlarged kidneys has been described with HIV nephropathy. Because similar patterns can be present with ATN, tumor infiltration or CMV, careful correlation with history and other imaging is required. Tumor and infection usually will demonstrate asymmetric involvement. Because of this nonspecificity, gallium scanning is usually not the primary modality to evaluate potential renal disease. It can be helpful in problem-solving situations and findings may be incidentally noted on a gallium survey.

WORTH MENTIONING

1. PET or FDG SPECT

These scans are being investigated for whole-body evaluation of AIDS patients. Fluorodeoxyglucose (FDG) localizes to tumors and infections to varying degrees. It also has been reported to differentiate cerebral toxoplasmosis from AIDS-related lymphoma. Like thallium, lymphoma demonstrates intense uptake of FDG, whereas toxoplasmosis has little or no uptake.

2. Radiolabeled antibodies

Radiolabeled antibodies that are injected intravenously and bind to leukocytes show promise for detecting infection and avoiding the problems associated with the preparation of tagged white blood cells.

3. Technetium-99m-DTPA aerosol scanning

Technetium-99m-diethylenetriamine pentaacetic acid (DTPA) aerosol scanning with calculated clearance curves can be useful in the evaluation of alveolar damage and can be completed within 30 min. Whereas the normal clearance curve is monoexponential, a rapid biphasic curve is seen with PCP and *Legionella* because of alveolar damage and capillary leakage. This test is performed rarely because an abnormal result is nonspecific and does not effectively direct clinical management.

PATIENT INFORMATION

I. GALLIUM SCAN

A. Test/Procedure

Your doctor has ordered a gallium scan to determine the source of your infection or to distinguish infection from possible cancer.

A small amount of radioactive gallium will be injected into a vein. You will be asked to return in 2–3 days for images. You also may undergo earlier imaging. During this imaging, you will be positioned next to a special machine called a gamma camera, which doesn't produce radiation but detects radiation coming from your body from the injected gallium. A series of pictures of your body will then be taken and you may have to return the next day for delayed pictures. Sometimes pictures over a series of days are needed for proper interpretation. The injection takes only a few minutes. Each imaging session may take from 30 min up to 3 hr.

This study also may be combined with a thallium scan for which you will receive additional information.

B. Preparation

You may eat and drink as usual and take your medications. You may be asked to take a gentle laxative to aid in clearance of the tracer from your bowel.

C. Radiation and other risks

The amount of radiation used is small and similar to that given by other diagnostic x-ray tests. The effective adult radiation dose to your whole body from this test is about the dose the average person living in the United States receives in 7 yr from cosmic rays and naturally occurring background radiation sources. Your radiation dose is about 50% of the yearly dose considered safe for doctors and technologists who work with radiation. You can be around other people and use a bathroom normally without risk to others.

D. Pregnancy

If you are pregnant or think you could be pregnant, inform your doctor so that this can be discussed with the nuclear medicine physician.

II. THALLIUM SCAN

A. Test/Procedure

Your doctor has ordered a thallium scan to help differentiate infection from possible cancer.

A small amount of radioactive material called a tracer will be injected into your vein. You will be positioned next to a special machine called a gamma camera, which doesn't produce radiation but detects radiation that is coming from the injected tracer in your body. A series of pictures of your body will then be taken and you may have to return for delayed pictures 2–4 hr later. If your brain is to be imaged, the imaging detectors will be brought close to your skull. This may cause claustrophobia, but you can close your eyes. Each imaging session may take 20–60 min.

The thallium study may be combined with a gallium scan for which you will receive additional information.

B. Preparation

You may eat and drink as usual and take your medications. If your abdomen is to be imaged, you may be asked to not eat or drink anything except water and to not take your medications for 4–8 hr before the examination.

C. Radiation and other risks

The amount of radiation used is small and similar to that given by other diagnostic x-ray tests. The effective adult radiation dose to your whole body from this test is about the dose the average person living in the United States receives in 8–11 yr from cosmic rays and naturally occurring background radiation sources. The radiation dose is about 50–70% of the yearly dose considered safe for doctors and technologists who work with radiation. You can be around other people and use a bathroom normally without risk to others.

D. Pregnancy

If you are pregnant or think you could be pregnant, inform your doctor so that this can be discussed with the nuclear medicine physician.

References

1. Vanarthos WJ, Ganz WI, Vanarthos JC, Serafini AN, Tehranzadeh J. Diagnostic uses of nuclear medicine in AIDS. *RadioGraphics* 1992;12:731–752.
2. Abdel-Dayem HM. Nuclear medicine applications in immunosuppressed patients, "AIDS." *Ann Nucl Med* 1996;10:369–373.
3. Ganz WI, Serafini AN. Role of nuclear medicine and AIDS: overview and perspective for the future. *Q J Nucl Med* 1995;39:169–186.
4. Prvulovich EM, Buscombe JR, Miller RF. The role of nuclear medicine in the investigation of patients with AIDS. *Br J Hosp Med* 1996;55:549–553.
5. Lorberboym M, Estok L, Machac J, et al. Rapid differential diagnosis of cerebral toxoplasmosis and primary central nervous system lymphoma by thallium-201 SPECT. *J Nucl Med* 1996;37:1150–1154.
6. Ruiz A, Post JD, Ganz WI, Georgiou M. Nuclear medicine applications to the neuroimaging of AIDS: a neuroradiologist's perspective. *Neuroimag Clin North Am* 1997;7:499-511.

8
The Central Nervous System

Nuclear imaging adds important information to the evaluation of cerebrovascular disease, seizures, dementia, brain tumors, brain death, the HIV-positive patient and cerebrospinal fluid flow dynamics. Nevertheless, nuclear brain imaging still is underused and has been handicapped by variability in technique, complexity and quality control issues. PET and SPECT can achieve high brain imaging resolution and provide a powerful window into cerebral function. Moreover, with the advent of coincidence detection systems and the increasing availability of fluorodeoxyglucose (FDG), new tools are becoming available to community hospitals. Recent software developments allow functional nuclear images to be fused with CT or MRI to enhance diagnostic accuracy and to guide biopsy.

SCANS AND PRIMARY CLINICAL INDICATIONS

CLINICAL QUESTIONS

CSF

PATIENT INFORMATION

8

SCANS

I. BRAIN PERFUSION SPECT IMAGING
A. Background

In the past, functional brain perfusion was confined to centers that could afford PET scanners and cyclotrons. The introduction of ^{99m}Tc brain perfusion agents has brought this technology to the community hospital. The strength of these studies is that the radionuclide is fixed in brain cells and can be imaged later, reflecting a snapshot of cerebral blood perfusion at the time of the injection.

B. Radiopharmaceuticals

Technetium-99m-exametazime (Ceretec), most commonly referred to as HMPAO, is used widely for cerebral nuclear imaging. It is injected intravenously and distributes in the brain proportional to blood flow. HMPAO crosses the blood brain barrier (BBB) as a lipophilic compound where it reacts with intracellular glutathione and converts to a secondary hydrophilic compound that cannot back diffuse out of the brain.

Technetium-99m-ethyl cysteinate dimer (ECD) (Neurolite) also crosses the BBB proportional to blood flow where the lipophilic moiety is converted by an unknown enzymatic reaction to a hydrophilic compound that is too polar to wash out. It has better blood clearance than HMPAO with resultant improved brain-to-background ratio but has similar overall accuracy except in some cases of stroke where ECD is preferred.

Xenon-133 is administered via inhalation or intravenously and imaged on a special gamma camera. It is not widely available.

C. How the study is performed

An intravenous line is started and the patient is injected with HMPAO or ECD (15–30 mCi [555–1110 MBq] adult dose). A constant environment usually is attempted by having the patient in a quiet, darkened room with no speaking or interacting with staff from 15 min before to 15 min after injection. After a variable delay of 15–90 min depending on the radiotracer and department protocol, the patient is placed on the scanning table and his or her head is immobilized. A single scan or a series of scans are then completed, which take 10–60 min. The data are computer processed and reconstructed in three orthogonal planes.

If the patient is being referred for seizure evaluation, certain modifications are necessary. Ictal or interictal studies may be attempted and electroencephalograph (EEG) monitoring becomes compulsory. Ictal injection usually is done in a specialized seizure monitoring unit, where the radiopharmaceutical can be administered as soon as possible after the onset of ictus. Imaging can be carried out after the acute event, because the brain image is essentially frozen at the time of injection.

D. Patient preparation

It is critical that the patient be able to lie still for the duration of the scan. Excessive motion and improper positioning can render an examination uninterpretable. If this may be a problem, the nuclear medicine physician should be informed so that modifications to scan acquisition may be contemplated, such as doing a series of shorter scans, rather than a long one. If the patient is agitated or confused, having a family member present may be helpful. If sedation is considered, it should not be given until 10–15 min after injection. A flowing intravenous line is needed in either case. Caffeine, alcohol and other drugs that may affect cerebral blood flow should be withheld for 24 hr before the examination. Neuropsychiatric and medication history and prior CT or MRI scans should be made available to the nuclear medicine physician.

E. Understanding the report

Uptake parallels perfusion to the brain (Fig. 1A). The report will state the extent and severity of any defect, correlate with morphologic imaging such as CT and MRI and comment if the examination was suboptimal due to motion or other technical problems. Expected changes of aging including mild atrophy and normal side-to-side asymmetry (up to 10–13%) are taken into account. Semiquantitative uptake ratios of regional cortical perfusion may be reported. The interpretation of the study is intimately connected to the reason for the study. The three most common indications are cerebrovascular disease, dementia and seizure workup. SPECT perfusion imaging and PET metabolism images often show similar radiotracer distribution patterns but with varying sensitivities.

1. Cerebrovascular disease. The brain perfusion scan is highly sensitive to lack of cerebral blood flow. A defect is seen immediately in acute stroke, and the

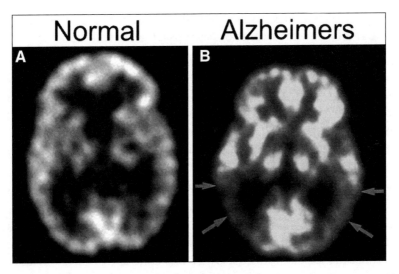

Figure 1. Single axial slice from a normal brain (A), contrasted with a patient with Alzheimer's dementia (B). Note relative decreased perfusion in the Alzheimer's brain in the parietal and temporal lobes (arrows).

penumbra of ischemia initially may be larger than the eventual completed infarct. The greater the severity of the perfusion defect, the more profound the ischemic event. Acutely decreased but not absent radiotracer activity correlates with some blood flow into the ischemic area from collateral circulation. This scan is best at detecting large vessel disease, and the lack of perfusion will parallel the vascular distribution of the insult. Hemorrhagic stroke cannot be differentiated from other types of infarct.

2. Dementia and other degenerative disorders. Different types of dementia can demonstrate classic patterns of hypoperfusion that probably are due to a combination of decreased blood flow and functioning neuronal mass. In the evaluation of dementia, patterns may overlap and confound results if the scan is evaluated in isolation. Alzheimer's dementia (AD) classically demonstrates symmetric decreased uptake in the bilateral posterior temporoparietal regions and, with more advanced disease, the frontal lobes (Fig. 1B). Frontotemporal degeneration (Pick's disease) is probably a heterogeneous group of disorders that have decreased frontal uptake, usually left greater than right, and may involve the temporal lobes. Multi-infarct dementia (MID) will show focal, asymmetric, wedge-shaped perfusion defects typically in occipital, temporo-occipital and temporoparietal cortex, which may be larger than the corresponding abnormality on CT scan. The defects often worsen with a Diamox (acetazolamide) challenge (see below), whereas AD defects may improve. AIDS dementia complex demonstrates a similar pattern with multifocal cortical or subcortical perfusion defects, especially in the frontal, temporal and parietal regions. The basal ganglia also may be involved. This can improve with appropriate therapy. A similar pattern also can be present in drug abusers and in patients with AIDS encephalopathy without dementia. Correlation should be made with the clinical situation, CT, MRI and the results of neuropsychiatric testing.

3. Seizures. SPECT with cerebral perfusion agents has found most clinical utility with partial complex seizures of the temporal lobe type. The pattern of localization depends on ictal status during radiopharmaceutical injection. A seizure focus during interictal scanning demonstrates hypoperfusion. Ictal scanning will show a seizure focus to be hyperperfused. Radiotracer injection in relation to the seizure is noted. Both an ictal and interictal scan can be performed on separate days and compared.

4. Other. A pattern has been described with herpes simplex encephalopathy of bilateral temporal lobe hyperperfusion. Most tumors and arteriovenous malformations (AVMs) will manifest as perfusion defects. Chronic post-trauma cases that are normal by CT and MRI may demonstrate various perfusion defects, presumably as a consequence of contusion. Other less constant patterns include frontal lobe hypoperfusion with schizophrenia, depression and chronic fatigue syndrome.

F. Potential problems

1. Lack of correlation. For all applications, correlation with CT or MRI is crucial, otherwise grave errors in interpretation can be made. Most tumors, infarcts and hematomas also will manifest as perfusion defects but should be suspected from the CT or MRI. As always, correlation with clinical information is important.

2. Age of infarct. Unless a prior scan is available, it is not possible to determine the age of an infarct or other perfusion abnormality.

3. Identifying ictus. For seizure locus identification, it is important to determine if the scan is performed during an ictal, interictal or peri-ictal period. Seizures may be silent. Without EEG monitoring during injection, what appears to be an interictal scan may actually be ictal, confounding proper interpretation.

4. Diaschisis. This is a phenomenon in which changes to blood flow in one segment of the brain affect uptake in uninvolved regions of the brain. Diaschisis most commonly occurs in the contralateral cerebellum.

5. Luxury perfusion. Metabolism may become uncoupled from blood flow 3–5 days after a stroke. Radiotracer may be deposited at an infarct due to increased flow, although the brain cells actually are nonfunctioning. This may obscure the stroke defect on the scan. It is seen with HMPAO but not ECD.

II. BRAIN DEATH SCAN
A. Background

Determining brain death is a difficult and emotionally challenging problem; nevertheless, it is important to be able to make this diagnosis to avoid needlessly prolonging artificial life support and to make donor organs rapidly available. No single test should be used to determine brain death. This is a clinical determination made by a qualified neurologist or neurosurgeon. EEG is used to confirm the diagnosis but can often be equivocal, especially in a noisy intensive care unit setting.

B. Radiopharmaceuticals

Technetium-99m-HMPAO or ECD are the same radiotracers used in brain perfusion SPECT.

Technetium-99m-pertechnetate or DTPA are traditional brain scanning radiotracers that do not cross the BBB unless it is disrupted. They normally are visualized only in vascular brain structures.

C. How the study is performed

The scan can be performed using one of two classes of radiotracers listed above. With pertechnetate or DTPA, a rapid angiographic flow phase is obtained after a bolus injection (20 mCi [740 MBq] adult dose) to determine if normal cerebral blood flow is present. With HMPAO or ECD (15–30 mCi [555–1110 MBq] adult dose), the angiographic phase may be omitted. For either class of radiotracer, delayed planar images are acquired at 10 min to 2 hr after injection. SPECT images also may be obtained in some institutions if the patient can be transported to the nuclear medicine department, although this is usually unnecessary for brain death determinations.

D. Patient preparation

No specific preparation is required except intravenous access. This examination should not be attempted unless the clinical criteria for brain death (e.g., persistent coma, apnea and absent brainstem reflexes) have been fulfilled.

E. Understanding the report

Interpretation depends on the agent being used. Lack of arterial blood flow to the brain is manifested by abrupt cut-off of vascular flow at the base of the brain, with only extracranial flow visualized. The adequacy of the injection bolus also may be described. Sometimes a "hot nose" sign is noted, in which there is activity in extracranial-to-intracranial collateral circulation about the midfacial region. On delayed images, lack of cerebral perfusion is manifested by intracranial photopenia (absent counts) and no venous sinus activity with pertechnetate or DTPA and no visualization of brain parenchyma with HMPAO or ECD (Fig. 2).

Generally, the term brain death is avoided. The report indicates whether cerebral blood flow is present or absent. If any brain activity is seen on delayed images, there is some cerebral perfusion; however, patients with absent perfusion to large areas of the brain have uniformly poor prognoses and follow-up examinations may be recommended.

F. Potential problems

1. Continuum of brain death. Brain death is a continuum. Ineffective arterial flow can persist despite true brain death, and a classically abnormal scan may not be present in some patients.

8

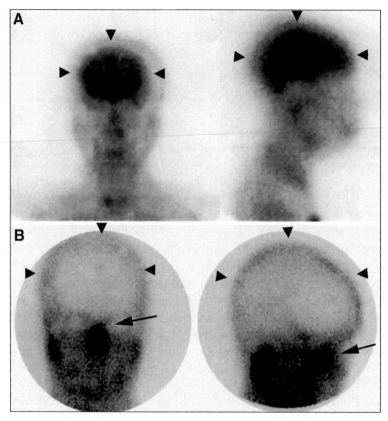

Figure 2. Planar anterior and lateral images from a normal brain scan (A) demonstrate cerebral uptake within the brain (arrowheads). Absence of cerebral activity in a brain death scan (B) is consistent with the clinical diagnosis of brain death (arrowheads). Note the "hot nose" sign (arrow) in the brain death study from collateral flow.

2. Barbiturates or hypothermia. False-positive scan results have been described for patients in barbiturate coma, those taking phenobarbital and those with hypothermia. Conversely, the scan can be performed in this setting, and, if cerebral perfusion is documented, the prognosis is usually good.

III. DIAMOX BRAIN STRESS SCAN
A. Background

The Diamox (acetazolamide) scan is designed to evaluate the physiologic (hemodynamic) significance of an anatomic vascular lesion such as carotid artery stenosis. What appears to be normal flow on a regular brain perfusion scan may in fact be compensated flow.

Acetazolamide is a carbonic anhydrase inhibitor that causes cerebral vasodilation and increased cerebral blood flow. The use of acetazolamide can unmask areas of low flow reserve by demonstrating regions of relative hypoperfusion compared with areas of the brain supplied by normal vessels or by comparing the Diamox scan to a baseline study. For example, a vascular territory supplied by a vessel with a high-grade stenosis will not demonstrate increased flow because the stenotic lesion cannot dilate. Thus, it will seem hypoperfused compared with normally supplied territories. This scan can be useful in the evaluation of the significance of carotid or other vascular lesions, in mapping potential vascular steal from an AVM and even in distinguishing AD from MID.

B. Radiopharmaceuticals

Technetium-99m-HMPAO or ECD are the same radiotracers used in brain perfusion SPECT.

8

C. How the study is performed

Diamox (1 g, adult dose) is injected by slow intravenous push. The radiotracer is injected 20 min later, and a scan is performed in the usual fashion. The protocol may vary. The baseline can be performed a day before or after or only if the stress scan is abnormal. Alternatively, a split-dose study can be completed, in which a low-dose baseline is performed (e.g., 9 mCi [333 MBq] adult dose), followed by infusion of Diamox with a high-dose (typically 2–3 times original dose or 27 mCi [1000 MBq] adult dose) scan to follow.

D. Patient preparation

Uncommon adverse effects that are usually self-limiting include mild vertigo, tinnitus, paresthesias, nausea and postural hypotension. Please contact your imaging section to determine the typical protocol so the patient will be prepared for a 1- or 2-day scan. Contraindications include known sulfa drug allergy. Diamox is to be avoided within 3 days of acute stroke. It also may induce migraine in those with a history of migraine.

E. Understanding the report

If cerebral blood flow is uniform after Diamox, the patient should have good cerebrovascular reserve. If asymmetry is present on the Diamox study, a baseline will have to be obtained to distinguish a preexisting abnormality from a Diamox-induced abnormality. If there is a flow reserve problem because of a carotid artery stenosis, flow to the affected region on the Diamox scan will be relatively decreased as compared with baseline. This can be expressed as a percentage of baseline. For the evaluation of MID versus AD, MID defects are often more pronounced after Diamox, whereas AD may normalize.

F. Potential problems

1. Adverse effects. Adverse effects of Diamox and contraindications are as described above.

2. *Balanced lesions.* Theoretically, completely balanced bilateral lesions may give a false-negative examination result unless absolute quantitation can be performed, but this clinical scenario is unlikely. Small or subtle changes may be missed, but these are probably of little clinical importance.

IV. FDG SCANNING
A. Background

PET scanning provides the most powerful evaluation of cerebral function because of high spatial resolution and ability to provide absolute quantitation. This technology has been confined to specialized centers because of the expense of an on-site PET scanner and a cyclotron but is becoming accessible at a lower expense to even small nuclear imaging departments because of the technology of coincidence SPECT. Furthermore, distribution networks are being put in place to deliver FDG from a centralized cyclotron.

B. Radiopharmaceuticals

Fluorine-18-FDG is the most commonly used PET radiotracer and the only PET neuroradiotracer with a long enough half-life to be shipped from a central source to a local facility. It is a glucose analog that is transported into viable cells where it is phosphorylated and irreversibly trapped. High-grade tumor will demonstrate intense FDG uptake, whereas cell necrosis has no uptake. Inflammation may show intermediate uptake.

C. How the study is performed

The patient is injected with FDG (10–20 mCi [350–750 MBq] adult dose) and imaged about 45 min later. The injection is done under similar conditions as a brain perfusion SPECT scan. EEG monitoring is required for seizure patients, because ictal and interictal uptake are quite different (interictal - hypometabolic; ictal - hypermetabolic). The entire process takes approximately 1–2 hr. Ictal PET is not practical and is logistically difficult. Interictal PET is most commonly performed.

D. Patient preparation

Whether with PET or coincidence detection, the patient usually is kept in a fasting state the day of the examination (water is permitted). If the patient is diabetic, the imaging center should be informed so that additional instructions may be provided. Otherwise, patient preparation issues are the same as those for brain perfusion SPECT imaging.

E. Understanding the report

FDG uptake is dependent on blood flow to and incorporation by active cells. It is taken up by higher-grade tumors in variable degrees compared with normal brain. Thus, a glioma may demonstrate greater, equal or less intensity when compared with adjacent brain parenchyma (Fig. 3). Most metastases have

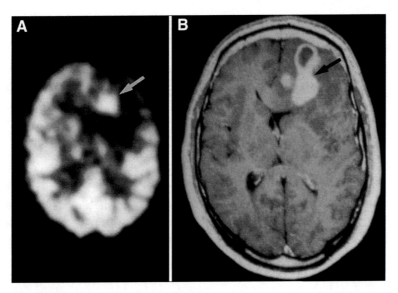

Figure 3. Corresponding axial slices from an FDG PET scan (A) and MRI (B) demonstrate a high-grade glioma in the left frontoparietal region (white arrow in A and black arrow in B).

increased uptake. Radiation necrosis should have no uptake. A cerebral infarct will manifest as a void in the vascular territory. Luxury perfusion is not a problem as it is with HMPAO. Similar patterns for dementia and neurodegenerative disorders are seen in PET and SPECT, but PET generally is more sensitive to subtle change. Interictal PET will demonstrate decreased uptake at the hypometabolic seizure focus.

F. Potential problems

Potential problems that may occur with FDG scans include problems 1–4 listed for brain perfusion SPECT imaging (see above). In addition, there are the following potential problems:

1. Lack of specificity. FDG is not a specific tumor marker. Inflammation may show moderate uptake. As these studies move from academic centers to the community with coincidence detection, more problems are likely to be uncovered.

2. Uptake in normal brain. Normal brain accumulates FDG. Differentiating abnormal uptake in low-grade tumors from normal brain may be difficult, especially in postsurgical or postradiation therapy patients.

3. Blood glucose and steroid use. Dexamethasone and blood glucose levels can affect FDG uptake and should be carefully controlled if repeat examinations are performed.

V. THALLIUM BRAIN TUMOR SCAN

A. Background

This scan has two primary uses: Differentiating recurrent neoplasia from radiation necrosis and discriminating AIDS-related lymphoma from toxoplasmosis in the AIDS patient (see Chapter 7, AIDS). Some centers have recommended the use of sestamibi because of improved tumor-to-background ratio, but its use is problematic because of choroid plexus uptake.

B. Radiopharmaceuticals

Like potassium, ^{201}Tl concentrates mainly in viable tumor, less so in inflammatory cells and almost negligibly in necrotic tissue. Although early imaging may demonstrate uptake in infection because of passive diffusion, this usually clears on delayed images. Thallium does not cross the BBB unless the barrier is disrupted.

C. How the study is performed

Thallium is injected intravenously (3–4 mCi [111–148 MBq] adult dose), and initial images are obtained at 10–30 min. SPECT of the brain is routine and may take up to 1 hr depending on equipment. Delayed 2- to 4-hr views are sometimes obtained. In the evaluation of tumor recurrence, some centers advocate comparing the thallium study with a brain perfusion SPECT. This can be performed concurrently or on different days.

D. Patient preparation

Thallium uptake is not affected by steroid use. No special preparation is required, and the patient may eat and drink as usual.

E. Understanding the report

Normal brain should have little or no thallium uptake. High-grade gliomas and lymphoma will be hot (Fig. 4). Infection or radiation necrosis usually will have no significant increase from background. A ratio of tumor-to-background uptake may be calculated. The higher the ratio, the greater the specificity for high-grade neoplasia. The study can be coregistered to the CT or MRI to facilitate surgery or gamma-knife therapy. If delayed images are performed, persistent retention with higher lesion-to-background ratio increases specificity for tumor.

F. Potential problems

1. False-negative results. If a lesion is necrotic, partially treated, near an area of normal uptake in the skull base or scalp or below the resolution of imaging (usually 1 cm), a false-negative scan may result.

2. False-positive results. There also have been reports of thallium uptake with abscess, with certain infections and rarely with radiation necrosis. Most of these false-positive occurrences do not demonstrate increased relative intensity on delayed images.

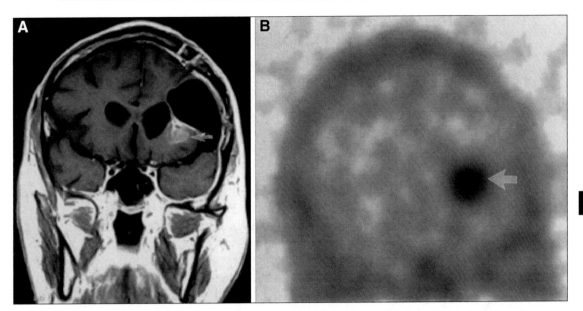

Figure 4. Coronal MRI slice (A) in a patient with an enhancing lesion (arrow) adjacent to encephalomalacia after radiation therapy for glioblastoma multiforme. Increased uptake (arrow) on a corresponding coronal slice from a subsequent thallium scan (B) is consistent with recurrent tumor, rather than radiation necrosis, which would manifest little or no uptake.

VI. CSF FLOW SCAN (RADIONUCLIDE CISTERNOGRAM)

A. Background

The radionuclide cisternogram images CSF flow. It can differentiate communicating hydrocephalus (and normal pressure hydrocephalus) from nonobstructive causes of ventriculomegaly, such as atrophy. It also can be used to diagnose whether a cyst communicates with the CSF space.

B. Radiopharmaceuticals

Indium-111-DTPA has good imaging characteristics, 3-day half-life and low radiation dosimetry, which make it an excellent marker for CSF-flow dynamic studies, which often require 24–72 hr imaging.

Technetium-99m-DTPA also is used to assess CSF flow in children.

C. How the study is performed

A lumbar puncture is performed, and ^{111}In-DTPA (250–500 μCi [9–18 MBq] adult dose) is introduced into the thecal sac by the clinician or the nuclear medicine physician. Planar views typically are obtained at 1–4 hr, 24 hr and up to 72 hr depending on department protocol. SPECT can be performed in selected cases.

D. Patient preparation

Preparation is the same as that for any lumbar puncture and may be performed prone or laterally and does not have to be done in the nuclear imaging department. Each facility has its own standard procedure. Some centers perform the lumbar puncture and radiotracer administration under fluoroscopic guidance. The patient and family should be told in advance about the lumbar puncture and the necessity for imaging that may take up to 3 days.

E. Understanding the report

Normally, the radiotracer reaches the basal cisterns by 1 hr, the frontal poles and Sylvian fissures by 2–6 hr, the convexities by 12 hr and the sagittal sinus by 24 hr. Clearance of radiotracer is underway by 24 hr. The ventricles are normally not filled but may demonstrate brief transient reflux. A grading system may be used.

F. Potential problems

1. Lumbar puncture. Gaining access via lumbar puncture is not always possible. Radiology assistance under fluoroscopy with the lumbar puncture is helpful with difficult cases. Extravasation of tracer will manifest as persistent activity at the lumbar puncture site and slow or no progression to the cranium.

2. Overlapping patterns. Often there is overlap of findings and no single classic pattern can be described.

VII. CSF LEAK SCAN

A. Background

CSF leaks manifest as rhinorrhea or otorrhea and can occur anywhere from the frontal sinus to the temporal bone, often at the cribriform plate. Most are the result of trauma. Meningitis can occur from a nonresolving leak, and surgery often is performed to seal such a leak. This scan is designed to aid in the presurgical localization of the leak. Though it does not provide as much anatomic detail as high-resolution CT after intrathecal myelographic dye, it has greater sensitivity, especially for intermittent leaks, and many departments combine the examinations for maximal chance of localization.

B. Radiopharmaceuticals

These are the same as for the CSF flow scan.

C. How the study is performed

Before the examination, labeled cotton pledgets often are placed into the nasal cavity or ears by the otolaryngology surgeon. Indium-111 DTPA is introduced into the thecal sac via a lumbar puncture (250–500 µCi [9–18 MBq] adult dose).

The patient lies supine or in Trendelenburg until imaging and is then positioned to maximize the leak. Planar or SPECT images are obtained at 1–4 hr. The patient also may be asked to perform the Valsalva maneuver to increase CSF pressure. The pledgets are usually withdrawn when a leak is detected or at 4–24 hr; they are subsequently weighed and counted for radioactivity. A plasma sample often is collected to calculate a pledget-to-plasma radioactivity ratio because CSF (and radiotracer) is absorbed into the bloodstream and will appear in normal nasal secretions. Further delayed views may be obtained up to 72 hr.

D. Patient preparation

As in the CSF leak study, the patient should be prepared for the lumbar puncture and extended imaging. He or she should also be informed about possible placement of nasal or ear pledgets.

E. Understanding the report

The nuclear imaging and the pledget counts, if obtained, are described along with a conclusion about the presence and location of a leak. A corrected pledget-to-plasma count ratio >1.5 indicates CSF leakage. If performed in conjunction with high-resolution CT, the functional and anatomic data can be amalgamated into a single report.

F. Potential problems

1. Lumbar puncture. As with the CSF flow scan, intrathecal access may be unobtainable, and extravasation could occur.

2. Pledgets falling out. It is not uncommon for pledgets to fall out spontaneously or if the nose is blown, thus confounding results. If this occurs, the patient is encouraged to at least keep the pledgets separated and individually wrapped until they can be given to the technologist. Labeling of pledgets before placement is important.

3. Nasal secretion radioactivity. As noted, normal nasal secretions will have some radioactivity from that absorbed into the bloodstream. Comparing pledget activity and obtaining pledget-to-plasma ratios are helpful. Pledget counts should be corrected for pledget weight.

VIII. CSF SHUNT PATENCY SCAN
A. Background

This is a useful test to determine whether ventriculoperitoneal, ventriculoatrial and other CSF shunts are patent. It also can be used to test patency of an Ommaya ventricular chemotherapy shunt and clearance of intraventricular chemotherapeutic agent. Although shunt patency often can be determined from examination of the patient and inspection of the flow reservoir, this test gives images of CSF flow and provides a definitive shunt patency evaluation.

B. Radiopharmaceuticals

Technetium-99m-DTPA or macroaggregated albumin (MAA) are used as marker agents to determine if shunt tubing is patent. Usually, the long half-life of ^{111}In is not required, and the excellent imaging characteristics of ^{99m}Tc are useful. If used in the evaluation of a ventriculoatrial shunt, MAA is taken up by the lungs, confirming patency (see Chapter 2, Pulmonary System and Thromboembolism).

Indium-111-DTPA is used when extended imaging may be required and for intrathecal injections.

C. How the study is performed

Technetium-99m-DTPA or MAA (0.5–1 mCi [18–37 MBq] adult dose) or ^{111}In-DTPA (250–500 μCi [9–18 MBq] adult dose) is injected into the shunt reservoir by the neurosurgeon or someone else trained in this technique. Serial images are taken over time, typically 30 min to 2 hr, traversing the course of the tubing. Radiotracer can be refluxed into the ventricular system by manually occluding the distal limb. A half-life clearance of reservoir or ventricular activity may be calculated.

D. Patient preparation

It is critical to ensure that the nuclear medicine physician is aware of the type and course of the shunt. The patient should be told about accessing the shunt, and someone trained in this procedure should be available.

E. Understanding the report

Normal flow through the tubing should be seen with significant reservoir clearance by 30 min. A ventriculoperitoneal shunt will have free distribution of radiotracer within the abdominal cavity. If the tip is intra-atrial, MAA is trapped in the lungs. The site of obstruction may be determined. Hold-up of radiotracer at the shunt tip in the peritoneum indicates a loculation. Extravasation also is described, if present, indicating a break in the continuity of the shunt. The time course of radiotracer migration and half-life reservoir or ventricle emptying time, if obtained, may be reported. For the evaluation of a ventricular chemotherapy shunt, the radiotracer should appear over the convexities by 24 hr if there is no obstruction to normal CSF outflow.

F. Potential problems

Unfamiliarity with shunt. One of the biggest errors is lack of understanding of shunt type and course. This can be especially complicated if multiple functioning and nonfunctioning shunts are present. Also, each type of shunt system has a different emptying curve. It is advisable for normal values to be established at individual facilities.

CLINICAL QUESTIONS

1 and 2. Has this patient had an acute stroke? What is the role of nuclear imaging in stroke evaluation and prognosis?

Cerebrovascular disease is the most common neurologic affliction and the second most common cause of dementia. The SPECT brain perfusion scan is highly sensitive for detection of vascular flow. In patients with a cortical stroke, 90% of brain SPECT scans are positive almost immediately, whereas only 20% of CT scans are positive at 8 hr. By 72 hr, CT and brain SPECT have the same sensitivity. Routine MRI also takes at least 4–8 hr to manifest ischemic change, although newer MR diffusion and perfusion technology can demonstrate near immediate abnormalities. Brain perfusion SPECT is so sensitive that it will map the penumbra of acute ischemia that is larger than the completed stroke. In addition, the patient can be injected during an acute event and imaged later. No other modality offers this advantage.

Yet, the place of brain perfusion SPECT in stroke evaluation is not settled. The use of this potentially valuable tool is hampered by the lack of on-call nuclear medicine at some hospitals, delay in performing and processing the study, as well as the need to obtain a CT scan in any case to exclude hemorrhage, tumor and other processes that can mimic a stroke.

Stroke is primarily a clinical diagnosis, and most interventional stroke algorithms do not use the brain perfusion SPECT scan in the acute evaluation. Thus, what is the place of this scan in the assessment of the potential stroke victim? First, not all strokes can be diagnosed with clinical certainty. There are situations in which the data are not clear and acute CT and routine MRI are negative. The brain perfusion SPECT scan can image flow, although small or lacunar strokes may be missed. In addition, the nuclear scan is helpful in categorizing stroke into large-vessel or small-vessel types and can help triage intervention. The ideal target group for thrombolysis includes those patients who have acutely decreased but not absent focal perfusion, implying collateral circulation. Complete absence of perfusion suggests lack of collateral circulation, and these patients are unlikely to benefit from acute intervention. The brain perfusion scan also can be used to monitor therapy and determine if reperfusion is occurring. Reperfusion increases the risk of bleeding and may necessitate an adjustment of thrombolytic dose. Finally, brain perfusion SPECT may be helpful in establishing prognosis. The larger and more severe the defect in the acute setting, the poorer the prognosis, although results of some studies have been mixed.

In summary, brain perfusion SPECT is not commonly used in the evaluation of acute stroke but may be useful in limited circumstances and may be increasingly used in the future in acute stroke intervention algorithms.

3. Does this patient have cerebral vascular spasm?

Clinical vasospasm or delayed ischemia is encountered in up to 30% of intensive care unit patients with subarachnoid hemorrhage and often complicates cerebral vascular surgery. Neurologic examination may be unreliable in this setting. Angiography is considered the gold standard and can be used for interventional angioplasty of spasmodic vessels, but it is invasive and may itself cause vasospasm. Moreover, angiography can only detect 68% of vasospasm found with brain perfusion SPECT, which can provide direct evidence of the presence and extent of cerebral vasospasm, even before symptoms. Transcranial Doppler is technically difficult, especially in the postoperative patient. It may not detect distal spasm and will not provide details of cerebral perfusion. Evoked potentials are not sensitive, although they are easy to perform and can be diagnostic. Brain perfusion SPECT can be combined in a protocol with physical examination and evoked potentials or transcranial Doppler for noninvasive screening to determine if angiography should be attempted. SPECT also can determine if a therapy has been successful or if more aggressive treatment is warranted.

4 and 5. Is cerebral flow reserve adequate? Does a borderline carotid artery stenosis warrant intervention?

MR angiography or duplex scanning are the screening tests of choice to determine if an anatomic carotid lesion is present. With intermediate stenosis, physiologic information often is needed to determine the hemodynamic significance of a vascular lesion. The Diamox brain stress scan of flow reserve is one of the most potentially useful examinations but it is underused. Whether testing the vascular implications of a borderline carotid lesion or as a preoperative assessment for vascular steal due to an AVM, this study is simple to perform and can provide added value to many clinical situations. The proper use of this technique requires teamwork with an interested neurologist or neurosurgeon. Its most valuable use is predicting those at risk from an asymptomatic carotid artery stenosis. It also can be used to document return to normal after intervention.

6. What type of dementia is present?

One half of patients with early dementia cannot be diagnosed clinically, yet an early diagnosis can help in finding a treatable cause and determine prognosis. AD is the most common type of dementia. Establishing a diagnosis is important to the patient and family and has implications for medical care. It is frustrating to be told that a loved one has dementia of an unknown type. MID is the second most common type of dementia. The progression of this disease is treatable with medical and surgical methods. Although many other causes of dementia, including AD, are not effectively treatable, therapies are being investigated and the ability to definitively diagnose these patients may have important future therapeutic implications.

CT scanning and routine MRI are crucial for proper interpretation of the brain SPECT and for the evaluation of structural lesions and multiple small infarcts. Yet, findings are often nonspecific. PET and brain perfusion SPECT are highly sensitive examinations in uncovering decreased metabolism associated with these conditions even with early symptoms and before atrophy is seen on CT or MRI. There can be overlap of findings with nuclear imaging between different causes of dementia. Yet, correlation with neuropsychiatric testing as well as anatomic imaging allow discrimination of subtypes with increased specificity. The probability of AD exceeds 80% when a specific abnormal pattern is correlated with memory loss. It should be noted that newer MRI volumetric techniques and MR spectroscopy are finding increased utility in the dementia workup.

One of the most important differentiations to make is between AD and MID and sometimes these conditions coexist. If there is any doubt, a Diamox challenge, in which defects of AD will improve and MID often gets worse, can be helpful. In addition, depression can sometimes masquerade as AD in the elderly. In a patient with moderate to severe dementia and a normal or near-normal brain perfusion SPECT, the probability of AD is low. In a patient with suspected HIV dementia, CT and MRI may not detect structural lesions, whereas SPECT can uncover perfusion abnormalities justifying early therapy.

7. Status after head injury and negative CT/MRI: What is the cause of continuing neuropsychiatric symptoms?

In the acute trauma setting, CT and MRI are the studies of choice. Yet, in the subacute/chronic symptomatic patient, especially after minor trauma and with normal anatomic imaging, brain perfusion SPECT is more sensitive in documenting abnormalities. This may have important medicolegal, prognostic and even therapeutic consequences. Negative anatomic imaging should not be accepted as an endpoint in the evaluation of the sequela of chronic head trauma. If there are abnormal findings on neuropsychiatric evaluation, functional imaging should be obtained. In one illustrative study, 97% of patients with a negative brain perfusion SPECT had resolution of symptoms by 3 mo; 95% of those with continued symptoms had an abnormal study at 3 mo.

8. Is nuclear imaging of value in the assessment of mental illness?

Nuclear imaging in mental illness has demonstrated mixed results and is still not useful in everyday clinical practice. It is considered a research tool and is used in the assessment of drugs in clinical trials.

9. Does nuclear imaging have a place in the initial evaluation of seizures?

MRI and CT scanning are considered the procedures of choice in the initial evaluation of new onset seizures without an identifiable cause. Nuclear imaging has an important place in the identification of a seizure focus for contemplated surgery as outlined below (see Clinical Question 10).

10. Can a seizure focus be confidently identified to allow for ablative surgery?

Although once of academic interest only, identification of a seizure focus has practical significance. Temporal lobectomy of an intractable seizure focus due to mesial temporal sclerosis leads to improvement in 80% of patients. Yet, presurgical evaluation is not uniform. All facilities that perform this surgery use some combination of imaging, EEG and functional testing. MRI is an important part of the workup. Obtaining surface EEG is also standard, but the results may not be conclusive or may not agree with the findings on MRI. A confirmatory test is then needed before such radical neurosurgery is contemplated. Some centers rely heavily on invasive depth electrodes, but this procedure is expensive and can be dangerous. Brain perfusion SPECT or FDG PET has an important ancillary role to play if depth electrodes are to be avoided and may uncover seizure foci undetected by MRI.

Ictal perfusion SPECT is the most sensitive nuclear examination for seizure focus localization, with approximately 90% success for partial complex seizures of the temporal lobe type. This study must be performed in a special monitoring unit requiring inpatient admission and by those well versed in the possible pitfalls. Interictal PET (and possibly coincidence SPECT) with FDG is the more common approach, has an approximately 70–80% success rate in seizure focus localization and can be performed on an outpatient basis. Interictal perfusion SPECT has the lowest localization rate (40–60%) but is the most widely available. Some authors recommend combining ictal and interictal perfusion SPECT. EEG monitoring is mandatory for all the above nuclear imaging procedures. Imaging of extratemporal partial complex seizures has less localization accuracy, and surgery is not as reliable. With primary generalized seizures, EEG, MRI and CT are not useful for localization.

Typical algorithms depend on the proclivities of individual neurosurgeons and test availability, but a useful scheme for the evaluation of potential temporal or extratemporal foci is to start with MRI and surface EEG. If these agree as to locus, surgery often can be performed with confidence. If these do not agree or if an additional confirmatory test is desired, ictal perfusion SPECT or interictal PET should be carried out. If these are not available, interictal perfusion SPECT can be attempted. If these scans are not revealing, depth electrodes can be considered.

11. Is brain death present?

A reliable and rapid means to confirm the diagnosis of brain death is important to help the family through their tragedy and to ensure that this diagnosis is made in a timely manner to enable organ donation. Formal definitions of brain death vary by institution. Physical examination performed by a neurologist or neurosurgeon to document persistent coma, apnea and absent brainstem reflexes remains the cornerstone of diagnosis. Any ancillary test such as the brain death scan should be used only to confirm this clinical diagnosis. EEG is important in this determination but can be plagued by artifact, especially in the intensive care unit setting. Four-vessel angiography is considered the traditional gold standard, but is too invasive and expensive for routine use.

The brain death scan has been recognized as an easy and reliable method to document lack of cerebral perfusion. It can be performed in many ways, and a facility usually has chosen a specific protocol. Technetium-99m pertechnetate or DTPA with planar imaging is the least sensitive to detect minimal cerebral blood flow, whereas ^{99m}Tc-HMPAO or ECD with SPECT is the most sensitive. High sensitivity may not always be an advantage, because comatose patients may be shown to have some cerebral blood flow even though minimal blood flow correlates with poor prognosis. These are issues that should be discussed by involved clinicians with the nuclear medicine physician in advance. The possibility of false-positive results from barbiturate use and hypothermia should always be kept in mind. It is not an unreasonable approach to perform repeat studies if the results are equivocal, because the patient's cerebrovascular status may be somewhere within a continuum of progressive loss of cerebral blood flow.

12. Is radiation necrosis or tumor recurrence the cause of enhancing brain lesions in a postradiation therapy patient?

Because high-grade brain neoplasia is being treated more aggressively with surgery, radiation and chemotherapy, patients are living longer. This has led to an increased need to determine when recurrent tumor may be present. Contrast-enhanced MRI is the first-line imaging examination. If it is negative, no further action is required unless clinical suspicion is high. Demyelination after radiation or chemotherapy and postsurgical change can demonstrate contrast enhancement on MRI that is indistinguishable from recurrent neoplasia up to 2 yr after therapy. Invasive biopsy does not have to be used for differentiation because of the excellent information that FDG or thallium brain scans can provide.

FDG and thallium brain scans have high sensitivity and specificity to differentiate radiation necrosis or post-therapy demyelination from recurrent neoplasia. Significant uptake is present only in neoplasia. Provided software is available, the nuclear scan can be coregistered to MRI or CT to direct biopsy. Each technique has advantages and disadvantages and similar overall accuracy. The type of scan provided is often an institutional preference.

13. Is global ventriculomegaly due to atrophy or communicating hydrocephalus?

CT or MRI is vital in the evaluation of potential hydrocephalus and the exclusion of an intraventricular (noncommunicating) cause. Ventriculomegaly due to central atrophy and that caused by potentially treatable extraventricular (communicating) hydrocephalus can appear similar on anatomic imaging. The CSF flow scan is a functional study that gives a physiologic picture of CSF flow dynamics and may identify communicating hydrocephalus. Early studies touted a positive scan as predictive of improvement with shunting, but later results have been mixed. The clinical implications of intermediate-grade abnormal studies are uncertain. The scan may be used to support a clinical decision to perform or withhold a shunt procedure. This is the type of study that some facilities may find useful, whereas others may bypass it altogether.

14. Is there a CSF leak present?

Although chemical and electrophoretic tests can be performed on nasal or ear secretions to determine if they are of CSF origin, often this does not provide enough information to plan surgery. High-resolution CT with intrathecal contrast is considered the first-line imaging examination and can localize the leak in up to 90% of cases. MRI is also increasingly used in some centers for attempted localization of the leak.

The nuclear CSF leak scan is an excellent physiologic test that can be combined with the CT examination. Because a lumbar puncture must be performed for the CT examination, it is logical to maximize the possibility of leak localization by adding the nuclear study. The nuclear CSF leak scan is especially important if an intermittent leak is present. Although the cost is greater to combine the studies, failure of surgery and possible meningitis present an even greater cost to the patient. The use of localizing pledgets for radiation counting increases the sensitivity and improves the accuracy of this examination.

15 and 16. Is the patient's ventricular shunt functioning properly? Can an Ommaya shunt be used for chemotherapy?

Although CT or MR brain scanning are the first line imaging tests with suspected shunt malfunction and physical examination with inspection of the reservoir is vital, there is no better test than the CSF shunt patency scan to determine physiologic shunt function and flow dynamics. Accurate image interpretation requires an understanding of the type and course of the shunt. The reservoir should be accessed by someone trained in this procedure. Most neurosurgeons prefer to inject their own shunts for this examination.

WORTH MENTIONING

1. Wada test

This examination is used at specialized centers where temporal lobectomies are performed for intractable seizures. The blood vessel supplying the area is selectively catheterized, and amobarbital is injected with HMPAO or ECD. Because the radionuclide and the amobarbital are injected through the same catheter, a subsequent SPECT scan will show the anatomic areas infused by the amobarbital. Neuropsychiatric testing is then carried out on the patient to determine the clinical deficit to be expected from surgery.

2. Balloon occlusion test

This examination is performed to determine if a carotid artery can be safely sacrificed as part of a surgical resection. A catheter is advanced into the appropriate carotid artery and a balloon inflated, occluding blood flow, while the patient undergoes EEG monitoring and neurologic evaluation. Either HMPAO or ECD is then injected intravenously. The patient subsequently undergoes SPECT scanning. Symmetric brain perfusion (or unchanged from a baseline study) implies that there is an intact Circle of Willis; these patients have been shown to do well after surgery.

3. Migraine

The use of nuclear imaging for migraine evaluation is the subject of research, but the results have been mixed.

4. Huntington's disease

Nuclear brain perfusion SPECT and PET techniques can demonstrate the early changes of decreased caudate and putamen uptake in Huntington's disease before atrophy manifests on CT or MRI or even before symptoms are present.

5. Parkinson's disease

Parkinson's disease is primarily a clinical diagnosis. Findings on brain perfusion SPECT have been mixed. PET scanning techniques using ^{18}F-fluorodopa can show decreased uptake in the putamen. CT and MRI are used to exclude confounding conditions such as tumor. Brain perfusion SPECT uptake patterns of Parkinson's disease patients with dementia can resemble those of AD or manifest frontal lobe hypo-perfusion.

6. Receptor binding tracers for seizure evaluation

Benzodiazapine and opioid receptor binding radiotracers show promise in the simple and accurate localization of seizure foci.

7. Radiolabeled neurotransmitters

Many radiolabeled neurotransmitter analogs and receptor binders have been developed. These continue to help researchers explore the mysteries of the brain and may one day allow better tailoring of psychotropic and antidepressant medication to disease subtypes.

8. Beta emitter therapy

Experimental therapies whereby beta-emitting antibodies are injected or infused directly into a cerebral glioblastoma may hold promise in the treatment of this fatal tumor.

9. Cerebrovascular flow reserve

Cerebrovascular flow reserve can be measured with a combination of brain perfusion SPECT and ^{99m}Tc-radiolabeled autologous red blood cells to obtain cerebral blood flow–to–volume ratios. This technique is not offered widely.

PATIENT INFORMATION

I. BRAIN PERFUSION SPECT IMAGING
A. Test/Procedure

Your doctor has ordered a brain perfusion SPECT scan to examine the blood flow to your brain to better understand your medical condition.

A small amount of radioactive material called a tracer will be injected into your vein. You may be asked to sit quietly in a darkened room without talking for 5–15 min before and after the injection. If this test is done for seizure evaluation, you may undergo EEG (brainwave) monitoring. You will be positioned next to a special machine called a gamma camera, which does not produce radiation but detects radiation that is coming from the injected tracer in your body. The imaging detectors will be brought close to your skull, which may cause claustrophobia but you can close your eyes at this point. A series of pictures of your brain will then be taken as the detectors spin around your head. The whole process may take 20–60 min. It is important that you are able to lie very still for the examination. If you cannot do this, please inform your doctor.

To test the blood flow to your brain, your doctor may have requested that a drug called acetazolamide (Diamox) be given to you in your vein. This increases blood flow to your brain, but it may not increase blood flow to areas of blood-vessel narrowing. If you have an allergy to sulfa drugs, please inform your doctor because Diamox is a sulfa drug. The scan will be performed as above with the tracer injected 20 min after the Diamox. You may undergo one or two scans, possibly on separate days, depending on the findings.

B. Preparation

You should refrain from alcohol and caffeine products like coffee, tea, and colas for 24 hr before the scan. Please review your medications with your doctor to determine if any of them should be withheld. It is also a good idea to have a list of your medications prepared in case this information is needed by the nuclear medicine staff. Otherwise, you may eat and drink as usual.

C. Radiation and other risks

The amount of radiation used is small and similar to that given by other diagnostic x-ray tests. The effective adult radiation dose to your whole body from this test is about the same as the amount the average person living in the United States receives in 1.5–4 yr from cosmic rays and naturally occurring background radiation sources. The radiation dose is about 10–25% of the yearly dose considered safe for doctors and technologists who work with radiation. You should urinate within 2 hr after the test to further decrease your radiation exposure. You can be around other people and use a bathroom normally without risk to others.

If Diamox is used, it can cause some self-limited adverse effects, such as altered taste of carbonated beverages, tingling in the fingers or hands, dizziness, ear ringing, loss of sensation or nausea. It also may cause migraine if you are prone to migraine headaches. Please make sure to get up slowly after the test, because Diamox may cause fainting if you get up too quickly.

D. Pregnancy

If you are pregnant or think you could be pregnant, inform your doctor so that this can be discussed with the nuclear medicine physician.

8

II. FDG SCANNING
A. Test/Procedure

Your doctor has ordered an FDG PET (coincidence SPECT) brain scan to examine the functioning of your brain to better understand your medical condition.

A small amount of radioactive sugar (FDG) will be injected into your vein. You may be asked to sit quietly in a darkened room without talking for 45–60 min. If this test is done for seizure evaluation, you may undergo EEG monitoring. About 45–60 min after injection, you will be positioned next to a special machine called a PET scanner or coincidence gamma camera, which doesn't produce radiation but detects radiation that is coming from the injected radioactive sugar in your body. Your head will either be advanced into the PET scanner, or the gamma camera coincidence detectors will be brought close to your skull, which may cause claustrophobia but you can close your eyes at this point. A series of pictures of your brain will be taken as the detectors spin around your head. The whole process may take 1–2 hr. It is important that you are able to lie very still for the examination. If you cannot do this, please inform your doctor.

B. Preparation

You will be asked to fast the day of the examination (water is permitted). Please ask your doctor about restrictions for any medications you are taking. If you are a diabetic, please make sure the PET center knows this, because special instructions may be provided.

C. Radiation and other risks

The amount of radiation used is small and similar to that given by other diagnostic x-ray tests. The effective adult radiation dose to your whole body from this test is about the same as the dose the average person living in the United States receives in 3–7 yr from cosmic rays and naturally occurring background radiation sources. The radiation dose is about 20–40% of the yearly dose considered safe for doctors and technologists who work with radiation. You can be around other people and use a bathroom normally without risk to others.

D. Pregnancy

If you are pregnant or think you could be pregnant, inform your doctor so that this can be discussed with the nuclear medicine physician.

III. THALLIUM BRAIN TUMOR SCAN

A. Test/Procedure

Your doctor has ordered a thallium brain tumor scan to help differentiate potential brain tumor from benign radiation therapy changes.

A small amount of radioactive material called a tracer will be injected into your vein. You will be positioned next to a special machine called a gamma camera, which does not produce radiation but detects radiation that is coming from the injected tracer in your body. The imaging detectors will be brought close to your skull. This may cause claustrophobia, but you can close your eyes. A series of pictures of your brain will then be taken as the detectors spin around your head. The whole process may take 20–60 min, and you also may undergo a delayed scan 2–4 hr later. It is important that you are able to lie very still for the examination. If you cannot do this, please inform your doctor.

B. Preparation

You may eat and drink as usual and take your medications.

C. Radiation and other risks

The amount of radiation used is small and similar to that given by other diagnostic x-ray tests. The effective adult radiation dose to your whole body from this test is about the same as the dose the average person living in the United States receives in 8.5 yr from cosmic rays and naturally occurring background radiation sources. The radiation dose is about 50% of the yearly dose considered safe for doctors and technologists who work with radiation. You can be around other people and use a bathroom normally without risk to others.

D. Pregnancy

If you are pregnant or think you could be pregnant, inform your doctor so that this can be discussed with the nuclear medicine physician.

IV. CSF FLOW OR LEAK SCAN

A. Test/Procedure

Your doctor has ordered a CSF flow scan (radionuclide cisternogram) to help understand the flow of cerebrospinal fluid within your brain or to see if there is a leak of this fluid.

After the administration of local anesthesia, a small amount of radioactive material called a tracer will be injected into the fluid around your spinal cord. You will be positioned next to a special machine called a gamma camera, which does not produce radiation but detects radiation that is coming from the injected tracer in your body. A series of pictures of your brain will then be taken at 1–4 hr, 24 hr and possibly at 48 and 72 hr. The pictures take less than 1 hr to obtain.

If you are undergoing this test to detect a leak of cerebrospinal fluid, cotton plugs may first be placed into your nose and you may be asked to lie in a position that encourages the leak. In addition, a special dye may be injected into your lumbar spine, along with the tracer and additional pictures also may be obtained on a different machine called a CT scan. Also, a blood sample may be withdrawn from your vein at the end of the procedure. If the cotton plugs fall out after you are sent home, please keep them separately wrapped in plastic bags and call the nuclear medicine department as soon as possible. The procedure may be stopped once the leak is detected.

B. Preparation
You may eat and drink as usual. If you are on blood thinners or aspirin, please tell the doctors because such medications must be stopped before the procedure begins. If you also are having a CT scan, there may be certain other medication restrictions. Please ask your physician about your medications.

C. Radiation and other risks
The amount of radiation used is small and similar to that given by other diagnostic x-ray tests. The effective adult radiation dose to your whole body from this test is less than the radiation dose the average person living in the United States receives each year from cosmic rays and naturally occurring background radiation sources. The radiation dose is about 5% of the yearly dose considered safe for doctors and technologists who work with radiation. You can be around other people and use a bathroom normally without risk to others.

The risks from the injection of radiotracer into your spinal canal are small and include bleeding, infection and headache. This procedure will be explained to you separately.

D. Pregnancy
If you are pregnant or think you could be pregnant, inform your doctor so that this can be discussed with the nuclear medicine physician.

V. CSF SHUNT PATENCY SCAN
A. Test/Procedure
Your doctor has ordered a CSF shunt patency scan to help determine if your shunt is blocked.

Your shunt reservoir will be injected with a small amount of radioactive material called a tracer. You will be positioned next to a special machine called a gamma camera, which does not produce radiation but detects radiation that is coming from the injected tracer in your body. A series of pictures will then be taken, usually from 30 min up to 2 hr.

B. Preparation

You may eat and drink as usual and take your usual medications.

C. Radiation and other risks

The amount of radiation used is small. The exact amount depends on the type of shunt and the radiotracer used, but it typically is far less than the average person living in the United States receives each year from cosmic rays and naturally occurring background radiation sources and a tiny fraction of the yearly dose considered safe for doctors and technologists who work with radiation. You can be around other people and use a bathroom normally without risk to others. The reservoir will be accessed with sterile technique, so there is only a small theoretical risk of shunt infection.

D. Pregnancy

If you are pregnant or think you could be pregnant, inform your doctor so that this can be discussed with the nuclear medicine physician.

References

1. Berger JD, Witte RJ, Holdeman KP, et al. Neuroradiologic applications of central nervous system SPECT. *RadioGraphics* 1996;16:777–785.
2. Mullan BP, O'Connor MK, Hung JC. Single photon emission computed tomography brain imaging. *Neurosurg Clin North Am* 1996;7:617–651.
3. Lewis DH. Functional brain imaging with cerebral perfusion SPECT in cerebrovascular disease, epilepsy and trauma. *Neurosurg Clin North Am* 1997;8:337–344.
4. Flowers WM, Patel BR. Radionuclide angiography as a confirmatory test for brain death: a review of 229 studies in 219 patients. *South Med J* 1997;90:1091–1096.
5. Tawes RL, Lull R. Value of single photon emission computerized imaging in the treatment of patients undergoing carotid endarterectomy. *J Vasc Surg* 1996;24:219–225.
6. Lorberboym M, Mandell LR, Mosesson RE, et al. The role of thallium-201 uptake and retention in intracranial tumors after radiotherapy. *J Nucl Med* 1997;38:223–226.
7. Masdeu JC, Brass LM, Holman BL, Kushner MJ. Brain single-photon emission computed tomography. *Neurology* 1994;44:1970–1977.
8. Messa C, Fazio F, Costa DC, Ell PJ. Clinical brain radionuclide imaging studies. *Semin Nucl Med* 1995;25:111–143.
9. Juni JE, Waxman AD, Devous MD, et al. Procedure guideline for brain perfusion SPECT using technetium-99m radiopharmaceuticals. *J Nucl Med* 1998;39:923–926. (Also *Society of Nuclear Medicine Procedure Guidelines Manual 1999*. Society of Nuclear Medicine: Reston, VA. 1999:105–110.)
10. Jacobs A, Put E, Ingels M, Bossuyt A. Prospective evaluation of technetium-99m-HMPAO SPECT in mild and moderate traumatic brain injury. *J Nucl Med* 1994;35:942–947.

9
The Thyroid

Abnormalities of thyroid anatomy or function usually present when the clinician suspects hyperthyroidism or hypothyroidism and confirms this suspicion with serum measurements of thyroxine (T4) or thyroid-stimulating hormone (TSH, thyrotropin) or when the clinician detects or questions the presence of a nodule or goiter on routine physical examination. Radionuclide evaluation of the thyroid often can contribute to the management of patients with diagnosed or suspected thyroid abnormalities.

The thyroid scan provides a means of documenting the location, shape and functional characteristics of thyroid tissue. The radioactive iodine (RAI) uptake complements the thyroid scan and can answer specific questions regarding thyroid function: Is a hyperthyroid gland taking up enough radioactive iodide to make therapy with radioiodine feasible? Is the patient's hyperthyroidism caused by a disorder associated with a low uptake such as subacute thyroiditis, struma ovarii or factitious hyperthyroidism? The functional and structural information provided by a thyroid scan and uptake combined with the physical examination and serum hormone measurements often permit an expeditious diagnosis and a logical approach to therapy or further diagnostic procedures.

SCANS AND PRIMARY CLINICAL INDICATIONS

CLINICAL QUESTIONS

Thyroid nodules

Hypothyroid newborn

^{131}I therapy for hyperthyroidism and nontoxic goiter

PATIENT INFORMATION

SCANS AND THERAPY

I. ^{123}I THYROID SCAN AND RADIOACTIVE IODINE UPTAKE

A. Background

Iodine-123-iodide is actively transported into the follicular cell (trapped) and bound to tyrosine (organified). Consequently, an ^{123}I scan shows the distribution of tissue that possesses both of these functions. An ^{123}I scan often is obtained to evaluate a questionable nodule, to determine the functional state of a nodule, to determine if a retrosternal mass represents a goiter and to confirm the presence of Graves' disease or nodular thyroid disease. The RAI uptake is used to evaluate the functional state of the thyroid gland and to help determine the dose of ^{131}I for subsequent radioiodine therapy.

B. Radiopharmaceuticals

Iodine-123 is an isotope of iodine, which is handled by the body exactly like nonradioactive iodine (^{127}I). Radioactive iodine is administered as ^{123}I-sodium iodide, which is absorbed readily by the intestine into the extrathyroidal iodide pool. Extrathyroidal iodide is transported rapidly across the membrane of the follicular cell where it is oxidized, bound to tyrosine (organified) and subsequently incorporated into thyroid hormone. Iodine-123 has a favorable 159 keV photon energy for routine imaging. There is no beta emission; consequently, the radiation exposure to the patient's thyroid is much lower than the radiation exposure after ^{131}I administration (see below).

C. How the study is performed

The typical adult patient swallows sodium iodide capsules containing 200–400 μCi (7.4–14.8 MBq) of ^{123}I and usually returns 24 hr later for imaging. The patient is imaged in the supine position with the neck extended. The imaging time takes 20–40 min depending on the local protocol and imaging equipment. If a 24-hr uptake is performed, a probe is placed over the thyroid to determine the percent of the administered dose present in the thyroid 24 hr after ^{123}I administration. In some centers, the ^{123}I uptake may be measured at 4 hr to facilitate determination of the treatment dose of ^{131}I. It is also possible to image the thyroid 4 hr after administration of the ^{123}I capsules.

D. Patient preparation

The patient may drink water but should not eat for 3–4 hr before radioiodine administration because food may delay or interfere with absorption of radioiodine. Patients should not be referred if they have had intravenous contrast within the preceding 4–6 wk. Thyroid hormone, antithyroid drugs, amiodarone and antibacterial soaps or mineral/vitamin supplements containing iodine also will decrease tracer uptake by the thyroid gland. Laboratory tests of thyroid function should be made available to facilitate interpretation of the scan and uptake.

E. Understanding the report

The report usually describes the configuration of the thyroid gland, comments on the homogeneity of uptake and notes the presence or absence of nodules. Nodules often will be described as cold (uptake in the nodule is less than the surrounding thyroid tissue) or hot (uptake in the nodule is greater than the surrounding thyroid tissue). The thyroid gland can be palpated while the patient is positioned under the camera. This procedure is advantageous because the examiner can determine whether a palpable nodule is hot or cold by placing a small radioactive marker on the nodule and noting its position on the scan. The routine scan does not provide an accurate measurement of thyroid size although an estimate of size may be included in the report.

The report also records the RAI uptake if an RAI uptake was measured. The RAI uptake can be affected by diet and medication (see Potential Problems, below). The normal 24-hr uptake usually falls between 10% and 30%. Patients with Graves' disease commonly have a 24-hr RAI uptake well in excess of 30% and a 4-hr uptake >15%. Patients with toxic nodular goiter may have a 24-hr uptake within the normal range, whereas the RAI uptake of patients with acute thyroiditis is usually <3% (see Clinical Question 2, below).

F. Potential problems

1. Exogenous iodine administration and variability of the iodide pool. Expansion of the extrathyroidal iodide pool by a high-iodine diet, iodine-containing contrast media or iodine-containing drugs (amiodarone, some vitamin pills, expectorants, kelp or mineral supplements) decreases the percentage of radioactive iodide in the extrathyroidal pool and consequently decreases the measured uptake of iodine. Because the 24-hr thyroid uptake is an indirect measure of thyroid function and is sensitive to changes in the extrathyroidal iodide pool, the 24-hr uptake should not be used as a primary test to determine if the patient is hypothyroid or hyperthyroid.

2. Cost of ^{123}I. Iodine-123 has a physical half-life of 13 hr and has to be ordered for a specific patient. Please emphasize to the patient the appointment must be kept or cancelled 2–3 days in advance. If the patient fails to show for the appointment, the ^{123}I will decay and the hospital, clinic or physician practice will need to pay for the radiopharmaceutical.

3. Exogenous thyroid hormone. Exogenous thyroid hormone will suppress the thyroid gland. T4 needs to be discontinued for approximately 6 wk before imaging. Cytomel (triiodothyronine) needs to be discontinued for approximately 2 wk.

4. What if a patient has a radioiodine or ^{99m}Tc-pertechnetate scan and is subsequently discovered to be pregnant? In general, radionuclides should not be administered to pregnant women if the test can be postponed safely until after delivery. Occasionally, a woman discovers she is pregnant some time after the administration of radioiodine or ^{99m}Tc-pertechnetate. Careful review of the available data during the first trimester of pregnancy seems to suggest at most a minimal risk. Radiation exposure is largely a function of transplacental delivery of radionuclide and of the radiation dose because of the proximity of the bladder. Radioiodine and ^{99m}Tc-pertechnetate both cross the placenta; however, because the fetal thyroid does not concentrate iodine during the first trimester, standard diagnostic doses deliver little radiation to the fetus before the 12th week of gestation.

II. ^{99m}Tc-PERTECHNETATE THYROID SCAN

A. Background

Technetium-99m pertechnetate is transported actively into the follicular cell (trapped) but it is not bound to tyrosine (organified). Images of the thyroid are obtained 10–30 min after injection and show the distribution of tissue that has the capacity to trap ^{99m}Tc-pertechnetate. Delayed images are not obtained because the unbound pertechnetate is not retained in the thyroid gland. Uptake measurements are not as well standardized as they are for ^{123}I, but they can be used to evaluate the trapping capacity of the thyroid gland.

B. Radiopharmaceuticals

Technetium-99m-pertechnetate functions as an anionic analog of iodide and is trapped by the thyroid cells but not organified; consequently, the scan images are exclusively a measure of trapping. A thyroid nodule that retains the capacity to trap iodide but has lost the capacity to organify will have normal or increased uptake (warm or hot nodule) on a pertechnetate scan but reduced uptake (cold nodule) on an ^{123}I scan. Technetium-99m-pertechnetate has a favorable energy for routine imaging, is cheaper than ^{123}I and results in a low radiation exposure to the thyroid.

C. How the study is performed

The adult patient receives an intravenous injection of 2–5 mCi (74–185 MBq) of ^{99m}Tc-pertechnetate, and images are obtained 10–30 min later; imaging takes approximately 20–40 min depending on the protocol and equipment. Some institutions also measure the uptake of ^{99m}Tc-pertechnetate shortly after administration to obtain an index of thyroid function.

D. Patient preparation

There are no dietary restrictions because, unlike ^{123}I, the drug is injected intravenously. Concurrent or recent administration of thyroid hormone, antithyroid drugs, amiodarone, mineral/vitamin supplements containing iodine or intravenous contrast will decrease tracer uptake by the thyroid gland, although the effect is usually less pronounced than it is for ^{123}I. Laboratory tests of thyroid function should be made available to facilitate interpretation of the scan and uptake.

E. Understanding the report

The report describes the configuration of the thyroid gland, notes the presence or absence of nodules and comments on the homogeneity of uptake. A pertechnetate uptake value may be reported along with its normal range.

F. Potential problems

1. Discordant nodules. There are reports of thyroid carcinomas, particularly follicular carcinomas, which will trap pertechnetate and appear as a warm nodule on the pertechnetate scan, whereas they do not organify as efficiently as normal thyroid and appear as cold nodules on an ^{123}I scan. The frequency of this occurrence is debated, but it is probably low.

2. Detection of retrosternal (substernal) goiter. An ^{123}I scan is preferable to a ^{99m}Tc-pertechnetate scan to diagnose a substernal goiter. Because pertechnetate scans are obtained shortly after injection, there is still blood pool activity, and it may be difficult to evaluate the presence of a substernal goiter because of the proximity of pertechnetate remaining in the great vessels.

III. [131]I THERAPY

A. Background

Iodine-131 therapy has a high success rate and carries minimal risk. More than 80% of patients are successfully treated with a single dose. Disadvantages are few but include a high likelihood of eventual hypothyroidism. The radiation dose to the thyroid after ^{131}I administration depends on the dose administered, the size of the gland, the homogeneity of distribution within the gland, the 24-hr uptake and the average length of time the ^{131}I remains in the thyroid gland. The treatment dose for Graves' disease usually is estimated based on the size of the gland, the 24-hr uptake and the desired dose of radiation to be delivered to the gland. There is no increased risk of cancer after ^{131}I therapy for Graves' disease (see Clinical Question 19, below). Patients with a toxic nodular goiter require larger doses of RAI than patients with Graves' disease to achieve a euthyroid state.

B. Radiopharmaceuticals

Iodine-131 is a beta- and gamma-emitting isotope of iodine that has been used in humans for more than 50 yr. The relatively high-energy photon of ^{131}I is not ideal for imaging with conventional gamma cameras, but adequate images of the tracer biodistribution can be obtained, particularly when higher doses are administered. The beta particle has an average path length of 0.8 mm, deposits all of its energy near its source and provides the basis for using ^{131}I to treat hyperthyroid states and thyroid cancer. Because of the relatively high radiation exposure resulting from its beta emission, ^{131}I is no longer recommended for routine diagnostic thyroid imaging and has no advantage over ^{123}I in substernal goiter.

C. How the procedure is performed

The procedure for RAI therapy is almost identical to the dosing procedure for an ^{123}I scan; however, a pregnancy test will need to be obtained in women of childbearing age. Instructions concerning risks and radiation safety practices are provided to the patient, the patient swallows a capsule containing the radioactive ^{131}I and is then allowed to leave. A typical dose for Graves' disease ranges from 8 to 20 mCi.

D. Patient preparation

Antithyroid drugs affect the RAI uptake, and they should be discontinued for at least 1 wk before therapy. The patient may drink water but should not eat for 3–4 hr before ^{131}I therapy. Alternative therapy should be chosen for pregnant patients; ^{131}I will cross the placenta, and the fetal thyroid is capable of accumulating iodide at 3 mo. A pregnancy test should be obtained before therapy in women of childbearing age. Contrast CT scans should be avoided for 6 wk before therapy. The patient also should be given instructions for post-therapy follow-up.

E. Understanding the report

The report indicates the reason for the ^{131}I therapy, the therapy dose administered, results of a pregnancy test if applicable and that a signed informed consent was obtained. The report often specifies that radiation safety precautions were explained to the patient and indicates the plans for the post-therapy follow-up appointment.

F. Potential problems

1. Hypothyrodism. Hypothyroidism may occur as part of the natural course of Graves' disease, but it is accelerated by RAI therapy (see Clinical Question 16, below).

2. Thyroid storm or exacerbation of hyperthyroid symptoms. The hyperthyroid state may be exacerbated, and there is the rare possibility of a thyroid storm occurring 1–2 wk after RAI therapy because of release of stored hormone. Symptoms usually can be managed with beta blockers. Patients at high risk for severe exacerbation of symptoms or thyroid storm after ^{131}I therapy include the elderly, patients with severe thyrotoxicosis and patients with underlying heart disease. These patients should be managed by inducing a euthyroid state with methimazole before ^{131}I treatment (see Worth Mentioning).

3. Fertility and birth defects. Treatment of hyperthyroidism with radioactive iodine does not cause a reduction in fertility and does not increase the risk of birth defects in children of parents treated before pregnancy.

4. Neck tenderness. The ^{131}I that concentrates in the thyroid gland may cause some neck tenderness within the first 2 wk after therapy. This resolves spontaneously and can be treated easily with acetaminophen.

CLINICAL QUESTIONS

1. Does a patient with hyperthyroidism have Graves' disease?

It is important to distinguish between hyperthyroidism associated with increased iodine uptake (Graves' disease, toxic nodular goiter) and hyperthyroidism associated with a low iodine uptake (thyroiditis, factitious hyperthyroidism, struma ovarii) because the treatment for these two categories of hyperthyroidism is different.

The diagnosis of Graves' disease usually can be made based on clinical and laboratory data. A thyroid scan and uptake can be helpful in confirming Graves' disease when hyperthyroidism presents without signs of proptosis, exopthalmos, thyroid acropachy or pretibial myxedema. The scan shows homogeneous uptake throughout both lobes (Fig. 1); the RAI uptake often is used to help calculate the dose of ^{131}I for patients with Graves' disease who are referred for ^{131}I therapy (see ^{131}I Therapy, above). Occasionally, Graves' disease can be confused with a toxic nodular goiter, but the two can be distinguished easily by the nuclear scan. This distinction is important because the RAI treatment dose for a toxic nodular goiter is 2–3 times higher than the treatment dose for Graves' disease.

2. Does a hyperthyroid patient have a silent, painless thyroiditis or subacute thyroiditis?

Occasionally, a subacute thyroiditis or silent, painless thyroiditis can be confused with Graves' disease. In all three settings, the patient may be clinically hyperthyroid with abnormal thyroid function tests. The thyroid scan and up-

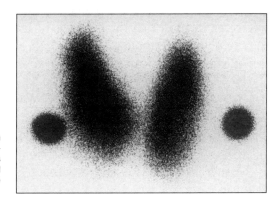

Figure 1. Graves' disease. An anterior view with a parallel hole collimator shows diffuse radioiodine uptake throughout the thyroid gland. Markers on each side of the thyroid are 10 cm apart and allow the size of the gland to be estimated. The 24-hr uptake was 67%.

take can be used to distinguish between Graves' disease or thyroiditis. Patients with subacute thyroiditis have a painful neck, but they may mistake the pain for the sore throat of an upper respiratory infection; by the time they present to the clinician with symptoms of hyperthyroidism, the neck tenderness may have resolved. Patients with subacute or silent, painless thyroiditis may have increased levels of circulating thyroid hormone that has been released from an acutely inflamed gland. Because of the inflammation, the thyroid is not able to trap and organify the ^{123}I and the 24-hr uptake is close to zero. Patients with Graves' disease typically have a high 24-hr uptake.

3 and 4. Is the patient's hyperthyroid state caused by Graves' disease or a toxic nodular goiter? Is it caused by toxic adenoma?

The scan can confirm the clinical impression of a toxic nodular goiter or toxic adenoma. The typical appearance is marked radiotracer uptake in the toxic nodule(s) with suppression of the rest of the gland. It is important to distinguish a toxic nodular goiter or toxic adenoma from Graves' disease because patients with a toxic nodular goiter or adenoma require higher doses of ^{131}I.

5. Is the patient's hyperthyroidism due to factitious hyperthyroidism?

The thyroid scan and uptake can be used to help confirm this diagnosis. If the patient is thyrotoxic due to exogenous hormone administration, the normal thyroid gland will be suppressed and the 24-hr RAI uptake will be close to zero. Silent, painless thyroiditis and factitious hyperthyroidism will have a similar scan presentation, but the two usually can be distinguished by a measurement of serum thyroglobulin or thyroid autoantibodies.

6. Is the patient's hyperthyroidism due to struma ovarii?

This is an extremely rare condition. Hyperthyroidism due to struma ovarii (adenomatous thyroid tissue in a unilateral ovarian teratoma) will suppress the normal thyroid gland. The 24-hr uptake will be close to zero. If this condition is suspected, request that the pelvis be imaged. Additional views of the pelvis are easy to obtain but are not routine.

7. Is the thyroid enlarged?

The volume of the thyroid gland cannot be determined by most standard ^{123}I or ^{99m}Tc-pertechnetate imaging procedures, although the volume can be estimated from measurements of length and width if a reference radioactive ruler or marker also is imaged. The scan should not be ordered simply to determine if the thyroid gland is enlarged without first confirming that this determination can be made.

8. Is a patient hypothyroid?

A thyroid scan with an uptake measurement rarely provides important information in the patient with a clinical diagnosis of hypothyroidism and a non-nodular gland. A measurement of TSH is usually sufficient.

9–11. How should a questionable thyroid nodule found on palpation be evaluated? Does a palpable thyroid nodule consist of functioning thyroid tissue? Does the patient have a solitary nodule or a multinodular goiter?

Fewer than 10% of palpable solitary thyroid nodules are malignant; however, the risk that a thyroid nodule is malignant is increased in children, adolescents and adults over age 60. The risk is substantially increased if the patient has had prior head or neck irradiation. When a solitary thyroid nodule is detected by physical examination of the neck, a FNAB usually is obtained to determine if the nodule is malignant. FNAB has become the cornerstone in the evaluation of solitary thyroid nodules detected on clinical examination and of dominant nodules within multinodular goiters. The procedure requires skill and experience as well as an experienced cytopathologist. Even in skilled hands, approximately 10% of biopsies are nondiagnostic.

Imaging tends to be reserved for those cases in which it is not certain if there is a nodule or if a palpable nodule is actually in the thyroid. Imaging also is used to distinguish between a questionable nodule and a prominent lobe or hemiagenesis of the thyroid, to distinguish between a solitary nodule and a multinodular goiter, to evaluate a thyroid mass when expert cytopathology is unavailable and to better evaluate a thyroid mass when the cytology is nondiagnostic.

The nuclear scan evaluates the thyroid gland for the presence or absence of a nodule. Placement of a small radioactive marker over the palpable nodule while the patient's neck is positioned under the camera clarifies the relationship of the suspected nodule to the thyroid gland. Unlike sonography, the nuclear scan also evaluates the functional state of a thyroid nodule. Hot nodules that accumulate ^{123}I to a greater degree than the rest of the thyroid gland are unlikely to be malignant and further biopsies or surgery can be avoided. For this reason, a scan can be particularly useful when FNAB (see below) is indeterminate. Cold (nonfunctioning or hypofunctioning) thyroid nodules have a 10–20% chance of being malignant (Fig. 2). Palpable nodules that accumulate ^{123}I to the same degree as the rest of the thyroid (warm nodules) are less likely to be malignant, but most clinicians also will biopsy these nodules depending on their size, consistency and clinical presentation. The presence of a multinodular goiter decreases the chance of a malignancy. The typical scan appearance of a multinodular goiter shows areas of increased and decreased uptake often involving both lobes; however, if there is a dominant cold nodule, FNAB usually is recommended.

Sonography clearly defines the thyroid gland, is more sensitive than a nuclear scan in detecting the presence of thyroid nodules and can determine if the nodule is intra- or extrathyroidal. Sonography often is used if the clinician is unsure if a nodule is present or is uncertain whether or not the nodule is located in the thyroid. Although the radiation dose from a ^{99m}Tc-pertechnetate or ^{123}I thyroid scan is quite low and there is no known risk, sonography avoids ionizing radiation and is often the initial imaging procedure in children with a questionable nodule in the neck. Sonography is the imaging procedure of choice in pregnancy. If a nodule is present, sonography can determine if the nodule is solid, cystic or mixed, but sonography cannot reliably exclude malignancy even in a cystic nodule, and biopsy usually is recommended. In settings in which a nodule or lymph node is difficult to palpate or if there are multiple nodules, ultrasound-guided biopsy provides the greatest certainty for correct sampling of the nodule. Ultrasound also can be used to determine if a nodule is increasing in size in a patient on suppressive therapy. Limitations include the necessity for a skilled operator, interoperator variability in nodule detection and the increasing prevalence and questionable significance of small thyroid nodules in the aging population. Thyroid ultrasound is so sensitive and nodules so prevalent that it may be difficult to interpret the results. In a recent study, two thirds of normal, middle-aged volunteers were found to have thyroid nodules by sonography, and 25% had at least one nodule >1.0 cm in diameter.

FNAB usually is obtained when a solitary thyroid nodule is detected by physical examination. If FNAB is unavailable or if the FNAB cytology is nondiagnostic, a thyroid scan can be useful in directing clinical management. A hot nodule is extremely unlikely to be malignant but a cold nodule has a 10–20%

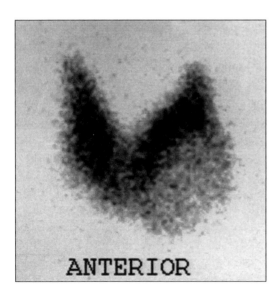

Figure 2. Cold nodule. An anterior pinhole view shows a cold nodule involving the inferior left lobe of the thyroid.

chance of malignancy and should be rebiopsied or excised. Sonography cannot reliably distinguish between a benign and malignant nodule.

If there is a question of a thyroid nodule or neck mass on physical examination, a thyroid scan or sonography should be obtained. Sonography can evaluate the thyroid as well as tissues adjacent to the thyroid, whereas the nuclear scan only evaluates the thyroid. Sonography also can be used to guide FNAB if the nodule is difficult to palpate. Sonography is more sensitive than the nuclear scan in detecting thyroid nodules, but sonography is so sensitive and nodules so prevalent in normal, middle-aged volunteers that it may be difficult to interpret the results. Unlike sonography, the scan evaluates the functional state of the nodule.

12. Is a neck or retrosternal mass a goiter?

The nuclear scan can often answer this question. A radioactive marker can be placed at the sternal notch, and the location of the thyroid or thyroid nodule can be determined relative to the sternal notch. A retrosternal goiter may be a manifestation of a multinodular goiter, which characteristically has areas of diminished radioiodide uptake. For this reason, scans to detect a retrosternal goiter often are performed with ^{123}I because the thyroid-to-background ratio is high at 24 hr and there is no blood pool activity in the great vessels to obscure a low level of uptake in the goiter. The absence of uptake does not exclude a nonfunctioning goiter.

13. FNAB shows a benign adenoma; will thyroid hormone arrest the growth of the adenoma or reduce its size?

A thyroid scan can be obtained after thyroid hormone administration to determine if a benign adenoma or hot nodule can be suppressed or if it is autonomous. This procedure occasionally is performed if thyroid hormone will be administered in an attempt to shrink the nodule or to prevent its further enlargement. If the uptake in the adenoma is not suppressed after thyroid hormone administration, the nodule is autonomous and will not be affected by exogenous hormone administration.

14 and 15. Does a hypothyroid newborn have a sublingual thyroid? Does a hypothyroid newborn have agenesis of the thyroid?

These congenital abnormalities usually are suspected when a newborn presents with an elevated TSH or a reduced T4. A scan can determine if the thyroid is present in a normal location and can simultaneously evaluate the patient for the presence of a sublingual thyroid.

16. Should hyperthyroid patients be treated with ^{131}I therapy?

Most adults are offered radioactive ^{131}I iodine (RAI) as the therapy of choice for thyrotoxicosis due to Graves' disease. It is the least expensive and safest form of therapy. The principal adverse effect is hypothyroidism; the incidence ranges from 20% to 40% at 1 yr and increases at 1–3%/year thereafter. PTU and methimazole may result in itching, a skin rash and, less commonly, arthralgias or elvated hepatic enzymes; the most serious adverse effects are life-threatening hepatic toxicity and a 0.3% risk of agranulocytosis. Agranulocytosis is idiosyncratic and is most apt to occur within the first few months of therapy. Patients receiving PTU or methimazole should be informed of the risks of these drugs and the early warning signs of toxicity. Surgery usually is reserved for patients with coexisting hyperparathyroidism and can be considered as an alternative to PTU/methimazole for patients with a severe opthalmopathy. Pregnancy is a contraindication to ^{131}I therapy.

It takes a higher dosage of ^{131}I to successfully treat a toxic nodular goiter or a toxic adenoma than it does to treat Graves' disease. The ^{123}I scan can distinguish a patient with a toxic nodule(s) from a patient with Graves' disease. The RAI uptake measurement can confirm that there will be adequate ^{131}I accumulation in the gland to expect a good response to therapy and justify the radiation exposure. Radioiodine results in a single-dose cure rate of approximately 80–90% in hyperthyroid patients with autonomously functioning thyroid nodules and a cure rate of 80–100% of patients with a toxic multinodular goiter, although more than one treatment may be necessary. In most patients, RAI therapy also results in a substantial reduction in thyroid (or nodule) volume. For most patients with a solitary toxic nodule, ^{131}I therapy is the treatment of choice but lobectomy or nodulectomy is also simple and effective.

17. Will ^{131}I therapy cause or exacerbate Graves' opthalmopathy?

Most patients with Graves' disease have some opthalmopathy consisting of orbital protrusion (exopthalmos) or larger extraocular muscles than normal subjects, but it is clinically evident in only 20–40% of patients. Patients without clinical opthalmopathy are usually unaffected by RAI therapy; however, there is probably a slight risk that RAI therapy may exacerbate clinically evident opthalmopathy. Preliminary data suggest this risk can be reduced by corticosteroid therapy, and some investigators recommend systemic corticosteroid therapy concurrent with RAI when patients have a clinically obvious opthalmopathy. Patients with a severe opthalmopathy should be treated with antithyroid drugs or surgery.

18. Is ^{131}I therapy a therapeutic option for euthyroid patients with compressive symptoms due to a large, nontoxic multinodular goiter?

Surgery often is considered standard therapy for patients with a large multinodular goiter leading to compression of the trachea, esophagus or great vessels. It relieves the compressive symptoms rapidly and effectively; however, it is not without risk. Complications include vocal cord paralysis, hypoparathyroidism, tracheomalacia, hemorrhage and recurrence of the goiter. The risk of surgical excision increases in elderly patients and those with cardiopulmonary diseases. Thyroid hormone is a second treatment option but thyroid suppression may not lead to shrinkage of the gland. Iodine-131 therapy is a viable alternative and can reduce the mean thyroid volume with amelioration of the compressive symptoms. Iodine-131 therapy can be repeated at intervals of several months to gradually reduce the size of the gland. Transient exacerbation of symptoms after ^{131}I administration is a theoretical possibility, but it does not appear to be a clinical problem. Iodine-131 therapy is a good alternative to surgery for patients with recurrent goiter, patients with medical contraindications to surgery and patients who prefer not to undergo surgery.

19. Can hyperthyroid patients be retreated with ^{131}I therapy?

Approximately 10–20% of patients with Graves' disease may need a second RAI treatment. The indications and risks are the same as for the initial therapy.

20. Will ^{131}I therapy for Graves' disease or toxic multinodular goiter increase the risk for cancer?

Multiple studies with 35 yr of follow-up show no evidence of an increased risk of carcinogenesis or cancer mortality after therapeutic use of ^{131}I for treatment of Graves' disease. Patients with toxic multinodular goiters often receive higher doses of ^{131}I, and the literature regarding subsequent cancer risk is sparse. There may be a slight increase in the risk of extrathyroidal cancers after ^{131}I therapy for toxic multinodular goiter, but this is debated.

21. Is there an increased risk of congenital abnormalities if a patient treated with ^{131}I becomes pregnant?

A 10-mCi dose of RAI delivers approximately 2 rads to the ovaries; this dose can be further reduced by hydration and frequent voiding. For comparison purposes, the ovaries receive approximately 0.7 rads from x-rays of the lumbar spine. The available data show no increased risk of congenital abnormalities in children of patients previously treated with [131]I.

22. When is it safe to have children after ^{131}I therapy?

As a precaution, most physicians recommend a wait of 6 mo for prospective mothers and fathers. The risk of miscarriage is reduced if the mother first achieves a euthyroid state.

23. Is it safe to treat a hyperthyroid child or adolescent with ^{131}I therapy?

Many physicians prefer a trial of antithyroid drugs in children or adolescents with Graves' disease, but there is no evidence of an increased risk of cancer, impaired fertility or abnormal offspring in children or adolescents treated with ^{131}I.

24. Should a patient with Graves' disease be made euthyroid with PTU or methimazole before ^{131}I therapy?

Elderly patients, patients who are severely thyrotoxic and those with cardiac disease are at increased risk if there is exacerbation of the hyperthyroid state due to release of preformed thyroid hormone after RAI therapy. Hyperthyroid symptoms often can be controlled with beta blockers, but the risk can be reduced substantially if the patient is pretreated with antithyroid drugs to achieve a euthyroid state and deplete the gland of stored hormone before ^{131}I therapy. Antithyroid drugs should be discontinued for 1 wk before RAI therapy.

25. Should Graves' disease patients referred for ^{131}I therapy be given a 30-mCi dose of ^{131}I to ensure a cure of the hyperthyroid state, reduce the need for retreatment and minimize the number of follow-up visits?

A 30-mCi (1110-MBq) dose used to be the maximum dose that the Nuclear Regulatory Commission permitted for outpatient therapies. It is sufficient to produce a hypothyroid state and minimize the recurrence of hyperthyroidism after RAI therapy. This arbitrary approach, however, gives the patient unnecessary additional radiation and increases the backgound radiation to the general public. The dose required to induce a hypothyroid state can be estimated from the gland size and the RAI uptake; for the vast majority of patients, it is substantially <30 mCi.

26. What advice typically is given regarding radiation safety after ^{131}I therapy?

With the exclusion of the thyroid gland, the radiation exposure to the rest of the body can be minimized if the patient remains well hydrated and urinates frequently for 24–48 hr. Most of the radioactive iodine will be eliminated in the urine, but some will be secreted in the saliva and sweat. The radiation exposure to others is extremely low, but it can be minimized by understanding that the radioiodine is eliminated from the body in urine, saliva and sweat and by following a few simple guidelines. Specific guidelines will be reviewed with the patient at the time of therapy. In general, the patient should sleep alone for several days after ^{131}I therapy. For several days after therapy, men should sit down when urinating, and the toilet should be flushed twice. Patients should not share utensils with other members of their household for a week because some radioiodine will be secreted in the saliva. Patients should not sit with a child in their lap for long periods until a week has elapsed after therapy. Patients should avoid sex for a week after RAI therapy. It is recommended that patients avoid pregnancy for 6 mo after radioiodine therapy in case they may need to be retreated.

WORTH MENTIONING

1. Technical note

A pinhole collimator provides better resolution of small structures such as the thyroid than a standard parallel hole collimator. Diagnostic accuracy is improved if the nuclear medicine department has a pinhole collimator and obtains oblique views to avoid the possibility of missing a small cold nodule just anterior or posterior to one of the lobes of the thyroid.

2. PTU or methimazole before RAI therapy?

PTU often is used to treat the hyperthyroid state and may be used to make the patient euthyroid before RAI therapy. Recent data suggest, however, that the use of PTU before RAI therapy may reduce the response rate after ^{131}I therapy. For this reason, methimazole is the recommended drug to treat hyperthyroid patients before RAI therapy.

PATIENT INFORMATION

I. RADIONUCLIDE THYROID SCAN
A. Test/Procedure

You have been referred for a thyroid scan. There are two types of thyroid scans. In one, you will swallow a capsule containing the radioactive iodide and return 24 hr later for a thyroid scan. You will lie on a table and pictures will be taken of your thyroid using a specialized camera; this will take 20–40 min. It is possible that you also will be asked to return. Alternatively, you may be given an injection of ^{99m}Tc-pertechnetate (a radioactive drug that is accumulated by the thyroid gland), and pictures of your thyroid will be obtained a few minutes after the injection.

B. Preparation

Diet. If your procedure will consist of swallowing a capsule containing radioactive iodide, you should not eat for 3 hr before the dose or 1 hr afterward. You may drink as much water as you want. If your procedure consists of an injection of ^{99m}Tc-pertechnetate, there are no dietary restrictions.

Medications. Thyroid hormone, antithyroid drugs, mineral or vitamin supplements containing iodine and recent intravenous contrast from a diagnostic x-ray procedure may interfere with your scan. If you are taking these medications or have had a recent x-ray examination using intravenous contrast, let your doctor know before the test.

C. Radiation and other risks

The radiation exposure is extremely low and is similar to that given by other diagnostic x-ray tests. The effective radiation dose to your whole body is about one third to one fourth of the background radiation that the average person in the United States receives each year from cosmic rays and other naturally occurring background radiation sources. The radiation dose is about 2% of the yearly dose considered safe for doctors and technologists who work with radiation. You can be around other people and use a bathroom without risk to others.

D. Pregnancy

If you are pregnant or think you could be pregnant, inform your doctor so that this can be discussed with the nuclear medicine physician.

References

1. Erjavec M, Movrin T, Auersperg M, Golouh R. Comparative accumulation of ^{99m}Tc and ^{131}I in thyroid nodules. *J Nucl Med* 1977;18:346–347.
2. Graham GD, Burman KD. Radioactive treatment of Graves' disease: an assessment of its potential risks. *Ann Intern Med* 1987;105:900–903.
3. Hamburger JI. Management of hyperthyroidism in children and adolescents. *J Clin Endocrinol Metab* 1985;60:1019–1024.
4. Bartalena L, Marcocci C, Bogazzi F, et al. Use of corticosteroids to prevent progression of Graves' ophthalmopathy after radioiodine therapy for hyperthyroidism. *N Engl J Med* 1998;321:1349–1352.
5. Hung W, Anderson KD, Chandra RS, et al. Solitary thyroid nodules in 71 children and adolescents. *J Pediatric Surg* 1992;27:1407–1409.
6. Imseis RE, Vanmiddlesworth L, Massie JD, et al. Pretreatment with propylthiouracil but not methimazole reduces the therapeutic efficacy of iodine-131 in hyperthyroidism. *J Clin Endocrinol Metab* 1998;83:685–687.
7. Nygaard B, Hegedus L, Hansen JM. ^{131}I treatment of nodular nontoxic goiter. *Eur J Endocrinol* 1996;134:15–20.
8. Bierwaltes WH, Widman J. How harmful to others are iodine-131 treated patients? *J Nucl Med* 1992;33:2116–2117.
9. Hermus AR, Huysmans DA. Treatment of benign nodular thyroid disease. *N Engl J Med* 1998;338:1438–1447.
10. Siegel RD, Lee SL. Toxic nodular goiter: toxic adenoma and toxic multinodular goiter. *Endocrinol Metab Clin North Am* 1998;27:151–168.
11. de Klerk JM, van Isselt JW, van Dijk A, et al. Iodine-131 therapy in sporadic nontoxic goiter. *J Nucl Med* 1997;38:372–376.

10
The Parathyroids

Eighty-five percent of primary hyperparathyroidism is due to a solitary parathyroid adenoma, 10% from hyperplasia, 4% from multiple adenomas and 1% from parathyroid cancer or other causes. Although the diagnosis of hyperparathyroidism is confirmed with biochemical testing, imaging studies are useful to help localize a hyperfunctioning adenoma and aid the definitive therapy of surgical removal.

SCANS AND PRIMARY CLINICAL INDICATIONS

I. Subtraction scan   Page 200
- To help localize a hyperfunctioning parathyroid adenoma before initial surgery in a patient with primary hyperparathyroidism

- To help localize a hyperfunctioning parathyroid adenoma in a patient with persistent hyperparathyroidism after parathyroid surgery

II. Single radiotracer dual-phase scan   Page 202
- To help localize a hyperfunctioning parathyroid adenoma before initial surgery in a patient with primary hyperparathyroidism

- To help localize a hyperfunctioning parathyroid adenoma in a patient with persistent hyperparathyroidism after parathyroid surgery

CLINICAL QUESTIONS

Hyperparathyroidism

PATIENT INFORMATION

10

SCANS

I. SUBTRACTION SCAN

A. Background

The ^{201}Tl/^{99m}Tc-pertechnetate subtraction scan was the first successful nuclear imaging procedure to localize parathyroid adenomas. Technetium-99m-sestamibi has virtually replaced thallium because it has imaging characteristics and higher sensitivity. Thallium-201 and ^{99m}Tc-sestamibi are taken up by the thyroid gland as well as hyperfunctioning parathyroid tissue, if present. Technetium-99m-pertechnetate and ^{123}I are taken up only by the thyroid and can be subtracted from the sestamibi or thallium scan, leaving resultant images of hyperfunctioning parathyroid tissue.

Subtraction scans have a higher sensitivity than the single-isotope dual-phase sestamibi scan, although this advantage has not been demonstrated consistently. Subtraction scans are more expensive to perform and are technically more difficult.

B. Radiopharmaceuticals

Technetium-99m-sestamibi (Cardiolite) was developed as a cardiac imaging agent but has found use in tumor imaging. It is given intravenously and accumulated by thyroid and parathyroid tissue in proportion to blood flow and metabolic rate, although activity in normal parathyroid glands is too low to be seen on an image.

Technetium-99m-tetrofosmin (Myoview) is another cardiac imaging agent that has biokinetics similar to sestamibi. It has been advocated for parathyroid imaging, but there is much less experience with its use.

Thallium-201 is a potassium analog that is given intravenously and transported into thyroid and parathyroid tissue in proportion to blood flow, although activity in normal parathyroid glands is too low to be seen on an image.

Technetium-99m-pertechnetate is trapped but not organified by functioning thyroid tissue and is not taken up by parathyroid glands. It is administered intravenously.

Iodine-123 is trapped and organified by functioning thyroid but is not taken up by parathyroid tissue. It usually is administered orally.

C. How the study is performed

Separate images using thyroid/parathyroid radiotracers and thyroid-only radiotracers are acquired either sequentially or simultaneously. The timing of the procedure depends on the radiotracers used for the thyroid/parathyroid phase and for the thyroid-only phase. Iodine-123 (200–500 µCi [7.5–20 MBq] adult dose) requires 4 hr to accumulate enough activity in the thyroid for adequate imaging, so the patient must arrive early to be given the radionuclide. Technetium-99m-pertechnetate (2–4 mCi [75–150 MBq] adult dose) can be administered and imaged before or after the ^{201}Tl (2–3.5 mCi [75–130 MBq] adult dose) or ^{99m}Tc-sestamibi (5–25 mCi [185–925 MBq] adult dose). Each method has its advantages and disadvantages, and the exact protocol is individualized according to departmental experience, preference, equipment and availability of radiotracers. Imaging of the neck and the mediastinum is standard.

Because of the different energies of ^{123}I, ^{99m}Tc tracers and ^{201}Tl, simultaneous acquisition of the thyroid-only and thyroid/parathyroid images is possible with the proper equipment, which can decrease time of imaging and prevent errors due to patient motion between scans. In addition to anterior planar imaging, which takes 5–10 min, multiple oblique views, pinhole images and SPECT can be performed, which may improve accuracy but add to imaging times. Thus, the entire study can take as little as 1 hr or as much as 6 hr.

D. Patient preparation

Thallium-201 and ^{99m}Tc-sestamibi imaging require no special preparation, but thyroid medications and recent (4–6 wk) intravenous iodinated contrast administration interfere with uptake of ^{123}I and ^{99m}Tc-pertechnetate by the thyroid gland. If the patient is on thyroid medications, the nuclear medicine physician should be consulted. In addition, patients are encouraged to fast (water and medications are permitted) for a few hours before the study to aid the absorption of ^{123}I. It is best not to schedule this study within the first few weeks after neck surgery because of confounding artifact from local inflammation. Providing a detailed medical and surgical history as they relate to the thyroid and parathyroid will aid in scan interpretation.

E. Understanding the report

The report will state the method used to obtain the scans. The thyroid-only images are subtracted either visually or with various computer algorithms from the combined thyroid/parathyroid images. Foci of activity on the thyroid/parathyroid images greater than the thyroid-only images, as well as remaining activity after subtraction, are consistent with parathyroid adenoma and/or hyperplasia. One or multiple areas of varying intensities may be described. Ectopic foci in the mediastinum also may be reported. If no abnormality can be confidently identified, this will be stated. The lesion(s) may simply be too small to detect.

F. Potential problems

1. Size of the lesion. Sensitivity for detection falls off for smaller lesions, especially those <500 mg.

2. False-positive and false-negative results. Thyroid adenomas, thyroid cancer and parathyroid cancer may simulate parathyroid adenomas. The relative uptake and washout of thallium/sestamibi and pertechnetate/^{123}I in areas of thyroid disease may be different, simulating or masking a parathyroid abnormality.

3. Parathyroid hyperplasia. Parathyroid imaging is less sensitive in the evaluation of hyperplasia. Four-gland hyperplasia with one dominant gland may appear as a single adenoma.

4. Patient motion and other technical difficulties. If sequential images are obtained, patient motion between scans may cause computer-subtracted images to be misaligned, simulating a parathyroid adenoma or hyperplasia. Computer subtraction techniques can be technically difficult and may lead to error.

5. Thyroid medications and recent iodinated contrast. These may interfere with ^{99m}Tc-pertechnetate or ^{123}I images necessary for thyroid subtraction.

II. SINGLE RADIOTRACER DUAL-PHASE SCAN

A. Background

Technetium-99m-sestamibi can be the sole imaging agent in a parathyroid scan. Although this method probably has slightly less sensitivity than subtraction techniques, it is easier to perform. The addition of SPECT increases detection rates, especially for ectopic foci.

B. Radiopharmaceuticals

Technetium-99m-sestamibi (Cardiolite) used as the only radiotracer relies on the fact that sestamibi washes out of normal thyroid tissue faster than it does from abnormal parathyroid adenomas and hyperplasia. This differential increases with time, so delayed images are usually compared with early ones. In addition, the presence of hypercalcemia decreases metabolism and suppresses sestamibi uptake in normal glands. As noted above, there is less experience with ^{99m}Tc-tetrofosmin (Myoview) in parathyroid scanning.

C. How the study is performed

The radiotracer (5–25 mCi [185–925 MBq] adult dose) is injected intravenously and a set of immediate images are obtained at 5–15 min, followed by delayed imaging at 2–5 hr. Imaging usually takes no more than 30 min for planar and pinhole images, or up to 1 hr if SPECT is also performed. Unlike subtraction techniques, no complicated postprocessing or subtraction methods are required.

D. Patient preparation

No preparation is needed. Iodinated contrast and thyroid medications will not interfere with this examination. As with subtraction techniques, it is best not to schedule this study within the first few weeks after neck surgery. A detailed thyroid and parathyroid medical and surgical history will aid in scan interpretation.

E. Understanding the report

Criteria for a positive scan include increased focal relative uptake compared with thyroid tissue on early images, delayed images or both. Some interpreters will consider a scan positive only if the early focus persists or becomes more prominent on delayed images. The location of the abnormality will be described as well as its appearance on early and delayed sequences. Ectopic foci also will be identified.

F. Potential problems

Lower sensitivity for small lesions, potential for false-positive and false-negative results and reduced sensitivity for parathyroid hyperplasia are potential problems (see Subtration scan, Potential problems, above). In addition, adenomas can have relatively rapid washout of radiotracer, with even faster washout from hyperplasia. Thus, the parathyroid abnormalities may only be visible on the early images. Strict positive criteria, requiring relatively increased visibility on delayed images, may result in a false-negative study.

CLINICAL QUESTIONS

1. Primary hyperparathyroidism: What is involved in the initial evaluation?

The search for a parathyroid adenoma or hyperplasia should only be undertaken after careful biochemical confirmation of disease. Traditionally, the next step in evaluation has been surgery. Results of studies at academic medical centers with experienced parathyroid surgeons indicate that careful neck exploration and identification of all four parathyroid glands yields a 92–95% cure rate. The most recent (1990) National Institutes of Health consensus conference dealing with this subject concluded that preoperative imaging localization was not indicated before initial surgery. Yet, preoperative imaging localization increasingly is used in clinical practice since the advent of the sestamibi techniques. A recent meta-analysis reported 91% sensitivity and 99% specificity of well-performed sestamibi preoperative localization scans. Because 85%

of primary hyperparathyroidism can be cured by removing a single adenoma, the preoperative use of sestamibi localization can lead to less extensive surgery, such as unilateral exploration, which has been demonstrated to save operative and patient hospitalization time and cost. Outpatient "key hole" surgery under local anesthesia also has been advocated in selected patients. These less-invasive techniques can be combined with preoperative methylene blue administration, which allows the surgeon to locate the parathyroid glands more easily. They also can be combined with intraoperative rapid serum parathyroid hormone measurements and the use of an intraoperative gamma detecting probe to confirm adenoma removal.

Confident preoperative localization may enable the surgeon to streamline his or her approach, even with a traditional four-quadrant exploration; for example, a likely adenoma can be removed quickly with simple visual inspection of the other glands instead of biopsies with frozen sections. The other major advantage of preoperative parathyroid adenoma scanning is identification of a potential ectopic adenoma in the mediastinum or elsewhere, remote from the surgical field, thus sparing the patient unnecessary neck surgery.

Once the decision has been made for preoperative localization, what type of study should be performed? Nuclear imaging, MRI, ultrasound, CT or angiography can be used. Nuclear imaging using ^{99m}Tc-sestamibi is a simple and reliable modality. It is the only technique that combines functional information and extensive anatomic coverage, allowing evaluation for adenomas in the neck and mediastinum. CT is a good problem-solving tool, especially in confirming mediastinal ectopia, but it is neither sensitive nor specific for juxta or intrathyroidal parathyroid tumors, requires iodinated contrast and is prone to artifact from the patient's shoulders. Ultrasound is excellent in experienced hands, but it is operator dependent and cannot evaluate for ectopic mediastinal foci. Some centers have reported superior results with MRI, but it is more expensive than nuclear scanning and is often used if the nuclear study is unrevealing or equivocal. Angiography and selective venous sampling may be helpful if performed by a radiologist who is expert in these techniques, but they are highly invasive and usually reserved for problem-solving situations when other tests are negative. Adenomas are easier to identify than hyperplasia with all modalities. If an ectopic mediastinal focus is seen on nuclear imaging, it should be correlated with CT or MRI before thoracotomy. Combining nuclear imaging with ultrasound or MRI yields the highest accuracy, but it is probably only cost-effective in high-risk or reoperative patients.

Although there has been consensus on the utility of sestamibi over thallium, there is none for subtraction versus dual-phase sestamibi scanning. It is more important that one protocol is chosen in a cooperative effort between nuclear imaging specialists and interested clinicians and that correlation is carried out with surgical and pathology results (Fig. 1).

In summary, although surgical exploration traditionally has been the next step after biochemical confirmation of primary hyperparathyroidism, preoperative localization of parathyroid adenomas with sestamibi scanning tech-

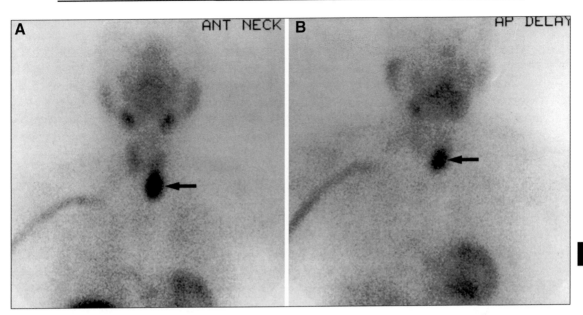

Figure 1. Immediate (A) and delayed images (B) from a dual-phase sestamibi parathyroid scan demonstrate an adenoma in the left inferior parathyroid gland (arrows).

niques increasingly is used to help streamline surgery and to detect ectopic adenomas.

2. Persistent hyperparathyroidism after surgery: Is it ectopic adenoma?

Persistent or recurrent hyperparathyroidism occurs in 5–8% of postsurgical patients. Reoperation can challenge the most experienced surgeon and carries a risk of higher morbidity and a lower success rate, due in part to 20–30% ectopia in this population. There is universal agreement that at least one imaging modality should be used preoperatively. Either nuclear imaging or MRI can evaluate the postsurgical neck and locate ectopic glands. The nuclear scan is preferred because it is just as sensitive as MRI but more specific and less expensive (Fig. 2). Imaging should take place after local inflammation from previous surgery has resolved. Some advocate combining nuclear scanning with MRI for maximal preoperative accuracy.

3. Is nuclear imaging effective for secondary hyperparathyroidism?

Secondary hyperparathyroidism, mostly due to renal failure, usually is treated medically. When surgery is performed, a subtotal parathyroidectomy or total parathyroidectomy with autologous parathyroid reimplantation is done. Imaging procedures are usually not useful preoperatively because they will not change the nature of the surgery.

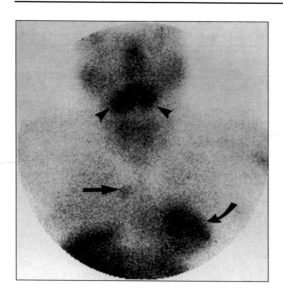

Figure 2. An ectopic adenoma (straight arrow) is localized in the mediastinum on this sestamibi dual-phase scan; this discovery spared the patient unnecessary neck surgery. Uptake also is present in the heart (curved arrow) and salivary glands (arrowheads).

WORTH MENTIONING

1. Autologous reimplantation

There is a 14% incidence of recurrent hyperparathyroidism in patients undergoing parathyroidectomy with autologous reimplantation. Nuclear imaging techniques can be helpful in determining if residual hyperfunctioning parathyroid tissue is present in the neck or if the transplanted tissue is hyperfunctioning.

2. PET

PET with various radiotracers such as fluorodeoxyglucose (FDG) is being investigated in parathyroid localization.

3. Antibody imaging

Research is ongoing in developing a parathyroid scan using monoclonal antibodies to human parathyroid surface antigen.

4. Coregistration

Digital fusion of SPECT and MRI may be helpful in correlating functional with anatomic localization.

5. Multiple endocrine neoplasia syndrome

Primary hyperparathyroidism can be part of a hereditary multiple endocrine neoplasia syndrome. If this is suspected, a full four-gland exploration should be performed.

PATIENT INFORMATION

I. THE PARATHYROID SCAN

A. Test/Procedure

Your doctor has ordered a parathyroid scan to determine the source of the problem with your parathyroid glands that may be causing your elevated calcium. A small amount of radioactive material called a tracer will be injected into your vein. Depending on how the scan is done, you may undergo one or two injections and you may be asked to swallow a pill containing a small amount of radioactive iodine. You will be positioned next to a special machine called a gamma camera, which doesn't produce radiation but detects radiation that is coming from the injected tracer in your body. A series of pictures of your neck will then be taken, and you may have to return for delayed pictures. The whole process may take 1–6 hr depending on the test specifics.

10

B. Preparation

Depending on how the scan is done, you may be asked to withhold medications that affect your thyroid gland, and to stop eating a few hours before the test (water and other medications are permitted). Otherwise, you may eat and drink as usual. Please ask your doctor to give you detailed instructions, especially if you are taking thyroid medications. Also inform the nuclear imaging physician or technologist if you have had a radiology study with intravenous contrast dye in the past 4–6 wk or have had surgery or other problems involving the thyroid or parathyroid glands.

C. Radiation and other risks

The amount of radiation used is small and similar to that given for other diagnostic x-ray tests. The effective adult radiation dose to your whole body from a typical examination is the dose the average person living in the United States receives in 1–3 yr from cosmic rays and naturally occurring background radiation sources. The radiation dose is about 5–15% of the yearly dose considered safe for doctors and technologists who work with radiation. You can be around other people and use a bathroom normally without risk to others.

D. Pregnancy

If you are pregnant or think you could be pregnant, inform your doctor so that this can be discussed with the nuclear medicine physician.

References

1. Greenspan BS, Brown ML, Dillehay GL, et al. Procedure guideline for parathyroid scintigraphy. *J Nucl Med* 1998;39:1111–1114. (Also *Society of Nuclear Medicine Procedure Guidelines Manual 1999.* Society of Nuclear Medicine: Reston, VA. 1999:19–24.)

2. Udelsman R. Parathyroid imaging: the myth and the reality. *Radiology* 1996;201:317–318.

3. Shaha AR, Sarkar S, Strashun A, Yeh S. Sestamibi scan for preoperative localization in primary hyperparathyroidism. *Head Neck* 1997;19:87–91.

4. Gordon BM, Gordon L, Hoang K, Spicer KM. Parathyroid imaging with ^{99m}Tc-sestamibi. *AJR Am J Roentgenol* 1996;167:1563–1568.

5. Ishibashi M, Nishida H, Hiromatsu Y, et al. Comparison of techenetium-99m-MIBI, techenetium-99m-tetrofosmin, ultrasound and MRI for localization of abnormal parathyroid glands. *J Nucl Med* 1998;39:320–324.

6. Denham DW, Norman J. Cost-effectiveness of preoperative sestamibi scan for primary hyperparathyroidism is dependent solely upon the surgeon's choice of operative procedure. *J Am Coll Surg* 1998;186:293–305.

7. Norman JG, Jaffray CE, Chheda H. The false-positive parathyroid sestamibi. A real or perceived problem and a case for radioguided parathyroidectomy. *Ann Surg* 2000;231:31–37.

10

11
The Skeletal System

Bone scanning evaluates bone physiology and skeletal anatomy and is one of the most common applications of nuclear imaging. SPECT provides improved sensitivity and even greater anatomic detail in a three-dimensional format. With continued technologic advances, the role of nuclear imaging is changing in patient workup and should be viewed as complementary to plain x-rays, CT and MRI in effective patient diagnosis. This chapter examines nuclear imaging as it relates to neoplasia, bone pain, skeletal trauma, bone viability and systemic diseases. Osteomyelitis is discussed in Chapter 6, Infection Imaging.

11

SCANS AND PRIMARY CLINICAL INDICATIONS

I. Bone scan Page 211

- To detect and follow up bone metastases

- To determine if a fracture is present

- To investigate the cause of unexplained bone or back pain

- To evaluate the significance of a bone lesion discovered on plain x-rays

- To diagnose avascular necrosis

- To investigate possible child abuse or the cause of limping in a child

- To determine the cause of joint prosthesis pain

- To establish viability of a bone graft

- To find the cause of delayed fracture healing

- To help diagnose and follow up activity of Paget's disease

- To ascertain if reflex sympathetic dystrophy is present

- To gauge the maturity of heterotopic ossification for surgical excision

II. Tumor imaging: Thallium, sestamibi, or fluorodeoxyglucose (FDG)

- To follow up the activity of a bone or soft-tissue tumor after therapy

CLINICAL QUESTIONS

Ordering the scan

Potential cancer

Pain

Preoperative and postoperative

11

SCANS

I. BONE SCAN

A. Background

The radionuclide bone scan is the cornerstone of skeletal nuclear imaging. Although the appearance of bones on plain x-rays depends on the skeletal mineral content, radionuclide bone scanning provides physiologic information, depicting blood flow to bone and bone metabolism or turnover. High sensitivity coupled with the ability to survey the entire skeletal system without added radiation give the radionuclide bone scan broad clinical utility. Although the bone scan lacks specificity, a specific diagnosis often can be made when the bone scan is correlated with plain films and other imaging. The standard bone scan typically is used for whole-body surveys such as those performed for metastatic disease. The three-phase bone scan can evaluate blood flow and soft-tissue uptake, in addition to bone uptake, and is used primarily to evaluate focal areas for suspected osteomyelitis, fracture and tumor.

B. Radiopharmaceuticals

Technetium-99m-diphosphonates are the agents of choice for bone imaging. The radiopharmaceutical is injected intravenously and is distributed via blood flow throughout the body. It passively diffuses into the extravascular and extracellular spaces and binds to the hydration shell around the bone crystal. Unbound radiotracer clears from the plasma via urinary excretion. Delayed images will demonstrate the radionuclide bound to the bone crystal, depicting the skeletal system. Imaging is delayed for 2–3 hr after injection to obtain the high bone-to-background ratio needed for optimal image quality. The greater the blood flow and metabolic activity of a particular bone region, the higher the up-take of radionuclide.

C. How the study is performed

There are two types of bone scans: the standard delayed scan and the three-phase scan. Typically, for both types of scans, the patient is encouraged to drink liquids and urinate frequently between the time of injection and delayed imaging to increase soft-tissue elimination of radiotracer. The patient also will be asked to empty the bladder before delayed whole-body imaging and will be given wipes to prevent urine contamination of skin and clothing.

Standard bone scan. The radiotracer is injected intravenously (20–30 mCi [740–1110 MBq] adult dose), and delayed views of the entire skeleton are obtained 2–5 hr later.

Three-phase bone scan. As the radiotracer is injected, rapid sequence flow images are obtained of the area in question (angiographic phase). Only one region can undergo flow imaging per scan (i.e., foot or hand, but not both). Ten-minute delayed static images are then acquired, which are called "blood pool" or "soft-tissue uptake" images. These first two phases usually take no longer than 30 min to complete. Delayed images of the region in question are then obtained, typically 2–5 hr later. It is not unusual for the entire skeleton to be imaged 2–5 hr later in addition to the area of clinical concern. Imaging may take as little as 10–20 min to complete or up to 2 hr if SPECT or other special views are required. Occasionally, further delayed images up to 24 hr later may be required.

D. Patient preparation

No special preparation is required, and there are no dietary restrictions. Good hydration may improve image quality, and the patient should be encouraged to drink fluids. In addition, he or she should be informed that this is not a quick examination and that a 2–5 hr delay between injection and imaging should be expected. As always, outside correlative studies should be made available to the nuclear medicine physician.

E. Understanding the report

A normal bone scan will demonstrate the axial and appendicular skeletal system. The nuclear medicine physician will be familiar with the expected appearance, including normal patterns in children who have increased uptake in physeal growth centers. In addition, thyroid cartilage, kidneys and bladder usually are seen (Fig. 1).

If the patient had a three-phase scan, angiographic blood flow and soft-tissue activity are described. The delayed bone uptake, which is imaged at 2–5 hr, de-

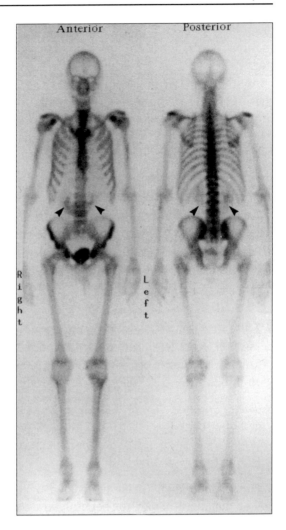

Figure 1. Anterior and posterior views from a normal bone scan with an incidentally noted horseshoe kidney (arrowheads).

pends on blood flow to the area and osteoblastic activity. A hot focus is one that demonstrates more uptake than expected. It is seen with such processes as fracture, osteomyelitis, neoplasia, later stage osteonecrosis and arthritis, including degenerative joint disease. Increased blood flow to the region also may cause adjacent but unaffected bone to have some degree of increased uptake. A cold lesion demonstrates less than expected focal uptake and may be seen with highly lytic lesions and tumor necrosis, early osteonecrosis, delayed sequela of radiation therapy and metallic foreign bodies.

Interpretative criteria. Interpretation depends on the clinical question to be answered and often relies on specific patterns of uptake. The report will delineate areas of increased or decreased uptake, correlate with other imaging if available (or recommend other imaging for correlation) and come to a conclusion about the clinical question. Soft-tissue or extra-osseous uptake, if present, also will be described. Soft-tissue uptake is caused by a host of factors, including inflammation and calcification, mucinous and other neoplasia, muscle necrosis, and myositis.

Another pattern that may be described is the so-called superscan in which there is intense diffuse abnormal uptake throughout the skeletal system, giving the appearance of a super-normal scan. This pattern may be caused by diffuse widespread blastic metastases such as from prostate cancer or metabolic bone disease such as hyperparathyroidism.

F. Potential problems

1. Lack of specificity. Although the bone scan is highly sensitive, increased uptake is the result of blood flow and osteoblastic activity. These are nonspecific processes that may be increased because of neoplasia, infection, trauma and arthritides. Pattern recognition by a trained nuclear medicine physician and correlation with other examinations transforms nonspecific uptake to a specific diagnosis.

2. Persistent uptake. Because bone scanning is sensitive, increased uptake may persist for years after trauma, infection and surgery. This potential for an abnormality to persist on bone scanning may make evaluation of that same region difficult if a baseline scan is not available for comparison.

3. The young and the old. Elderly patients may take 2–7 days to manifest a positive bone scan after fracture because of delayed osteoblastic response. Infants younger than 1 mo of age do not have as avid skeletal tracer uptake compared with older children and adults.

4. Flare phenomenon. In the period of 3–6 mo after chemotherapy, hormonal therapy or radiation therapy for bone metastases, increased uptake in known lesions and even foci of new uptake may be seen because of a healing response rather than worsening disease. This is most commonly seen in breast and prostate cancer. Serial scanning and correlating scan findings with the patient's condition will allow differentiation of the flare phenomenon from increased disease.

5. Etidronate. This bisphosphonate may block uptake of the bone imaging radiopharmaceutical and lead to a poor quality or nondiagnostic bone scan.

II. TUMOR IMAGING: THALLIUM, SESTAMIBI OR FDG

A. Background

Thallium and sestamibi have been used to evaluate tumor extent and response to therapy, taking advantage of their propensity to localize in high-grade neoplastic cells and not in tumor necrosis. Sestamibi results in more detailed images, but there is more clinical experience with thallium scanning in tumors.

FDG scanning probably will replace thallium and sestamibi for tumor evaluation. Although PET scanning is only available at limited locations, coincidence SPECT systems adapted to gamma cameras and centralized delivery of FDG are making this technology more widely available. FDG is a glucose analog that localizes to a greater extent in active tumor and not in necrotic regions but suffers from a certain lack of specificity. Uptake has been described with inflammation, fracture and other benign processes. Absolute quantitation can be performed that can characterize and stage tumors. (See Chapter 15, Introduction to Cancer and FDG Imaging for more details.)

CLINICAL QUESTIONS

1 and 2. Should I order a standard bone scan or a three-phase scan? Should I get a whole-body scan or a scan of a limited area?

The answer to these questions is specific to each clinical situation and may depend on particular institution protocols. In general, a whole-body scan is indicated in a patient with a history of neoplasia, multiple sites of trauma or unexplained bone pain in patients older than 50 yr of age. With problems such as possible focal osteomyelitis, a three-phase scan clearly is indicated. For focal local trauma or pain, a three-phase scan often is helpful but not critical because the important information will be present on delayed images. A whole-body scan does not expose the patient to any additional radiation but requires a little extra time and is more expensive than a limited-area scan.

3 and 4. Does a patient have skeletal metastases? When should I get a bone scan for cancer staging?

Thirty percent of patients with cancer will develop skeletal metastases. This is the most common indication for the radionuclide bone scan. There is no better examination for rapidly and cost-effectively surveying the entire skeletal system for the presence of osseous metastases. It is an easy test to undergo, has no contraindications and is sensitive. Most metastatic processes will manifest an abnormality on bone scan, either increased or decreased uptake. Yet, bone scanning is not necessary or indicated in all neoplastic evaluations.

The finding of multiple asymmetric foci of increased uptake in the axial and appendicular skeleton is characteristic of osseous metastases (Fig. 2). Other processes may have multifoci of increased uptake that can be mistaken for metastatic disease. Correlation with plain x-rays and other imaging modalities, pattern recognition and the judicious use of follow-up studies are important in arriving at the proper diagnosis.

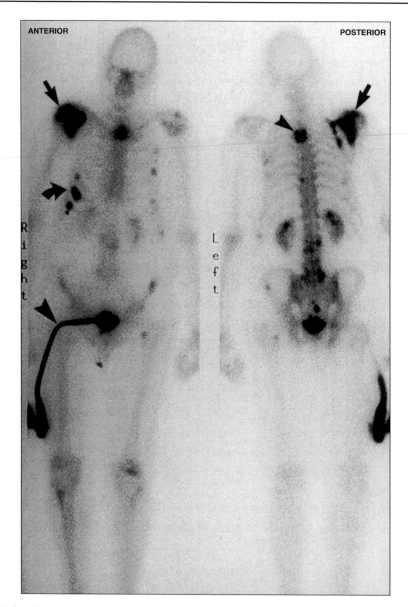

Figure 2. Anterior and posterior images from a bone scan in a patient with prostate cancer demonstrate extensive osseous metastases, including intense uptake in the right shoulder (arrows), right anterior ribs (curved arrow) and upper thoracic spine (small arrowhead). Foci of less intense uptake also are noted elsewhere in the spine and ribs, sacrum, left iliac bone and proximal left femur. A suprapubic bladder catheter is present (large arrowhead).

Bone scanning in prostate, breast, lung and other cancers. The initial evaluation of prostate cancer traditionally has included bone scanning because of its high sensitivity. With the advent of prostate-specific antigen (PSA) serum testing, the role of the bone scan has changed. If the PSA is <10 ng/ml, there is a low likelihood of bony metastases. The recommendation is to obtain a bone scan to exclude metastatic disease if the PSA is >10, if there is a high Gleason histologic grade, a high clinical stage or symptoms suggestive of metastatic disease. A baseline bone scan can be helpful in patients with a history of trauma or arthritis to enable comparison with subsequent bone scans that may be obtained because of new pain or rising PSA.

Breast cancer also metastasizes frequently to bone, including local invasion of the sternum. The role of the bone scan in this disease has been somewhat controversial. The recommendation is not to obtain a bone scan in an asymptomatic patient with a small, low-stage, primary tumor. If the patient has bone pain, has laboratory values suggestive of metastatic disease or is in clinical stage 3 or 4, a bone scan should be obtained.

In non–small-cell bronchogenic cancer, a bone scan is recommended if curative surgery is contemplated and there is no evidence of other metastatic disease or if there is clinical or laboratory evidence of bone metastases. Small-cell lung cancer frequently metastasizes to bone, and a bone scan often is included as part of the routine workup.

For renal cell cancer, routine bone scanning in the absence of clinical and laboratory findings is not indicated but should be used when the patient is symptomatic or when a change in therapy is contemplated. Many surgeons advocate nephrectomy even in the presence of bone metastases.

Neuroblastoma is another nonprimary bone neoplasm in which bone scanning commonly is performed for screening in conjunction with the use of metaiodobenzylguanidine (MIBG) or Octreoscan (see Chapter 16, Neuroendocrine Tumors). If there is focal skeletal pain, plain x-rays should first be obtained, followed by CT or MRI as necessary.

The possibility of thyroid cancer bone and soft-tissue metastases is investigated routinely with ^{131}I. Bone scanning may be useful in specific clinical situations. Bone scanning is not routine for lymphoma or leukemia. Gallium or FDG scanning is more useful to detect osseous and soft-tissue lesions for lymphoma. The bone scan is standard in the metastatic workup of Ewing's sarcoma and osteosarcoma. (Multiple myeloma is discussed in Clinical Question 6, below.)

Bone scanning versus MRI in the evaluation of bone metastases. Each has advantages and disadvantages, and they should be considered complementary, rather than competing modalities. The most important advantage of bone scanning is that the entire skeletal system can be surveyed with ease and little expense. This cannot be done with MRI. Bone scanning can be performed when there are contraindications to MRI such as a pacemaker and certain vascular clips. Bone scanning more easily evaluates the skull, ribs and extremities. MRI is considered more sensitive and specific for most marrow processes, although other imaging modalities as well as biopsy may be required. In scanning the spine and pelvis, MRI is more accurate in differentiating benign from malignant abnormalities. For patients with acute neurologic deficits and a history of cancer, urgent MRI is necessary to evaluate for spinal cord compression, which may require emergency radiotherapy or surgery.

Summary. Bone scanning should be used routinely to aid in the evaluation of stage 3 and 4 breast cancer, prostate cancer with PSA >10, non–small-cell bronchogenic cancer when curative surgery is considered, neuroblastoma, Ewing's and osteosarcoma and small-cell lung cancer. It is also useful and efficient for any clinical stage cancer in a patient with nonlocalizable or diffuse bone pain or laboratory findings suggestive of bone metastases. If the patient has focal bone pain or local back pain or neurologic symptoms, primary evaluation with plain x-rays or MRI is probably more cost-effective. MRI may be required urgently to determine if spinal cord compression is present. For cancer that can spread to bone, a negative bone scan has important prognostic implications and can serve as a baseline in case of future bone pain, especially in patients with a history of trauma or arthritis.

5. Can the bone scan be used to follow up the activity of skeletal metastatic disease?

The activity of metastatic disease can be followed up with bone scanning. Plain x-rays may demonstrate lesions even after successful treatment because the bone may continue to remodel. If there is absent activity on a formerly positive bone scan after treatment, this is a strong indicator of disease regression. Irradiated bone initially may show increased uptake due to osteitis but then decreased uptake in the radiation port for up to several years afterward. (See Potential Problem 4, Flare Phenomenon, above.)

Follow-up intervals are usually institution- and protocol-specific. After radical prostatectomy for prostate cancer, PSA should drop to near zero. Thus, routine follow-up bone scanning usually is performed only in face of a rising PSA or new bone symptoms. Also, PSA may not be a reliable indicator of progressive disease when the patient is on hormonal therapy. For other types of cancer including that of the breast, bone scanning is the first choice for routine follow-up in asymptomatic patients, as well as in those with diffuse bone pain or abnormal laboratory values. In a patient with focal back pain or neurologic symptoms, MRI should be the initial modality.

6. Is bone scanning appropriate for multiple myeloma?

The bone scan is most sensitive in detecting hot lesions with an osteoblastic component. Yet, multiple myeloma lesions tend to be lytic, and many lesions elicit little, if any, osteoblastic response. These cold multiple myeloma defects are less conspicuous on bone scanning. Thus, the plain x-rays are still considered most appropriate for multiple myeloma. A bone scan may be helpful for local pain when plain x-rays are negative, but MRI is considered far more sensitive for focal questions. MRI is also the best method to evaluate the spine.

7 and 8. What is the significance of an incidentally discovered bone lesion on plain x-rays? What is the likelihood that a solitary lesion on bone scan represents a metastasis in a patient with a known or suspected malignancy?

X-rays, CT and MRI are the mainstays of noninvasively diagnosing a bone tumor. The likelihood that a solitary lesion on bone scan represents a metastatic focus varies with clinical history, as well as location and appearance of the abnormality. Correlation with plain x-rays is important in making this distinction. For example, in a patient with a known malignancy, a solitary lesion on a bone scan in a vertebra or in the pelvis will represent metastatic disease 60–70% of the time, but this likelihood decreases to almost zero if the abnormality correlates to a benign finding on plain x-rays such as degenerative disease.

Benign and malignant bone lesions run the gamut from faint to intense uptake on bone scanning. Although bone scanning alone may not distinguish a benign from malignant process, it can be helpful in evaluating a potential abnormality and in determining if there are single or multiple lesions. For example, a bone scan may be performed to differentiate a bone island that has little or no uptake from a blastic metastasis that will exhibit greater uptake and often presents as one of many lesions.

9. Is nuclear imaging helpful in the staging and follow-up of primary bone tumors?

Primary bone tumors such as osteosarcoma and Ewing's sarcoma are more common in the pediatric age group. MRI is considered the procedure of choice in preoperative staging of local bone and soft-tissue involvement. Although the three-phase bone scan is sensitive because of intensely increased flow, soft-tissue and delayed uptake, it overestimates local extent of disease. Because bone scanning is sensitive in detecting skip lesions and metastatic foci, it is included as part of the standard workup.

Bone scanning may demonstrate nonspecific increased uptake in the tumor bed after surgery, chemotherapy or radiation therapy. Flare phenomenon also may occur. (See Potential Problem 4, Flare Phenomenon.) Persistent increased uptake at the treatment site 6–12 mo after therapy, compared with a post-therapy baseline, is considered suspicious for local recurrence. A negative scan has good prognostic implications. CT and MRI are not optimal for monitoring local recurrence because of the difficulty in distinguishing necrosis and fibrosis from recurrent tumor. Thallium, sestamibi or FDG tumor imaging seem to provide an excellent means to monitor response to therapy, in conjunction with a pretherapy baseline scan. Successful treatment and decreased tumor burden correlates with decreased to absent uptake on these tumor-imaging scans.

10. What is the cause of a patient's bone pain?

Bone scanning is an excellent screening examination for bone pain, especially diffuse pain or ill-defined symptoms. Yet it should not be used in isolation. Each situation must be judged on the basis of individual history and physical examination. With focal pain, especially after trauma, it is mandatory to begin the evaluation with a plain x-ray. A plain x-ray is relatively inexpensive and may obviate bone scanning. If the plain x-ray is not revealing, bone scan may be an appropriate next study to evaluate for traumatic fracture, stress fracture, avascular necrosis, primary tumor, occult metastasis (especially in patients over 50 years old), infection, shin splints, avulsion fractures and a host of other possibilities. MRI may be more accurate and cost-effective in some situations, especially if a soft-tissue component is strongly suspected. CT may allow definitive characterization of an abnormality on plain x-rays.

A bone scan is uniquely suited to determine the true cause of the patient's pain in the presence of other possible causes such as degenerative disease or old trauma discovered on plain x-rays. For example, pain often is referred to the pelvis region and upper chest/shoulders. Just because a patient has degenerative disease of the hips, does not mean that a sacral insufficiency fracture may not be present that can be classically defined with bone scan. In summary, although one generally should begin with plain x-ray evaluation, the bone scan is an excellent tool for screening because of its sensitivity and may suggest other studies.

11. Bone pain: Is a post-traumatic fracture present?

The nuclear bone scan is highly sensitive in the evaluation of fractures, yet it is not the optimal examination for the rapid and efficient workup of acute trauma. In the setting of acute trauma, plain x-rays should be obtained first. Yet fractures may not be immediately apparent on plain films; the patient can be treated clinically and a follow-up x-ray obtained in 3–5 days.

If a definitive diagnosis is needed immediately, such as establishing the presence of a hip fracture in an elderly patient, MRI is the next logical test. It is sensitive and specific for not only cortical fracture but also bone bruising, as well as soft-tissue injury. If MRI cannot be performed, a bone scan is an excellent choice. Potential false-negative results must be kept in mind though. Although the majority of fractures will manifest a positive three-phase bone scan immediately, it may take up to a week for the scan to become positive in a small percentage of the elderly. The best route of evaluation must be decided on a case by case basis with an understanding of the mechanism of injury.

In a polytrauma situation, bone scan provides excellent whole-body screening and may reveal fractures that initially were missed in the heat of the acute workup (Fig. 3). In addition, bone scanning is more helpful in the regional survey of certain problem areas such as the pelvis and lower extremities, which may be difficult to evaluate because of referred pain. CT scanning also can be useful when plain x-rays are not definitive and is often used in the secondary evaluation of spine and hip fractures, as well as for presurgical planning.

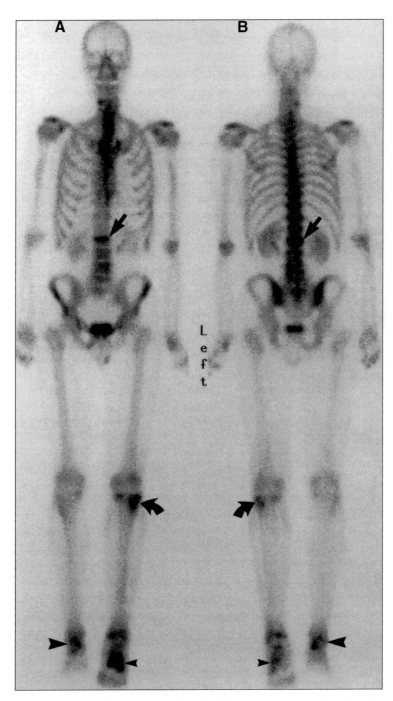

Figure 3. Injured hiker with complaint of "hurting all over." At initial emergency room evaluation, a left ankle fracture was diagnosed with plain x-rays. After experiencing multifocal pain days after the trauma, the patient underwent bone scanning. Anterior (A) and posterior (B) views revealed additional fractures at L2 (arrows), proximal left fibula (curved arrows), left foot (small arrowheads) and right ankle (large arrowheads).

12 and 13. Delayed fracture healing: Is bone scan helpful? Can bone scanning be used to date fractures?

With the clinical question of nonunion, the appearance of the bone scan can help the orthopedic surgeon plan therapy. Reactive nonunion will demonstrate intense activity at the fracture sight and predicts a good response to electrical stimulation. A photon deficient gap may represent atrophic nonunion (which does not respond well to electrical stimulation) and may indicate pseudoarthrosis, interposed soft-tissue or infection, or an impaired blood supply.

Although not usually indicated, the three-phase bone scan can be used to date fractures. The first phase should be positive for the first 3–4 wk, the second phase is positive for the first 8–12 wk, and the delayed phase may be positive for many years after healing, but typically normalizes by 2 yr.

14 and 15. Bone pain: Is a stress or insufficiency fracture present? Bone pain: Is a tibial stress fracture or shin splints present?

In the clinical setting of suspected stress or insufficiency fracture, bone scanning is nearly 100% sensitive and specific and is the preferred whole-body and regional screening choice. If there is focal pain, plain x-rays should be obtained first and may obviate bone scanning. MRI is highly sensitive but less specific. CT is less sensitive and is not a practical method for an extensive regional survey. CT and MRI are excellent problem-solving modalities when the bone scan is equivocal.

The term stress reaction may be used to describe bone remodeling and repair covering the continuum of injury from early periosteal reaction to an overt fracture; it usually manifests as uptake in all three phases of the bone scan with focal intense delayed uptake. There also are characteristic patterns of stress injury/fracture depending on location. In the tibia, increased uptake on all three phases with delayed fusiform uptake in the upper tibia, sometimes extending across the bone, allows differentiation of stress reaction from shin splints, which have less intense, superficial and elongated posteromedial uptake on delayed imaging only (Fig. 4). Sacral insufficiency fractures often manifest with an H-shaped delayed uptake extending across the sacral alae. In addition, a whole-body survey can easily be performed with bone scanning, and may uncover unsuspected additional foci of stress injury.

16. Bone pain: Is AVN present?

Both MRI and bone scanning have been used in the evaluation of AVN in the hips. In the first 7–10 days, AVN will demonstrate a cold defect on delayed bone scan images, but will then transition to increased uptake in the reparative phase. (Flow images are generally not helpful.)

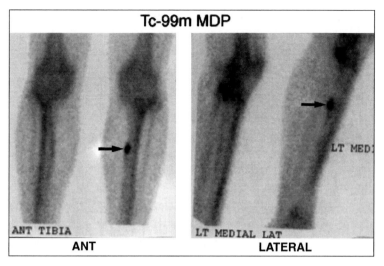

Figure 4. Young female patient with painful left leg after training for an athletic event. Anterior and lateral bone scan images of the lower extremities demonstrate a left tibial stress fracture (arrows).

In the adult hip, AVN usually becomes symptomatic in the reparative phase. Therefore, increased uptake will be seen. Although bone scanning has high sensitivity, it has poor specificity and suffers from relatively poor spatial resolution. MRI is considered the state of the art in the evaluation and grading of hip AVN. Plain x-rays should be obtained first, because classic findings of AVN may obviate more advanced imaging. If MRI cannot be performed, a negative bone scan can exclude anything but the smallest focus of osteonecrosis. It is a rapid and simple examination to perform in the elderly, many of whom cannot hold still for MRI, and may incidentally discover a fracture or other abnormality elsewhere in the pelvis.

In a child in whom there is suspicion of Legg-Calvé-Perthes disease, symptoms usually manifest early, and classic findings of a perfusion defect in the anterolateral femoral head are sought. Imaging should include pinhole views and be performed at a center experienced in pediatric evaluation. It is easier to perform bone scanning than MRI on a child, and the examination is highly sensitive and specific for not only AVN, but also osteomyelitis. Scanning of the entire lower extremities also can be completed without extra radiation exposure.

MRI or bone scanning may be used elsewhere in the skeletal system depending on body part, age of patient and clinical history.

17. Back pain: How is spinal pathology determined?

Bone scanning and MRI play complementary roles in back pain, depending on patient age and clinical presentation. If pain can be localized, initial plain x-rays may be diagnostic. Bone scanning is excellent in evaluating low back, pelvic and hip pain, especially in the elderly, because pain may be referred. It is also useful in surveying the entire back in children, who are more apt to present with nonlocalized pain. Bone scanning with SPECT is highly sensitive in screening for spondylolysis and for osteoid osteoma and can be used to focus subsequent CT and MRI investigations.

For most adult chronic back pain in which disc abnormalities are sought, MRI is the procedure of choice. Bone scanning can be helpful in the differentiation of benign from malignant disease to find if there are multifocal abnormalities characteristic of metastases. CT and MRI are the preferred methods to evaluate individual lesions. In a patient with neurologic symptoms, MRI is also the technique of choice. A myelogram can be performed if MRI is not available or contraindicated.

For the postoperative spine, recurrent or residual disc questions should be evaluated with MRI, but for evaluation of bone grafting and complications such as pseudoarthrosis, bone scan and CT are preferred. Metal fixation devices can interfere with MRI or CT, although they do not present as much of a problem with the bone scan. A normal bone scan is helpful postoperatively. Increased uptake at the lumbar fusion site after 1 yr is consistent with a complication such as pseudoarthrosis. The bone scan also may localize adjacent areas of spinal instability.

18. Bone pain: How can osteoid osteoma be identified?

Bone pain at night relieved with aspirin is the classic history with osteoid osteoma but is not universally present. Plain x-rays should be obtained first, and a positive finding will allow detailed evaluation with CT scanning to look for the nidus. If plain x-rays are unrevealing, a wide region can be surveyed with bone scanning to help focus the search because pain may be referred. This lesion typically demonstrates intense activity on all three phases of a bone scan and may show a focus of more intense uptake within the hot area called the double density sign. Findings should be confirmed with CT before surgery or other intervention is contemplated.

19. How can persistent pain after orthopedic prosthesis be evaluated?

Three-phase bone scanning is useful in the postoperative hip evaluation, although a plain x-ray should be obtained first. The bone scan can help diagnose loosening and heterotopic bone. When combined with radiolabeled white blood cell or gallium scanning, infection also can be investigated (see Chapter 6, Infection Imaging). There are characteristic increased uptake patterns with which the nuclear medicine physician will be familiar. These are based on the type of prosthesis and the time since surgery.

Uptake involving knee replacements and other prostheses is variable. For example, persistent uptake around normal total-knee replacements has been described for years after surgery. Yet a negative scan correlates with a low likelihood of complication. Serial scanning also may be required in some instances of equivocal studies.

20 and 21. Is a bone graft viable? Is a bone fusion solid?

The three-phase bone scan is an excellent technique to noninvasively monitor graft viability. Autologous grafting with revascularization will demonstrate increased uptake on all three phases and should become uniform to adjacent bone as the graft is incorporated. Allografts usually are photon deficient but will fill in with serial imaging.

22. Can bone scanning help with the presurgical evaluation of heterotopic ossification?

The three-phase scan is useful for tracking the maturity of heterotopic ossification. This process manifests with increased flow and uptake even before plain x-ray evidence of calcifications is present. Surgery is delayed until activity is similar to that of adjacent bone. Once this maturity has been ascertained, resection can be performed with less chance of recurrence. Alternatively, a bone marrow scan can be performed that will show uptake in mature heterotopic bone to indicate timing of surgery.

11

23. Is child abuse present?

A combination of bone scanning and plain x-rays is critical in the evaluation of potential child abuse. Bone scanning is useful for surveying the entire skeleton without added radiation, especially for difficult-to-evaluate areas on plain x-rays such as scapula, ribs and sternum. Plain x-rays are helpful to date the fractures, determine type and treatment and exclude bone diseases such as osteogenesis imperfecta. Skull fractures are also easier to document on plain x-rays because they may not evoke a significant osteoblastic response. The bone scan is especially useful with infants who cannot communicate areas of pain, and it can be used to direct plain x-ray evaluation. Of course, negative bone scanning and plain x-rays should not deter additional investigations because not all child abuse involves bone damage.

24. The limping child: Is bone pathology present?

Plain x-rays of the area in question should be obtained first. Limping may be caused by a variety of processes including AVN (Legg-Calvé-Perthes disease), stress reactions and post-traumatic fractures from the lower spine to the pelvis, benign and malignant tumors and infections. If plain x-rays are unrevealing, or a suspected area cannot be identified, bone scanning is the best screening method to survey extensive areas easily, inexpensively and with great sensitivity.

25. Is nuclear imaging helpful with metabolic bone disease?

Bone scanning is not useful for the initial diagnosis of metabolic bone diseases of calcium metabolism such as primary or secondary hyperparathyroidism. Yet, such processes can be suggested from a superscan appearance. Bone scanning is best used to survey for suspected complications of these metabolic diseases such as pseudofractures and brown tumors.

26. Is bone scanning helpful with Paget's disease?

Baseline and serial bone scanning is useful in surveying for Pagetic involvement, in screening for complications such as fracture and sarcoma and in monitoring the efficacy of therapy. The bone scan will be hot in the early osteolytic and osteosclerotic active phases and becomes cooler in later osteosclerotic disease. A sudden increase in activity from baseline images is suspicious for fracture or neoplastic transformation. Paget's disease is 70% polyostotic, and bone scanning can be used to find unsuspected sites before disease can be detected on plain x-rays. Bone scanning is also useful in diagnosis when x-rays are equivocal.

27. Is bone scanning useful to evaluate arthritis?

Bone scanning is sensitive for most arthritic processes, but it is not specific. Usually arthritis will cause diffuse periarticular uptake. A whole-body bone scan survey can be performed in one sitting, and it can be used in the identification of areas that represent active disease and in the assessment of response to treatment. Yet nuclear imaging has not found widespread use because most clinicians can assess the arthritides effectively with a combination of clinical history, physical examination, laboratory tests and plain x-rays. The bone scan may be valuable as a problem-solving tool in some situations, such as those that involve documenting joint pain from osteoarthritis even before the joint appears abnormal on plain x-rays.

28. Is reflex sympathetic dystrophy present?

There is no pathological standard or well-defined clinical criteria for reflex sympathetic dystrophy. Bone scan patterns depend on the extremity and the stage of the disease. From 0–6 mo, increased flow and delayed periarticular uptake is characteristic. At 6 mo to a year, perfusion returns to normal, but the delayed uptake pattern persists. After a year, decreased flow and normalization of delayed uptake is described. Plain x-ray evaluation is neither sensitive nor specific, and MRI is of little value. Although the above patterns have been described in the hand, there is much less agreement on diagnostic criteria in the foot and knee. Thus, with early scanning, in appropriately screened patients, the three-phase bone scan has high sensitivity and specificity in diagnosing reflex sympathetic dystrophy of the hand. With longer duration of symptoms and in other extremities, nuclear imaging is not as helpful, reflecting confusion about this disease process.

WORTH MENTIONING

1. Bone marrow (sulfur colloid) scan

Because bone marrow is so well imaged by MRI, use of the sulfur colloid scan is limited. Some applications include correlation with radiolabeled white blood cell scans for potential prosthesis infection, the differentiation of osteomyelitis from bone infarcts in patients with sickle cell anemia and the evaluation of marrow expansion processes such as myelofibrosis with myeloid metaplasia. Any marrow-replacing process such as tumor, infarct or abscess that is of sufficient size and focalization will result in a cold defect.

2. Amputation

Bone scanning can help the surgeon delineate viable from nonviable bone in preparation for amputation.

3. Rhabdomyolysis

Bone scanning is a sensitive indicator of muscle death, demonstrating increased uptake in soft tissue. Technetium-99m-pyrophosphate has been used for infarct imaging of the heart and brain. Pyrophosphate imaging also may be helpful to assess the degree of muscle necrosis after electrical injury.

4. Multiple myeloma

Thallium, sestamibi and FDG scanning show promise in whole-body evaluation of multiple myeloma lesions.

5. ^{18}F fluoride

Fluorine-18-fluoride, a positron emitter, was once the most commonly used bone scanning agent but was replaced by the more practical technetium diphosphonates. With the increasing availability of PET and coincidence detection systems, this radionuclide may find more use because it produces higher resolution images and is quantifiable. It can also be combined with FDG scanning.

6. Osteoid osteoma

A special nuclear probe may prove useful during surgery to localize the osteoid osteoma nidus, which will concentrate radiotracer.

7. Radiation synovectomy

Beta-emitting radiopharmaceuticals have been used for a number of years to alleviate the pain and swelling of rheumatoid arthritis and other arthritides including psoriatic arthritis and hemophiliac synovitis. The procedure consists of a direct injection of the radiopharmaceutical into the joint capsule, where it is in contact with the inflamed, hyperplastic synovium. As the radionuclide decays, the beta particles deliver a therapeutic dose of radiation to the synovium. The response rate is reported to be high and benefits to the patient include increased joint movement and reduced swelling, effusion and pain.

Most of the radiopharmaceuticals are colloids, and leakage from the joint appears to be minimal. No detectable damage to the articular cartilage has been determined from a recent MRI study. A number of different radionuclides and colloid preparations have been studied widely in Europe and Australia and, to a lesser degree, in the United States. The most commonly used agent is ^{32}P chromic phosphate, but as of 2000 no therapeutic agent has been approved by the United States Food and Drug Administration, and this procedure is not widely available in the United States.

11

PATIENT INFORMATION

I. BONE SCAN
A. Test/Procedure
Your doctor has ordered a bone scan to detect possible bone problems.

A small amount of radioactive material called a tracer will be injected into your vein. You will be asked to return 2–5 hr later, and you will be positioned next to a special machine called a gamma camera, which does not produce radiation but detects radiation that is coming from the injected tracer in your body. A series of pictures of your body will then be taken, which typically takes about 30 min but may take up to 2 hr if special views are required. Sometimes, images also are acquired during the initial injection of tracer.

B. Preparation
No special preparation is required. You may eat and drink as usual and take your medications. You will be asked to drink as much fluid as possible before and after the procedure. Most of the radioactive material not going to the bones leaves your body through the urine. You should empty your bladder as often as you can after the injection and again just before the pictures are taken.

C. Radiation and other risks
The amount of radiation used is small and similar to that given by other diagnostic x-ray tests. The effective adult radiation dose to your whole body from this test is approximately the same the dose the average person living in the United States receives in 2–3 yr from cosmic rays and naturally occurring background radiation sources. The radiation dose is about 15% of the yearly dose considered safe for doctors and technologists who work with radiation. Please

urinate frequently for the day after the test to lessen radiation exposure. You can be around other people and use a bathroom normally without risk to others.

D. Pregnancy

If you are pregnant or think you could be pregnant, inform your doctor so that this can be discussed with the nuclear medicine physician.

References

1. Johnson RP. The role of bone imaging in orthopedic practice. *Semin Nucl Med* 1997;27:386–389.
2. Zrasnow AZ, Hellman RS, Timins ME, Collier BD, Anderson T, Isitman AT. Diagnostic bone scanning in oncology. *Semin Nucl Med* 1997;27:107–141.
3. Connolly LP, Treves ST. Assessing the limping child with skeletal scintigraphy. *J Nucl Med* 1998;39:1056–1061.
4. Fournier RS, Holder LE. Reflex sympathetic dystrophy: diagnostic controversies. *Semin Nucl Med* 1998;28:116–123.
5. Campanacci M, Mercuri M, Gasbarrini A, Campanacci L. The value of imaging in the diagnosis and treatment of bone tumors. *Eur J Radiol* 1998;27(S1):S116–S122.
6. Donohue KJ. Selected topics in orthopedic nuclear medicine. *Orth Clin North Am* 1998;29:85–101.
7. Weissman BN. Imaging of total hip replacement. *Radiology* 1997;202:611–623.
8. Anderson MW, Greenspan A. Stress fractures. *Radiology* 1996;199:1–12.
9. Clunie G, Ell PJ. A survey of radiation synovectomy in Europe. *Eur J Nucl Med* 1995;22:970–976.

11

12
Bone Density

Osteoporosis is a reduction in bone mass and abnormal internal bone architecture. Osteoporotic bone carries an increased risk of fragility fracture. The goal of bone densitometry is to identify those at high risk for fractures so that therapeutic interventions can be instituted to prevent fractures. The bone densitometry measurements can be translated into an estimate of fracture risk. Dual-energy x-ray absorptiometry (DXA) measurements predict fracture risk as well as or even better than cholesterol tests predict risk of heart disease and better than high blood pressure predicts stroke.

SCANS AND PRIMARY CLINICAL INDICATIONS

I. DXA   Page 232

- To diagnose osteoporosis

- To assist in decision for hormonal replacement or other therapy and to motivate patients to be compliant

- To assess fracture risk for premenopausal patients who have risk factors for osteoporosis

- To assess response to therapy

- To evaluate bone density of patients on corticosteroids or being considered for corticosteroid therapy, hyperparathyroidism and primary hyperthyroidism and that of patients receiving thyroxine suppression

CLINICAL QUESTIONS

PATIENT INFORMATION

SCANS

12

I. DXA
A. Background

Approximately 1 in 4 women older than 50 yr and 1 in 8 men older than 50 yr have osteoporosis. Osteoporosis is the cause of 1.5 million fractures each year, including approximately 300,000 broken hips and 700,000 spine fractures in persons older than 50 yr. The cost is about $13.8 billion a year. Women are the major victims of osteoporosis; they have smaller frames and lower peak bone mass (occurs at ages 25–35 yr) than men. At menopause, estrogen dwindles, along with its inhibition of bone resorption and facilitation of calcium absorption. Because of the fall in estrogen, all women lose bone density after menopause at accelerated rates, approximately twice as rapidly as age-matched men.

More than 90% of the gain in bone mass from childhood to adulthood occurs during a 2–3 yr window centered around the adolescent growth spurt, with a bit more gain until the true peak is reached around age 30. The DXA definition of osteoporosis is based on comparison of the patient's DXA to the peak measurements of 30 yr olds. The average woman loses 20% of her bone mass between ages 35 and 70.

B. How the scan is performed

The patient lies quietly on the table for about 10 min while the detector and x-ray tube scan the lumbar spine and/or the hips.

C. Patient preparation

No special preparation is needed, and no restriction of diet or medications is required. The patient should not have had any recent radiographic contrast material, particularly barium, as it may falsely elevate the bone density measurements. Any internal hardware, such as orthopedic hip prostheses or lumbar metal rods will interfere. Specialized software programs to measure bone mineral density (BMD) in regions around a hip prosthesis may be available at some centers.

D. Understanding the report

Defining osteoporosis quantitatively using bone density. Osteoporosis can be defined in terms of a statistical unit of bone density measurements called a T score. The T score expresses the difference between the patient's bone density and that of a healthy 30 yr old (peak bone mass) of the same sex and race as the patient. T scores are expressed as standard deviation (SD) units below or above the mean sex- and race-matched normal 30 yr old. The T score minus 2.5 SD units (World Health Organization [WHO] definition) or 2.0 SDs (National Health and Nutrition Examination Survey [NHANES]) are defined as osteoporosis by those two groups. Both groups agree that for T scores of −1 or higher, bone density is normal. For T scores of −1 to −2.0 (NHANES) or −1 to −2.5 (WHO), the borderline category of osteopenia is defined.

These diagnostic criteria are useful for epidemiologic purposes, but they should not be used to decide if treatment should be given to a particular patient. Rather, bone density should be used along with other relevant information about the patient to decide about management. For example, a 45-yr-old woman and an 80-yr-old woman with the same bone density probably would be treated differently. The relationship between bone mass and fracture risk is a doubling of fracture risk for every SD of reduction in bone mass. Thus, the risk of a hip fracture, for example, can be estimated from BMD measurements.

The BMD report specifies the equipment used and the anatomic region examined. The actual measurements in grams per centimeter (bone mineral content) and grams per square centimeter (bone density) are reported. It compares the patient's BMD to that of members of his/her sex- and race-matched age group (Z score) and to the young normals (T score). The report gives an estimate of fracture risk and lists the problems, if any, that may falsely elevate or alter the accuracy of BMD measurement for the patient. Figure 1 shows the bone density for the lumbar vertebral spine (A) and the hip (B) for two patients measured on different manufacturers' DXA scanners, with the accompanying graph that plots the patient's bone density on the appropriate sex- and race-matched file.

E. Potential problems

Several pitfalls are associated with measuring and using bone mineral densitometry.

1. Falsely elevated measurements. Falsely elevated measurements can result from degenerative bone production or soft-tissue densities (vascular calcifications, other soft-tissue densities related to calcification in an enlarged uterus, tumors, radiographic contrast material in bowel or cerebrospinal fluid). Other

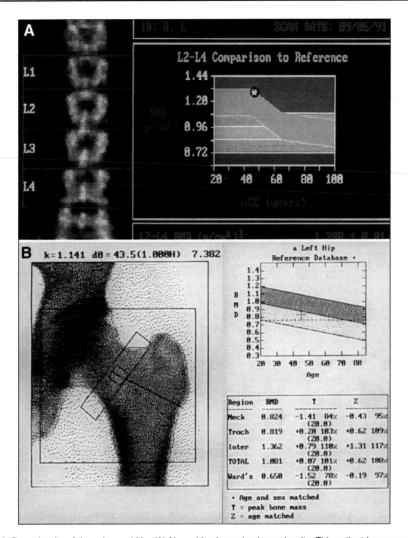

Figure 1. Bone density of the spine and hip. (A) Normal lumbar spine bone density: This patient has normal bone density measured on a Lunar scanner. Her lumbar bone density is 1.29 g/cm²; T score and Z score are positive values. (B) Normal hip bone density. This patient has normal hip bone density measured on a Hologic scanner. On the left, the regions of interest for the femoral neck, trochanter (greater trochanter), intertrochanteric, Ward's (the small square) and the total hip (sum of all regions) are shown. On the right, the plot of the patient's measurement on an age-versus-bone density graph is shown. This patient's T score is +0.07, based on the total hip measurement of 1.08 g/cm².

causes relate to region-of-interest assignment: inclusion of ribs in upper lumbar spine regions or misplacement of assignment of regions of interest over appropriate bone structures, e.g., L1–L4 and hip regions, including neck, trochanteric and total hip.

2. Lateral spine BMD. Lateral spine BMD, in contrast to the conventional frontal projection, can eliminate the undesirable osteoarthritic degenerative changes that are localized primarily at the periphery of the vertebral bodies, as well as the posterior elements. Reference databases for lateral vertebral body bone density have been generated; however, there are other problems, such as the increased and heterogeneous thickness of soft-tissue in the cross-table lateral view, which degrades accuracy and precision of the measurement.

3. Reference databases for T scores, Z scores. Use of inappropriate reference databases for the patient, e.g., a patient of Asian origin compared with a Caucasian patient database, can lead to misinterpretation of the measurement.

4. Use of inappropriate precision to determine significance of a BMD change. Manufacturers' quoted precisions may apply to their own machines, but each machine may be slightly different and each technologist may have his or her unique impact on measured precision values. In general, with DXA equipment, if the precision is 1% or slightly greater, a change of almost 3–4% is needed to be designated as significant with 95% confidence. Over a period of a year, hormone replacement therapy (HRT) or bisphosphonates (Fosamax [alendronate]) may result in a change of up to 3%, and therefore it would seem reasonable to follow up bone density measurements at no less than 18-mo intervals to determine if there is a response to therapy, or even more importantly, no response. Precision may be slightly worse in patients with extreme osteoporosis because of increased difficulty in identifying bone edges for region-of-interest assignment. Patients with scoliosis, who may be more difficult to position well, also may have worse precision. Figure 2 shows the bone density measurements plotted for a man with osteoporosis who was treated with Fosomax. The measurements show nearly a 5% increase in bone density in the spine and 6.3% increase in the hip over a year, a significant increase.

5. Measuring spine BMD in older patients. Using the spine in subjects older than 65 yr with no other sites measured is not advised because of the artifacts caused by frequent osteoarthritic changes in older patients.

6. BMDs on different instruments. BMD results may be slightly different on different machines. To optimize precision, patients should have their sequential studies performed at a single center and on the same machine. Use of different manufacturers' instruments to follow up a patient without correcting the measurements (applying a conversion factor) so that comparisons can be legitimately made should be avoided. Unfortunately, often those corrections are not available.

CLINICAL QUESTIONS

1. What are the risk factors for osteoporosis?

Generic risk factors for osteoporosis (men and women) include: Caucasian or Asian race, thin bones and small stature, family history of osteoporosis, smoking, alcohol abuse, immobility, hypertension, hyperparathyroidism, steroid med-

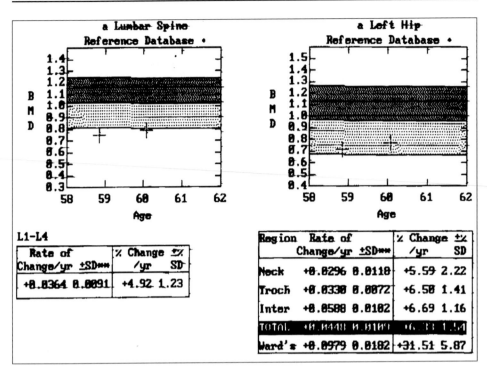

Figure 2. Treated osteoporotic patient: Two bone density measurements approximately 1 yr apart are plotted, showing a significant increase of about 5% in the spine and 6.3% in the hip over 1 yr. These increases are significant for instruments with precision of 1%, or even 2%.

ications, anticonvulsant medications, cancer, suppressive thyroxine therapy, bowel resection and Crohn's disease.

Postmenopausal women. The single most common cause of osteoporosis is estrogen deficiency in postmenopausal women. Estrogen therapy prevents (or reduces) postmenopausal bone loss and fractures and can improve BMD. Of all postmenopausal white women, 20–30% are osteoporotic; after age 80, 70% are osteoporotic. BMD evaluation is appropriate for postmenopausal women before the occurrence of fractures, because the object is to prevent the fractures by identifying individuals at high risk and instituting appropriate therapy. Assessment of fracture risk is not indicated for healthy young people. Women who are on estrogen or other pharmacologic treatment for osteoporosis should have a baseline BMD measurement and follow-up at intervals not less than 1.5 yr and up to 5 yr, depending on BMD results, therapy and risk factors.

Perimenopausal women. Assessment of fracture risk with bone densitometry is particularly helpful for managing women who are undecided about postmenopausal estrogen treatment. It also may be useful for women with major clinical risk factors. It is probably appropriate for all perimenopausal women as an aid in identifying their risk for fracture.

Premenopausal women. BMD measurement is appropriate in patients with medical problems known to increase bone loss, such as hyperthyroidism, suppressive thyroxine therapy, bowel disease, liver disease, amenorrhea, bulimia and anorexia.

Men. Osteoporosis is a substantial problem for older men (75 yr); 25% of all hip fractures occur in men. There are also increasing reports of vertebral fractures associated with masculine osteoporosis. Decreased testosterone (associated with aging, steroids, stress and primary endocrine abnormalities) is a contributing factor. Even though men have higher bone mass and larger bones than women, the persistent loss of bone mass with increasing age results in osteoporosis in men. Men are subject to the same risk factors as women, except for menopause.

2. At what age should men and premenopausal women be screened for osteoporosis?

Premenopausal women and men should be screened at any age when significant risk factors are evident, particularly long-term corticosteroid therapy or hyperparathyroidism. Men who have not had a BMD measurement probably should be screened at age 70, in advance of the reported age for high incidence of fractures in men (75 yr).

12

As premenopausal women approach the perimenopausal age, 45–50, they should have a BMD measurement to provide them with important data that they need for decisions about HRT and other osteoporosis preventive therapy that will be made when they become menopausal. Some investigators advocate that the bone density T score be used to determine if and when osteoporosis therapy should be initiated. If the T score is lower than 2.5 SDs below the mean for sex- and race-matched young adult normals, the patient should be treated. Some investigators recommend that therapy be initiated when the T score is 1.5 SDs below the peak normal level.

3. Suspected osteoporosis: What tests (DXA, ultrasound, quantitive CT) should be ordered?

Standard x-rays are insensitive indicators of osteoporosis of bone. Depending on which bone is imaged, 30–60% of bone mass must be lost before reduced density is evident on an x-ray. Radiographic absorptiometry based on computer analysis of phalangeal density on a hand film using a known density standard allows quantitation and may be useful to assess fracture risk but does not have the same precision or value as DXA. Quantitative CT measures trabecular bone in the vertebral spine but involves higher radiation exposures. It has the advantage of being able to limit the measurement to the trabecular vertebral body bone, minimizing the unwanted effects of degenerative changes. The precision of quantitative CT measurements is not as favorable as DXA, and it is problematic to compare a DXA measurement with a quantitative CT measurement.

Because most BMD measurements are performed with DXA equipment, accurate follow-up is more accessible to the patient if DXA is used.

Ultrasound does not measure bone mass. Instead, it measures speed of sound through bone (broadband ultrasound attenuation), which is a function of bone structure, and stiffness, based on speed of sound and broadband ultrasound attenuation. The advantage offered by ultrasound is that the instruments are small, mobile and less expensive than the gold standard, DXA, and do not involve use of any ionizing radiation. Quantitative ultrasound instruments available in the United States make only peripheral measurements of the calcaneus or tibia for diagnosis of osteoporosis and for follow-up. The disadvantage of ultrasound is its poorer precision compared with DXA. Thus, follow-up studies to detect significant changes in BMD and response to therapy are better done with DXA.

Peripheral bone density testing can be done by quantitative CT of the wrist, peripheral DXA of the wrist or phalanges, quantitative ultrasound of the calcaneus, tibia or phalanges, x-ray absorptiometry of the calcaneus and conventional x-ray absorptiometry of the fingers.

The most reliable test for estimating fracture risk and following response to therapy over time is the BMD measurement using a DXA machine for hip and spine. More expensive screens can be obtained with quantitative CT. Less expensive screens for fracture risk can be obtained using ultrasound or radiographic absorptiometry machines, both of which are small and portable. Radiographic absorptiometry machines, which only require that a finger be inserted into a hole, have been distributed in some shopping malls for the public to use for a fee. These modalities are adequate to screen for fracture risk, but, for the best follow-up, the patient will need to obtain a baseline DXA study.

4. Does a bone density measurement at any one site reflect fracture risk at other sites?

Epidemiologically important fractures (i.e., those associated with particularly high cost to our society) include those of the hip, spine and forearm. Can we assume that decreased bone mineral content in one skeletal site reflects fracture risk at all sites? Correlations between the hip and spine diminish with increasing age because of degenerative changes primarily in the spine. Thus, many investigators recommend using hip measurements in patients older than 60–65 yr but advocate spine measurements, particularly in younger patients, as the best indicator of early osteoporosis and risk for vertebral fractures because of the higher trabecular bone content of vertebral bodies. Most centers, therefore, generally use hip and anterior-posterior spine measurements with DXA. Prediction of hip fracture is best based on BMD of the hip, with proximal radius and calcaneus giving next best predictions. Prediction of vertebral fracture (in patients older than 65 yr) is best based on BMD measurements of the calcaneus, spine or proximal radius.

Ongoing multicenter trials indicate that bone sites may show differences in magnitudes of BMD decreases as the patient's age advances. Furthermore, drug therapies may affect BMD and fracture incidences differently at the various sites.

Table 1. When to Use Bone Densitometry*

Appropriate patients	Purpose of scan	Timing to follow-up
Perimenopausal and post-menopausal women with no history of fracture	Baseline* • Postmenopausal women not on HRT or other therapy	
	• Perimenopausal women at higher risk, e.g., Caucasian or Asian	
	Assist in decision for HRT and motivate compliance in taking HRT	2 yr
	Assist in decision for other therapies (bisphosphonate, calcitonin, raloxifene-selective estrogen receptor modulator [SERM])	2 yr
Women or men of any age with history of fragility fracture	Assess response to therapy	2 yr
Premenopausal women with significant risk factors	Motivate compliance	2 yr
Patients on HRT, alendronate, calcitonin, raloxifene	Assess response to therapy	
Patients on corticosteroid therapy	Baseline and assess response to therapy	1–1.5 yr
Patients with hyperthyroidism	Basleine and assess response to therapy	1.5 yr

HRT, hormone replacement therapy; FDA, United States Food and Drug Administration.

*Medicare covers all FDA-approved bone density technologies for the following patients: estrogen-deficient women at clinical risk for osteoporosis, individuals with vertebral abnormalities (vertebral fractures), individuals receiving or planning to receive long-term glucocorticoid therapy, individuals with primary hyperthyroidism, individuals being monitored for response to an approved osteoporosis drug therapy.

PATIENT INFORMATION

I. DUAL-ENERGY X-RAY ABSORPTIOMETRY SCAN

A. Test/Procedure

Your doctor has requested that you have a bone density test to measure the strength of your bones. For 15–20 min you will lie on a table as instructed by the technologist, while an x-ray tube and detector device scan your hips and spine. It is best to wear nothing but a hospital gown from the waist down. The computer will process the data recorded and express your bone density measurements for each area scanned. Your measurements will be compared with those of hundreds of others of your same sex and race to determine your bone density relative to statistically expected values.

B. Preparation

Diet and medications. No special preparation is needed for this test. You may continue your usual diet and prescribed medications. If you have had any dye (contrast material) x-ray studies (iodine or barium for a gastrointestinal x-ray study) in the past week, please let the technologist know. If you have ever had dye injected into your spinal canal, please let the technologist know.

The only interferences with this test are recent x-ray contrast material or metallic screws, nails or prostheses placed in the vertebrae or hips during orthopedic surgery. Calcium deposits overlying the vertebrae or hips also may interfere. Any metal or dense object in clothing or on the surface of your body at the time of the test can interfere with the accuracy of the test.

C. Radiation risk

The only risk of this procedure is that associated with the very small amount of radiation to your spine and hips. This has been calculated to be equivalent to the radiation we all get from the natural background radiation while living on earth for a few days. No precautions are necessary, as the amount of radiation is so low.

D. Pregnancy

If you are pregnant or think you might be pregnant, please inform your doctor so that this can be discussed with the nuclear medicine physician.

References

1. Miller PD, Bonnick SL, Rosen CJ. Consensus of an international panel on the clinical utility of bone mass measurements in the detection of low bone mass in the adult population. *Calcif Tissue Int* 1996;58:207–214.
2. Black DM. Why elderly women should be screened and treated to prevent osteoporosis. *Am J Med* 1995;98:67S–75S.
3. Wahner HW, Looker A, Dunn WL, Walters LC, Hauser MF, Noval C. Quality control of bone densitometry in a national health survey (NHANES III) using three mobile examination centers. *J Bone Miner Res* 1994;9:951–960.
4. Mazess R, Chestnut CH, McClung M, Genant H. Enhanced precision with dual-energy x-ray absorbtiometry. *Calcif Tissue Int* 1992;51:14-17.
5. Cummings SR, Black DM, Nevitt MC, et al. Bone density at various sites for prediction of hip fractures. The Study of Osteoprotic Fractures Research Group. *Lancet* 1993;341:72–75.
6. Cummings SR, Nevitt MC, Browner WS, et al. Risk factors for hip fracture in white women. Study of Osteoporotic Fractures Research Group. *N Engl J Med* 1995;332:767–773.
7. Looker AC, Johnston CC Jr, Wahner HW, et al. Prevalence of low femoral bone density in older U.S. women from NHANES III. *J Bone Miner Res* 1995;10:796–802.

13
Women's Health

Nuclear medicine makes important contributions to women's health, particularly in the areas of coronary artery disease, diagnosis and staging of breast cancer and detection of osteoporosis.

I. CORONARY ARTERY DISEASE

Coronary artery disease (CAD) (see Chapter 1, Cardiovascular Diseases) is the leading cause of death for women in the United States. Women with CAD are generally about 10 yr older than men when they get the disease. Many of the risk factors associated with CAD in women (except for menopause) are the same as those for men (smoking, hypertension, obesity, etc.), but some risk factors carry much higher mortality for women. For example, diabetic women have three times the cardiovascular (and all-cause) mortality as diabetic men. In CAD, in particular, in most large trials conducted during the past 30 yr, women represented only 10–20% of participants. Thus, although we have large amounts of data on coronary disease, the data are primarily regarding men. The conclusions about risk factors and management of CAD derived from studies composed predominantly of men are not necessarily applicable to women. As this problem has become increasingly recognized, large new studies to address diseases in women have been launched. The National Institutes of Health-sponsored Women's Health Initiative will have 25,000 postmenopausal women enrolled and followed for 10 yr to study CAD, the effects of estrogen therapy on CAD, osteoporosis, breast cancer and more.

Published data document sex-related bias in workup of CAD, with women referred less frequently for stress myocardial perfusion studies and less frequently to cardiac catheterization after noninvasive testing. Earlier reports implicated diminished accuracy of stress myocardial perfusion tests in women; improvements in the imaging and testing methods have largely nullified those problems. In fact, dual-isotope (stress technetium, rest thallium) studies have shown greater discriminative value in identifying high-risk women compared with high-risk men. Generally, risk stratification is similar for both sexes.

Stress electrocardiogram is frequently less effective for testing women for CAD because women often do not stress as well as men on a treadmill: typically women are older, and they may not be accustomed to treadmill stress. Myocardial perfusion can be adequately performed with pharmacologic stress (dipyridamole or adenosine) for patients unable to stress on a treadmill. Thus, many women can be more easily and effectively tested for CAD with pharmacologic myocardial perfusion than with stress electrocardiogram examinations.

II. BREAST CANCER

Mammoscintigraphy and PET are useful for imaging breast cancer (see Chapter 20, Breast Cancer) in high-risk patients (those who carry the known breast cancer genes or have mothers or sisters with breast cancer) with problematic mammograms. PET is also useful in evaluating remote metastases.

Lymphoscintigraphy to assist in identifying the sentinenal lymph node is gaining acceptance among patients, surgeons and imagers as the staging procedure for early breast cancer (<5 cm). The scan can identify the sentinel lymph node(s) that subsequently can be located easily with the intraoperative gamma probe at surgery. This procedure spares women the cost and morbidity of a full axillary dissection. Data indicate 97% accuracy of the sentinel lymph node histopathology (using immunohistochemical stains) to diagnose micrometastases or macrometastases, compared with axillary node dissection. On the other hand, the sentinel node is often the only node to reveal micrometastases of all nodes removed in a full dissection and reveals micrometastases not detected by routine axillary dissection. Improved detection probably results from more thorough histopathology and multisectioning of the sentinel node, which cannot be done for 10–30 nodes submitted with a full axillary dissection.

III. OVARIAN CANCER

A labeled antibody product and PET can be used to detect metastatic spread from ovarian cancers (see Chapter 22, Ovarian Cancer). Both nuclear techniques are more sensitive than CT scans and can be a cost-effective tool in patient management.

IV. OSTEOPOROSIS

Osteoporosis (see Chapter 12, Bone Density) affects most postmenopausal women (after age 80, 70% of Caucasian women are osteoporotic and 20–30% of all postmenopausal women are osteoporotic). Fractures related to osteoporosis are costly for our society and for the individuals; 55% of hip fractures occur after age 79 and are associated with 2–5 times increased likelihood of death in the 12 mo after the hip fracture.

Bone density measurement (see Chapter 12, Bone Density) is the single most predictive indicator available to warn of increased risk of an individual for fracture due to osteoporosis. The bone density measurement is used by physicians to indicate the need and the level of urgency for instituting therapy for osteoporosis aimed at fracture prevention and to follow patients on therapeutic regimens to document adequate response, to determine the need (if any) to alter the therapy and to motivate patient compliance.

V. WOMEN AND RADIATION EXPOSURE FROM DIAGNOSTIC NUCLEAR MEDICINE TESTS

The radiation associated with diagnostic nuclear medicine tests is similar to that of other diagnostic procedures involving radiation, such as x-rays. There is a difference, however, between tests in which x-rays are transmitted through the region being imaged—chest, abdomen, pelvis and bone x-rays and CT examinations, for example—and administration (usually by oral or intravenous routes) of a radioactive material, which usually localizes primarily in one part or organ of the body, for example a lung scan, bone scan, thyroid scan. Sometimes there is more generalized distribution of the radionuclide throughout the body, as in a tumor scan using ^{18}F-fluorodeoxyglucose or ^{67}Ga. More detailed discussion of radiation dose and exposure considerations, including risks, is presented in Chapter 28, Radiation, Radiopharmaceuticals and Imaging Devices.

Potential exposure of in utero fetus

Women of childbearing age who could be pregnant at the time of a nuclear medicine test and not know that they are will be questioned about their last menstrual period and will usually be asked to undergo a pregnancy test before a therapeutic procedure. Before diagnostic tests, they are requested to let the technologist or the physician know if they think that they may be pregnant (there are prominently displayed signs in every nuclear medicine department asking women to let the technologist know if they think they might be pregnant). The consequences of radiation exposure to a fetus or embryo from a diagnostic nuclear medicine test are usually insignificant. Nonetheless, if the diagnostic test is an elective procedure as opposed to an urgent procedure, it can be postponed and rescheduled if the patient is pregnant, even if only for peace of mind. Some physicians recommend that radiation procedures be scheduled during the first ten days of a woman's menstrual cycle, when pregnancy is unlikely. The same considerations should be exercised for all radiation diagnostic tests (chest x-rays, bone x-rays, etc.). (See Chapter 28, Radiation, Radiopharmaceuticals and Imaging Devices.)

The issues of nuclear medicine tests for nursing mothers are discussed in Chapter 2, Pulmonary System and Thromboembolism. Basically, if the radio-tracer is excreted into breast milk, nursing should be discontinued for the time necessary for the radiation levels in the milk to decrease to lower than three times background levels.

13

14 Pediatrics

14

Most nuclear medicine imaging procedures also are used to image infants, children and adolescents. In addition to the standard studies, specialized tests are available to address clinical problems that are more likely to occur in a pediatric practice. This chapter lists topics that relate more specifically to the pediatric patient and provides the chapter, question and page number where each topic is located. The chapter also addresses two important issues that may arise when a pediatric patient is referred for a nuclear medicine scan: Parental concern regarding radiation exposure and the patient's inability to lie still for the examination.

I. PARENTAL CONCERN REGARDING RADIATION EXPOSURE

Several points can be made to reassure the parents.

A. Low dose

The dose of a radioactive tracer administered to a pediatric patient is usually substantially less than the dose administered to an adult patient. The administered dose is adjusted based on body weight or body surface area.

B. Minimal risk

The radiation risk from a diagnostic study is quite low and can be compared with the risk from radiation originating from cosmic rays and natural background radiation sources that we all experience from living on the planet earth. The risk from most diagnostic studies falls in the range of a few months to a few years of background radiation exposure.

C. Relative risk

The risk of the test is much less than the risk of not performing the test.

II. THE PATIENT MAY NOT BE ABLE TO LIE STILL FOR THE EXAMINATION

Some imaging procedures require the patient to lie still for 15–30 min while the image is being acquired. A patient may be too young to comprehend the necessity of lying absolutely still for the duration of the examination. An older child may be reluctant to cooperate because of pain, hyperactivity, developmental disabilities or an exaggerated fear of the procedure. In a dedicated pediatric facility, sedation is rarely a problem because the referring physicians and the imaging physician communicate closely and have developed protocols to address sedation needs. In facilities that deal primarily with adults, sedation of pediatric patients may require the approval of and a prescription by the referring physician. If your patient may need sedation, advanced communication with the imaging center may avoid unnecessary patient delay and frustration.

For infants and young children less than 15 kg, chloral hydrate is recommended by the American Academy of Pediatrics as an "effective sedative with a low incidence of acute toxicity when administered orally in the recommended dosage for short-term sedation." In older, larger or mentally handicapped children, chloral hydrate often doesn't suffice as the only sedation and additional medication may need to be included in the sedation regimen.

III. SELECTED PEDIATRIC TOPICS

A. Cardiac

Quantitation of right-to-left shunt. Chapter 1, Background.

B. Lung

Aspiration secondary to reflux. Chapter 5, Clinical Question 9.
Breast-feeding after a V/Q scan? Chapter 2, Clinical Question 8.

C. Genitourinary tract

Dilated renal pelvis on antenatal sonography. Chapter 3, Clinical Question 5.
Testicular torsion. Chapter 3, Clinical Question 16.
Congenital abnormality/renal function. Chapter 3, Clinical Question 17.

Acute pyelonephritis. Chapter 3, Clinical Question 18.
Ureteral reflux. Chapter 3, Clinical Questions 19–21.

D. Hepatobiliary tract
Aspenia, polyspenia. Chapter 4, Clinical Question 14.
Biliary atresia/neonatal hepatitis. Chapter 4, Clinical Question 6.
Right upper quadrant mass/choledocal cyst. Chapter 4, Clinical Question 10.

E. Gastrointestinal tract
Meckel's diverticulum. Chapter 5, Clinical Question 5.
Reflux/aspiration. Chapter 5, Clinical Questions 7 and 9.

F. Infection/inflammation
Sickle cell disease (bone infarction versus infection). Chapter 6, Clinical Question 11.

G. Central nervous system
Cerebrospinal fluid shunt patency. Chapter 8, Clinical Question 16.
Seizure site. Chapter 8, Clincial Questions 9 and 10.
Brain death. Chapter 8, Clinical Question 11.

H. Thyroid
Neonatal hypothyroidism (sublingual thyroid, agenesis). Chapter 9, Clinical
Questions 14 and 15.
Graves' disease. Is ^{131}I therapy safe? Chapter 9, Clinical Question 21.

I. Skeletal system
Primary bone tumors. Chapter 12, Clinical Question 9.
Osteoid osteoma. Chapter 12, Clinical Question 18.
Child abuse. Chapter 12, Clinical Question 23.
Neuroblastoma, Ewing's sarcoma, osteosarcoma. Chapter 12, Clinical Question
4.
Limping child. Chapter 12, Clinical Question 24.

J. Radiation
Risk of cancer from low-level radiation. Chapter 28, Clinical Questions 6 and 7.

References
1. American Academy of Pediatrics Committee on Drugs and Committee on Environmental Health. Use of chloral hydrate for sedation in children. *Pediatrics* 1993;92:471–473.
2. Mandall GA, Cooper JA, Majd M, et al. Society of Nuclear Medicine procedure guideline for pediatric sedation in nuclear medicine. In: *Society of Nuclear Medicine Procedure Guidelines Manual 1999.* Society of Nuclear Medicine: Reston, VA. 1999:139–143.

14

15
Introduction to Cancer and FDG Imaging

Approximately 25% of people in the United States will get cancer during their lifetime, and 15% will die of the disease. Cancer can be treated more effectively when metastatic disease can be localized or excluded; it often can be cured if detected early. Nuclear medicine techniques play an important role in the detection of malignant disease and in the management of the patient with known or suspected cancer. The oncology sections in this book are indexed at the end of this chapter, but they are not intended to be exhaustive. They focus on the role of nuclear medicine in the management of the most common types of cancers.

15

Fluorine-18-fluorodeoxyglucose (FDG) has become an important radiopharmaceutical for the detection of neoplastic disease. Until recently, however, FDG imaging was only available in specialized PET centers equipped with a dedicated cyclotron facility for the production of ^{18}F, the synthesis of FDG and a PET imaging system to image the high-energy coincident photons of positron emitters. In 1999, the Health Care Financing Administration (HCFA) approved reimbursement for diagnostic FDG imaging for the management of patients with recurrent colorectal cancer, staging of lung cancer, evaluation of the solitary pulmonary nodule after a CT scan and staging of lymphoma and recurrent malignant melanoma. Although not yet approved for reimbursement in the United

States, FDG scans are also useful in the management of many other types of cancers (see references 1 and 2), and wider applications have been approved for reimbursement in other countries.

As the utility of FDG imaging has become more widely recognized, medical cyclotron facilities have been established throughout the United States to make FDG more available to the general community. In addition, hybrid imaging systems have been developed to image standard photons emitted by traditional radiopharmaceuticals as well as the high-energy photons of positron emitters such as ^{18}F. These hybrid systems permit FDG imaging to be performed in hospitals or clinics that do not have the volume of PET studies to justify purchase of a dedicated PET system. Dedicated PET, SPECT and hybrid SPECT/PET coincidence systems are described in Chapter 28. Because FDG is used to image many cancers, the FDG scan is discussed below to avoid repetition. Details of FDG imaging that relate to specific cancers are discussed under the radiopharmaceutical section of each specific cancer.

FDG SCAN

A. Background

Positron emitters allow the production of radiopharmaceuticals that closely mimic endogenous molecules. FDG is the most commonly used PET tracer in oncology and permits in vivo evaluation of glucose metabolism. Many positron emitters have a short half-life (seconds to a few minutes), but ^{18}F has a relatively long physical half-life of 110 min. Although still short, the 110-min half-life allows time for the radiopharmaceutical to be shipped from the cyclotron where it is produced to neighboring sites where it can be used for imaging. In addition to the specific tumors approved by the HCFA, FDG PET is increasingly used in the following settings:

1. Initial (preoperative) staging of cancer
2. Differentiation between scar and residual tumor
3. Demonstration of suspected recurrences
4. Monitoring response to therapy. In susceptible tumors, FDG uptake can be markedly diminished or even completely suppressed after one or two cycles of chemotherapy. The early determination of therapeutic resistance is also important, because it can avoid the toxicity of an ineffective therapy and allow selection of a new therapeutic regimen.
5. Prognosis.

Tumors with intense FDG uptake or a high standardized uptake valve (SUV) (see Understanding the report, below) tend to be more aggressive and enlarge more rapidly.

B. The radiopharmaceutical

FDG is an analog of glucose and is used as a tracer of glucose metabolism. FDG enters the cell by the same transport mechanism as glucose and is intracellularly phosphorylated by hexokinase into FDG-6-phosphate. In tissues with a low concentration of the enzyme glucose-6-phosphatase (brain, myocardium and most malignant cells), FDG-6-phosphate cannot be further metabolized, and it accumulates within the cell in proportion to the cell's rate of glycolysis. In addition to brain and myocardium, normal FDG uptake may be observed in the stomach and bowel. Unlike glucose, FDG is excreted by the kidneys into the urine.

Tumor cells demonstrate increased glucose metabolism compared with normal cells; this increase is due, in part, to a greater number of glucose transporter proteins and elevated levels of intracellular enzymes that support glycolysis. Increased FDG uptake has been demonstrated in many malignant tumors, although variation in uptake exists among tumor types. The relatively high tumor-to-background ratio coupled with the superior resolution of PET systems has resulted in the high reported sensitivities and specificities of FDG imaging.

C. How the study is performed

Emission images are obtained approximately 1 hr after the intravenous injection of approximately 10–20 mCi (370–740 MBq) of FDG. During the 60-min distribution period after FDG injection, the patient should be relaxed and avoid talking, chewing, excessive swallowing or other muscular activity to minimize FDG uptake in laryngeal muscles or muscles of mastication; this is particularly important in the evaluation of the patient with head and neck cancer. Some centers also will place an irrigating catheter in the bladders of patients with suspected pelvic tumors to minimize interference from FDG in the urinary bladder.

The imaging session lasts from 30 to 90 min, depending on the instrumentation and the number of sites to be imaged. Dedicated PET systems can correct for soft-tissue attenuation using transmission scanning from an external source. Correction for soft-tissue attenuation improves lesion detection and allows calculation of the SUV (described in Understanding the report, below).

D. Patient preparation

1. Hydration. Patients should be encouraged to drink water to maintain hydration, promote diuresis and minimize FDG activity within the renal collecting system.

2. Food restrictions. Patients should be fasting except for water for at least 4 hr before the study to maximize FDG uptake by the tumor cells. If there is a question of lung cancer, patients should avoid food or sugar-containing beverages for 12 hr, if possible, before the study to minimize cardiac uptake of FDG. When glucose concentrations are low, the heart tends to use fatty acids rather than glucose as a metabolic substrate. FDG activity in the heart is reduced, and it is easier to evaluate possible metastatic disease in the lung and mediastinum.

15

E. Understanding the report

The report describes any areas of increased uptake that are indicative of or suspicious for tumor and compares the FDG scan with any available conventional imaging tests such as CT/MRI.

The report also may mention the SUV or standardized uptake ratio (SUR). The SUV or SUR normalizes the FDG accumulation in a suspicious lesion to the injected dose and the patient's body weight. This normalized value can be used to help determine if the questionable lesion is a tumor or a benign abnormality. To place the SUV in perspective, a recent FDG PET study analyzed 51 patients with pulmonary abnormalities that could not be characterized by chest radiograph or CT as benign or malignant. The SUV of the benign lesions was 1.5 ± 0.9 compared with an SUV of 6.8 ± 3.7 in the malignant lesions.

F. Potential problems

1. Genitourinary tract activity. FDG is excreted by the kidneys into the bladder. Bladder activity may interfere with the evaluation of a pelvic mass, and some centers place an irrigating catheter to minimize this problem.

2. Gastrointestinal activity. There may be prominent uptake in the cecum as well as activity in the esophagus, stomach and intestine; occasionally gut activity can present a problem in interpretation.

3. Muscle activity. Muscle tension, hyperventilation with increased diaphragmatic exertion and stress-induced tension in the trapezius and paraspinal muscles may result in increased FDG uptake in the active muscle groups. In anxious patients, a muscle relaxant such as diazepam may be given.

4. Sites of inflammation. Inflammation can be associated with increased FDG uptake, particularly when there is granulomatous inflammation such as tuberculosis, sarcoid, histoplasmosis and aspergillosis. Uptake can be intense enough to be confused with tumor. For this reason, FDG imaging usually is delayed for several days after surgical trauma or biopsy procedures.

PATIENT INFORMATION

FDG SCAN
A. Test procedure

Your doctor has ordered an FDG scan to evaluate the possibility of tumor spread or recurrence or the response of the tumor to therapy. A small amount of radioactive sugar called FDG will be injected into a vein. Approximately 45–60 min after the injection, you will lie on a table, and images will be obtained using a special machine, either a PET scanner or coincidence gamma camera. This machine does not produce any radiation but detects radiation coming from the injected sugar in your body. The injected sugar preferentially accumulates in tumor tissue. The whole process may take from 1 to 2 hr depending on the type of camera and how much of your body needs to be imaged. It is important that you are able to lie still for the examination. If you cannot do this, please inform your doctor.

B. Preparation

You typically will be asked to fast (water is permitted) for 12 hr before the examination. Please ask your doctor about any medications. If you are a diabetic, please inform the nuclear medicine department because special instructions may be provided.

C. Radiation risks

The amount of radiation used is small and similar to that given by other diagnostic x-ray tests. The effective adult radiation exposure to your whole body from this test is approximately equal to the dose the average person living in the United States receives in 3–7 yr from cosmic rays and naturally occurring background radiation sources. The radiation dose is about 20–40% of the yearly dose considered safe for doctors and technologists who work with radiation. You can be around other people and use a bathroom normally without risk to others.

15

D. Pregnancy

If you are pregnant or think you could be pregnant, inform your doctor so that this can be discussed with the nuclear medicine physician.

SPECIFIC CANCERS AND THERAPIES

SPECIFIC CANCERS

THERAPIES

References

1. Delbeke D. Oncological applications of FDG PET imaging: brain tumors, colorectal cancer, lymphoma and melanoma. *J Nucl Med* 1999;40:591–603.
2. Delbeke D. Oncological applications of FDG PET imaging. *J Nucl Med* 1999;40:1706–1715.

15

16
Neuroendocrine Tumors

Pheochromocytomas, carcinoid tumors, neuroblastomas and a variety of neuroendocrine and other tumors often accumulate radioiodinated metaiodobenzylguanidine (MIBG), Octreoscan and fluorodeoxyglucose (FDG) and can be detected and localized by nuclear scans. In addition to diagnosis, many patients have been helped by therapies using high doses of ^{131}I-MIBG to target and irradiate tumors, similar to the use of ^{131}I in the treatment of thyroid cancer.

SCANS, THERAPIES AND PRIMARY CLINICAL INDICATIONS

I. MIBG diagnostic scan   Page 256

- To diagnose and localize suspected neuroendocrine tumor(s)

- To search for metastases, bilateral tumors, extra-adrenal tumor (if CT fails to identify an adrenal tumor) in patients with pheochromocytoma

- To localize and identify carcinoid tumor(s)

- To localize and identify neuroblastoma tumor(s) in children

- To determine if high-dose ^{131}I-MIBG therapy may be beneficial

II. Octreoscan imaging   Page 259

- To identify metastases from neuroendocrine tumors diagnosed by serum or urine biochemical indicators and for indications in I (above), except the last

CLINICAL QUESTIONS

PATIENT INFORMATION

16

SCANS

I. MIBG DIAGNOSTIC SCAN
A. Background

Neuroendocrine tumors are relatively rare in adults; they mainly consist of pheochromocytomas, carcinoids, paragangliomas, neuroblastomas and medullary thyroid cancer. In the pediatric population, neuroblastoma is the most common solid tumor in infants younger than 1 yr and the most common extracranial solid tumor of childhood.

Neuroendocrine tumors derive from pluripotent stem cells or differentiated neuroendocrine cells and share a characteristic histologic pattern, secretory products and some cytoplasmic proteins. They were thought to derive from neural crest cells according to the amine precursor uptake and decarboxylation (APUD) theory, which is no longer accepted.

The sensitivity and specificity for uptake on scans varies, depending primarily on the tumor type. MIBG scan sensitivity in neuroblastoma is 90%, and specificity approaches 100%. In pheocromocytoma, sensitivity is also approximately 90%. The sensitivity is higher with ^{123}I-MIBG than with ^{131}I-MIBG, but ^{123}I is not generally available. In carcinoid tumors, sensitivity is also good, 80%, whereas sensitivity is relatively poor for medullary thyroid cancer, 30–55%. Reports of ^{131}I-MIBG imaging in cases of multiple endocrine neoplasia (MEN) type 2B have shown ^{131}I-MIBG accumulation, with aggressive tumor behavior in some cases and mild uptake in others. Thallium, the myocardial perfusion imaging agent, accumulates in many tumors and has been reported to image some medullary thyroid carcinomas successfully when MIBG or Octreoscan have failed.

B. Radiopharmaceuticals

Iodine-123-MIBG and ^{131}I-MIBG are accumulated in catecholamine storage granules. Radiolabeled MIBG, which structurally resembles norepinephrine, images the adrenal medulla (particularly in pathologic conditions) and sympathetic nervous tissue. MIBG is accumulated by tumor cells that possess the type-1 amine uptake mechanism (e.g., pheochromocytomas) (Fig. 1). Drugs that interfere with the type-1 uptake mechanism or the storage of MIBG may decrease MIBG uptake into tumor cells or speed its exit from the cells. Tumor uptake is proportional to the number of neurosecretory granules within the tumors.

C. How the scan is performed

Intravenous injection of 1 mCi (37 MBq, adult dose) ^{131}I-labeled MIBG (10 mCi ^{123}I-MIBG) is followed at 24 hr (for ^{123}I) or 72 hr (for ^{131}I) with whole-body imaging. SPECT is added for ^{123}I imaging, but not with ^{131}I, which does not provide sufficient counts for SPECT imaging.

D. Patient preparation

Diet. There are no dietary restrictions.

Medications. Many drugs interfere with MIBG uptake by the neuroendocrine tumor cells. To obtain a diagnostic scan, the patient must stop any drugs listed in Table 1 for the recommended period of time.

The patient is given a saturated solution of potassium iodide (2 drops, twice a day) or Lugol's solution (5 drops, twice a day) for 1–3 days before receiving the ^{123}I- or ^{131}I-MIBG to minimize thyroid uptake of radioactive iodide, which may dissociate from the MIBG molecule. Even with careful measures to block iodide uptake by the thyroid, some ^{123}I-MIBG is usually evident in the thyroid.

E. Understanding the report

The report describes the rationale for performing this scan, the tumor type suspected or previously diagnosed, the procedure and the findings. Abnormal foci

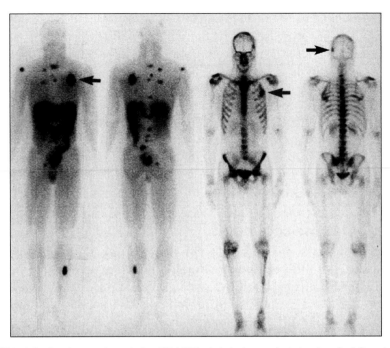

Figure 1. Metastatic pheochromocytoma: Iodine-131-MIBG whole-body scan (anterior view, far left, and posterior view, middle left) and ^{99m}Tc-methylene diphosphonate (MDP) whole-body bone scan (anterior view, middle right, and posterior view, far right). The MIBG scan shows multiple foci of tumor in the thorax, mediastinum, sacroiliacs, vertebral spine, proximal left humerus and left tibia. The bone scan shows bone metastases in a right anterior upper rib (arrow), lumbar, thoracic and sacral vertebrae, sacroiliac bones, and left skull (arrow), which is seen only faintly on MIBG scan, and left tibia, which is less well seen than on the MIBG scan.

16

of ^{123}I- or ^{131}I-MIBG anywhere in the body on the scan are likely to represent tumor in these patients.

If the ^{123}I- or ^{131}I-MIBG scan shows prominent localization in metastatic tumor sites, high-dose ^{131}I-MIBG therapy can be performed if clinically warranted. Although ^{131}I-MIBG is United States Food and Drug Administration (FDA)-approved for diagnostic imaging, high-dose ^{131}I-MIBG therapy is an off-label use. Only a few centers in the United States can perform ^{131}I-MIBG therapy under a physician's Investigational New Drug (IND) Application.

F. Potential problems

1. Drug interference. Drug interferences may cause false-negative results (see Table 1).

2. Poor ^{131}I-MIBG image quality and low sensitivity for liver metastases. The image quality of ^{131}I-MIBG scans is not as good as most nuclear medicine studies because of the difficulty in imaging the unfavorable higher energy photons and the low counts associated with ^{131}I diagnostic studies. Liver metastases, particularly, may be more difficult to visualize with ^{131}I-MIBG because of normal liver uptake of MIBG around the tumors.

TABLE 1. Drugs and MIBG Uptake

Drugs that interfere with MIBG uptake

Cocaine

Tricyclic antidepressants—should not take these for 6 wk before MIBG test:
Desipramine, amitriptyline (Elavil), amoxapine (Asendin), doxepin (Adapin, Sinequan), imipramine, pamole (Tofranil, Imavate, Janimine, Presamine, SK-Pramine, Tipramine), maprotoline (Ludiomil), nortriptyline (Aventyl, Pamelor), protriptyine (Vivactil), trimipramine maleate (Surmontil), trazodone HCl (Desyrel)

Phenylpropanolamine/pseudoephedrine/phenylephrine

Catecholamine agonists
Sympathomimetics, amphetamines and amphetamine-like compounds

Reserpine (because it depletes the catecholamine stores in the neurosecretory storage granules)

Antipsychotics
Phenothiazines (Thorazine, Compazine, Mellaril, etc.) and thiothixines

Calcium channel blockers
Adrenergic blockers
Long-acting beta-blockers: labetalol and possibly metoprolol (labetalol should be discontinued for at least 3 wk before scanning; the absence of salivary and parotid activity can serve as a clue that patients may be on this medication)

Possibly some foods
Those containing vanillin and catecholamine-like compounds such as chocolate and blue-veined cheeses

Drugs that do not affect MIBG uptake

Alpha-blockers (clonidine, phenoxybenzamine, hentolamine, prazosin)
Alpha-methyldopa
Angiotensin-converting enzyme inhibitors
Aspirin, acetaminophen
Digoxin
Diuretics
Hypnotics
Minor tranquilizers
Morphine and other opioids

16

II. OCTREOSCAN IMAGING
A. Background

Most neuroendocrine tumors express a high density of somatostatin receptors. Somatostatin is a neuropeptide first found in the hypothalamus about 25 yr ago. A somatostatin analog (pentetreotide) labeled to a radionuclide, ^{111}In, effectively localizes tumors on nuclear scans. The high tumor-to-background count ratios have facilitated the use of hand-held gamma detecting probes in the operating room to localize somatostatin-receptor–positive tumors intra-operatively.

B. Radiopharmaceuticals

Indium-111-pentetreotide (Octreoscan), a structural analog of somatostatin, is effective in imaging neuroendocrine tumor sites with high densities of somatostatin receptors. Scan sensitivities are reported at 80–95% for many tumors, but for some tumors may be considerably lower, depending on the abundance of somatostatin receptors.

C. How the study is performed

After intravenous injection of 6.0 mCi (222 MBq; adult dose) ^{111}In-pentetreotide, whole-body imaging is obtained, usually at 4–6 hr and at 24 hr. SPECT also may be valuable for better localization of lesions.

D. Patient preparation

1. Diet. There is no dietary restriction. The patient should be well hydrated for the test and should drink fluids liberally for faster renal excretion of the tracer.

2. Medication. Treatment with unlabeled octreotide may diminish accumulation of the Octreoscan in the tumor because of occupancy of somatostatin receptors by unlabeled octreotide. Therefore it may be advisable for the patient to discontinue taking octreotide for 3 days before the Octreoscan injection, or the sensitivity of the test may be reduced.

E. Understanding the report

Abnormal foci visualized on the scan, anywhere in the body, may represent tumor (Fig. 2). In addition to neuroendocrine tumors, a variety of other tumors (neuroblastomas, astrocytomas, pituitary tumors, meningiomas), breast tumors, malignant lymphomas (Hodgkin's and non-Hodgkin's), renal cell cancers, and small-cell lung carcinomas may have somatostatin receptors and will be imaged.

F. Potential problems

1. Nonspecificity. Active sarcoidosis and chronic inflammation can show abnormal focal uptake on scans, as well as a wide variety of tumors, as discussed above.

2. Normal organ uptake. Cells in normal tissues express somatostatin receptors, including thyroid, pituitary, salivary glands, spleen, liver, kidneys and bladder. Gallbladder is seen in patients who have not fasted and intestinal activity is often present. Normal uptake occasionally can obscure detection of a small tumor.

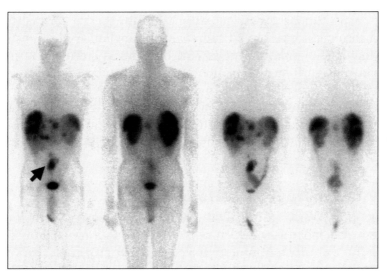

Figure 2. Metastatic carcinoid tumors: Octreoscan images were obtained at 4 hr (anterior view, far left, and posterior view, middle left) and 24 hr (anterior, middle right, and posterior, far right). Images show multiple foci of tumor uptake of the Octreoscan in liver, abdomen (arrow, probably mesenteric nodes or mass) and lower thoracic vertebra. Normal uptake is seen in the kidneys and bladder.

3. Iodine-131-MIBG therapy. Octreoscan imaging does not predict utility of ^{131}I-MIBG for therapy. Thus, if therapy using ^{131}I-MIBG is a consideration, a diagnostic MIBG scan, not Octreoscan, is needed.

16

III. FDG IMAGING

The reader is referred to Chapter 15, Introduction to Cancer and FDG Imaging, and the chapters on lung and colorectal cancers for discussions on the background, procedures and reporting of FDG tumor imaging studies. Clinical Question 1 (below) discusses FDG scans relative to the alternatives for neurodendocrine tumors.

IV. ^{131}I-MIBG THERAPY

A. Background

Neuroendocrine tumors usually respond poorly to chemotherapy. Since 1983, 600–1000 patients with metastatic neuroendocrine tumors have been treated worldwide with high-dose ^{131}I-MIBG therapy. The protocols used in Europe and the United States have varied in regard to administered dose, frequency of treatment and criteria for patient acceptance for therapy. Nonetheless, published reports show good results, much better than those with chemotherapy. The subjective response rate for ^{131}I-MIBG-treated metastatic neuroendocrine tumor is approximately 75%. Clinically, 84% of patients have stabilization of disease progression when treated with 1–6 doses ranging from 30 to 1356 mCi. A recent review of 24 institutions' experience with ^{131}I-MIBG therapy for malignant adrenal pheochromocytomas or extra-adrenal paragangliomas in 116 patients reported symptomatic improvement in 76% of patients, hormonal responses in 45% of patients and tumor regression in 30% of patients. Patients with soft-tissue metastases responded better to ^{131}I-MIBG therapy than those with bone metastases. Investigators also have reported symptomatic improvement in 70% of patients with metastatic carcinoid; tumor burden reduction and hormone reduction is seen in 20%. Better responses are reported with higher doses of ^{131}I-MIBG.

B. How the therapy is performed

High doses of ^{131}I-MIBG (usually 200–300 mCi) are prepared by the University of Michigan Radiopharmacy, which sells the doses to a few approved institutions (i.e., those at which FDA permits its use under physicians' IND protocol; the protocol also must be approved by the local institutional review board). The administration of the ^{131}I-MIBG is performed with close radiation safety supervision in an isolated, monitored, hospital room where the patient is kept until the physician and radiation safety officer decide it is safe to release the patient, in accord with Nuclear Regulatory Commission (NRC) or state regulations.

Hospitalization may range from 0 to 7 (or more) days, depending on state regulations and how rapidly the patient excretes the ^{131}I-MIBG and reaches the allowable level (5 mR/hr) for mixing with the general public. The NRC permits the patient to be discharged earlier if the physician is certain that members of the general public will not be exposed to significant radiation from the patient, based on his/her home sleeping and living environment and willingness to remain isolated for a prescribed period of time.

C. Patient preparation

Diet. The patient is encouraged to eat and drink lots of fluids to facilitate excretion of ^{131}I-MIBG via the kidneys and bowel.

Medications. It is critically important that the patient discontinue all medications that could interfere with tumor uptake of ^{131}I-MIBG (see Table 1).

Pregnancy. Pregnancy is a contraindication to this therapy. This high-dose radiation therapy will likely damage an embryo or fetus.

D. Understanding the report

The report describes the procedures, results and the fact that the patient was counseled on radiation safety and realistic expectations from the therapy. The patient is counseled that this therapy is not a cure but is palliative. The patient may not feel any positive results for 2–3 wk, or may never have positive results. Most patients are symptomatic but, rarely, patients may become quite ill, including nausea, weakness and loss of appetite, possibly due in part to tumoricidal activity). Patients may experience mild to dramatic relief from diarrhea (carcinoid), headaches, palpitations and hypertension.

E. Potential problems

1. Hematologic toxicity. Bone marrow depression is the most serious and likely toxicity. Thrombocytopenia, leukopenia and anemia have all been reported. Bone marrow depression can occur as early as 7 days after treatment and last as long as 17 wk. The seriousness of the depression correlates with extent of bone marrow or bone involvement with tumor and the amount of previously received chemotherapy. Patients who have had chemotherapy for metastatic neuroendocrine tumors are more likely to have bone marrow depression after ^{131}I-MIBG therapy.

2. Hepatic toxicity. Although rare, in cases of extensive liver metastases hepatic toxicity with severe liver failure (even death) has been reported.

CLINICAL QUESTIONS

1. Suspected neuroendocrine tumor or neuroblastoma: Which test (MIBG, Octreoscan or FDG) is preferred and why?

Iodine-123- or ^{131}I-MIBG, Octreoscan and FDG all effectively localize in neuroendocrine tumors wherever they may be situated in the body. The sensitivities of MIBG and Octreoscan are roughly similar, with the exception of neuroblastoma, in which MIBG may be preferred, but MIBG carries the disadvantage of requiring avoidance of all medications that interfere with MIBG cellular uptake (see Table 1). This may be inconvenient if the patient is taking a long-acting beta blocker, a tricyclic antidepressant or other ongoing medication important for daily well-being. Octreoscan is more convenient to use than MIBG and comparable in price. FDG is an effective method for whole-body tumor imaging, but is less effective in well-differentiated tumors. It is probably slightly higher in cost than Octreoscan. Of the three (MIBG, Octreoscan and FDG), the simplest to use, probably the most widely available, and equally effective for most neuroendocrine tumors is Octreoscan.

2. Suspected pheochromocytoma: Should a nuclear scan be obtained? If so, which scan?

Patients who present with hypertension that is difficult to control may harbor a pheochromocytoma. Biochemical diagnosis of pheochromocytoma depends on identifying increased levels of serum catecholamines or of metanephrines and catecholamines in a 24-hr urine collection. If elevated catecholamines or metanephrines, hormonal products of the adrenal glands, are present, the first imaging examination should be a CT study to visualize the suspected adrenal

16

tumor, determine its size and identify bilateral pheochromocytomas, which occur in 10% of patients who have pheochromocytoma. Larger tumors (>6 cm) are at higher risk for being malignant (10% are malignant), whereas small tumors can be surgically removed easily through a laparoscope. Larger tumors might warrant a whole-body nuclear scan to search for metastases. If the CT scan fails to demonstrate an adrenal tumor, a whole-body nuclear scan might be ordered to search for an extra-adrenal pheochromocytoma (which occurs in 10%).

Because the sensitivity of MIBG and Octreoscan are equally high for pheochromocytoma, either would be acceptable, depending on availability and expertise or experience of the nuclear physician. FDG scans are sensitive in metabolically active neuroendocrine tumors and could be used. Octreoscan and FDG have the advantage over MIBG of not requiring discontinuing medications that interfere with incorporation of MIBG into the tumor.

3. Suspected metastatic carcinoid tumor: Which test should be ordered?

Patients with carcinoid tumor may come to clinical attention because of uncontrolled diarrhea, intermittent abdominal pain or even intestinal obstruction. The diagnosis is not usually suspected before surgery but is established by biopsy. The biggest impediment to making the diagnosis is not thinking of the carcinoid syndrome or not considering it because of its rarity. Once considered, the diagnosis usually can be confirmed by urine 5-hydroxyindoleacetic acid, the breakdown (waste) product of serotonin. Bronchial carcinoid tumors may be asymptomatic and come to attention on a chest x-ray, leading to biopsy, or they may be symptomatic if secreting serotonin or causing bronchial obstruction. The most frequent sites for carcinoids are the gastrointestinal tract (75%) and the bronchopulmonary system (25%). Within the gastrointestinal tract, most occur in the small bowel (~30%), appendix (~20%) and rectum (10–15%). A cumulative analysis of all types of carcinoid tumors indicates that 45% of patients already have metastases at the time of diagnosis. The overall 5-yr survival rate of all carcinoid tumors regardless of site is about 50%.

Because of the high likelihood of metastases at the time of diagnosis, diagnostic whole-body imaging with Octreoscan (Fig. 2) or MIBG is warranted to define and localize metastastases. Tumors that can be seen on the Octreoscan study are likely to respond to treatment with octreotide, a first-line therapy to control symptoms and discomfort. Also, sensitivity of Octreoscan is probably slightly higher than MIBG for carcinoid tumors.

4. If bone metastases are suspected, would a bone scan be the best test?

The bone scan is probably the best tool for identifying bone metastases. It should be regarded as complimentary to the MIBG, Octreoscan or FDG. In children with neuroblastoma, both bone scans and MIBG scans generally are done.

5. When should a patient be offered ¹³¹I-MIBG therapy?

High-dose ¹³¹I-MIBG should be considered for patients with metastatic neuroendocrine tumors that concentrate ¹²³I- or ¹³¹I-MIBG (Fig. 1) and show uncontrolled progression or increasingly uncontrollable symptoms. Iodine-131 MIBG therapy is palliative, not curative. Seventy to 86% of patients get relief from debilitating diarrhea caused by carcinoid tumors and hypertension due to pheochromocytomas after ¹³¹I-MIBG therapy. Biochemical documentation of catecholamine hypersecretion should precede diagnostic imaging and ¹³¹I-MIBG therapy and should be monitored subsequently. At the time of discharge from the hospital, the patient should have a post-therapy whole-body scan to document the biodistribution of the therapeutic ¹³¹I-MIBG.

Chemotherapy has not been effective in metastatic carcinoid or pheochromocytoma, and its use may increase the risk of bone marrow depression if the patient subsequently receives high-dose ¹³¹I-MIBG. Surgical removal of primary tumors and some metastases often is recommended. Other therapies to be considered for carcinoid patients include hepatic resections of tumors, hepatic artery embolizations and unlabeled octreotide

6. What is the best diagnostic imaging test for patients with suspected medullary thyroid cancer?

None of the available diagnostic agents effectively images medullary thyroid cancer; sensitivities are in the 40–60% range, at best. Medullary thyroid cancer is the rarest of all thyroid malignancies; it occurs as a solitary tumor or as part of multiple endocrine neoplasia syndrome. In multiple endocrine neoplasia type 2B, medullary thyroid cancer is associated with pheochromocytoma, ganglioneuromatosis and marfanoid habitus.

Technetium-99m-dimercaptosuccinic acid (DMSA) has been advocated as an effective adjunctive agent for imaging thyroid medullary cancer and improves sensitivities when added as a second imaging test to the Octreoscan or MIBG. DMSA as prepared for renal scans is not in the chemical form needed for imaging medullary thyroid cancer. If therapy with high-dose MIBG is to be considered, an MIBG diagnostic scan must be done (see Clinical Question 5, above).

7. If the clinical presentation or laboratory data suggest gastrinoma or insulinoma, what test should be performed?

Endocrine tumors of the pancreas arise from pancreatic and duodenal neuroendocrine cells; they are slow-growing, uncommon tumors. The clinical presentation of functioning tumors is determined by the action of the secreting hormone (elevated serum gastrin and elevated gastric acid levels for gastrinoma and elevated insulin for insulinoma). Nonfunctioning insulinoma and gastrinoma tumors are the most common of this group. They usually present because of their mass effect. CT and ultrasound imaging studies have relatively poor sen-

16

sitivity for finding the primary lesion, unless it is large. Octreoscan imaging identifies these tumors because of the presence of somatostatin receptors in ~75%, is more frequently successful than MIBG imaging and is the recommended first-line nuclear scan. FDG imaging is successful if the tumor is relatively undifferentiated, but these tumors often are well differentiated. Endoscopic and intraoperative ultrasound have shown promising results, and intraoperative gamma probe localization of Octreoscan uptake in these tumors has been reported. Surgical resection is the only curative treatment; resection of hepatic metastasis can improve survival.

WORTH MENTIONING

1. NeoTect imaging

NeoTect is a ^{99m}Tc-labeled somatostatin analog. It was recently approved by the FDA for small-cell lung cancer imaging. It is reported to compare favorably with FDG PET for determining or excluding malignancy in solitary pulmonary nodules (see Chapter 18, Lung Cancer).

2. New therapies for neuroendocrine metastatic tumors

Octreotide labeled with ^{90}Y, a beta-emitting radionuclide, is in clinical trials in Europe. It holds promise as an effective, more easily managed alternative or adjunct to high-dose ^{131}I-MIBG therapy. Indium-111 pentetreotide also has been used therapeutically in multiple high-dose regimens with some success.

3. Use of intraoperative ^{131}I gamma detection probe

Hand-held surgical probes to detect radioactivity localized in a tumor can be used for a variety of tumors, including metastatic neuroendocrine tumors. Indium-111 Octreoscan, after having been imaged in a tumor on a nuclear scan, which provides a road map for the surgeon, can be localized intraoperatively using the probe. The technique requires some training for the surgeon. The scan is important as it indicates where normal tracer deposition exists.

PATIENT INFORMATION

I. MIBG DIAGNOSTIC SCAN
A. Test/Procedure

Your doctor has ordered an MIBG scan to localize and define the extent of spread, if any, of a neuroendocrine-type tumor that you (may) have. You will receive an intravenous injection of a radioactive form of iodine labeled to MIBG, which is accumulated by neuroendocrine tumor cells. Depending on the type of MIBG, you will have pictures taken of your whole body by a special camera to detect the radiotracer in your body at 24 or 72 hr. Imaging will take 1–2 hr.

B. Preparation

Diet. There are no dietary restrictions for this test.

Medications. There are medication restrictions, because several drugs may interfere with the MIBG localization in tumors. You need to carefully review all your medications with your doctor 4–6 wk before this test to see if you need to discontinue any of them.

Other. If any members of your family (siblings, parents, grandparents) have had tumors of neuroendocrine type (thyroid, adrenal, carcinoid, etc.), please inform your physician and the nuclear medicine technologist.

C. Radiation risk

The amount of radiation used is small and similar to that given by other diagnostic x-ray tests. The radiation exposure to your whole body from this test is about the same as the average person living in the United States receives each year from cosmic rays and naturally occurring background radiation sources.

The radiation dose is about 5–10% of the yearly dose considered safe for doctors and technologists who work with radiation. You can be around other people and use a bathroom normally without risk to others.

16

D. Pregnancy

If you are pregnant or think you could be pregnant, inform your doctor so that this can be discussed with the nuclear medicine physician.

II. OCTREOSCAN IMAGING
A. Test/Procedure

Your doctor has ordered Octreoscan imaging to localize and define the extent of spread, if any, of a neuroendocrine type tumor that you (may) have. You will receive an intravenous injection of a radioactive drug, Octreoscan, which binds to neuroendocrine tumors. You will have pictures taken of your whole body by a special camera to detect the radiotracer and tumor deposits wherever they may be in your body. This will take 1–2 hr.

B. Preparation

Diet. There are no dietary restrictions for this test. It is advisable to drink water liberally.

Medication. If you are taking octreotide, it may interfere with the scan. Please make sure the doctors are aware if you are taking octreotide.

Other. If any members of your family (siblings, parents, grandparents) have had tumors of neuroendocrine type (thyroid, adrenal, carcinoid, etc.), please inform your physician and the nuclear medicine technologist.

C. Radiation risks

The amount of radiation used is small and similar to that given by other diagnostic x-ray tests. The radiation exposure to your whole-body from this test is about seven times the dose the average person living in the United States receives each year from cosmic rays and naturally occurring background radiation sources. The radiation dose is about 50% of the yearly dose considered safe for doctors and technologists who work with radiation. You can be around other people and use a bathroom normally without risk to others.

D. Pregnancy

If you are pregnant or think you could be pregnant, inform your doctor so that this can be discussed with the nuclear medicine physician.

References

1. Seregni E, Chiti A, Bombardieri E. Radionuclide imaging of neuroendocrine tumors: biological basis and diagnostic results. *Eur J Nucl Med* 1998;25:639–659.
2. Bongers V, de Klerk JM, Zonneberg BA, de Kort G, Lips CJ, van Rijk PP. Acute liver necrosis induced by iodine-131-MIBG in the treatment of metastatic carcinoid tumors. *J Nucl Med* 1997;38:1024–1026.
3. Sisson JC, Frager MS, Valk TW, et al. Scintigraphic localization of pheochromocytoma. *N Engl J Med* 1981;305:12–17.
4. Loh KC, Fitzgerald PA, Matthany KK, Yeo PB, Price DC. The treatment of malignant pheochromocytoma with iodine-131 metaiodobenzylguanidine (^{131}I-MIBG): a comprehensive review of 116 reported patients. *J Endocrinol Invest* 1997;20:648–658.
5. Troncone L, Rufini V, Montemaggi P, Danza FM, Lasorella A, Mastrangelo R. The diagnostic and therapeutic utility of radioiodinated metaiodobenzylguanidine (MIBG). 5 years of experience. *Eur J Nucl Med* 1990;16:325–335.
6. Hoefnagel CA, Schornagel J, Valdes Olmas RA. [131I]metaiobenzylguanidine therapy malignant pheochromocytoma: interference of medication. *J Nucl Biol Med* 1991;35:308–312.
7. Yamamoto Y, Isobe Y, Nishiyama Y, et al. Iodine-131 MIBG imaging in multiple endocrine neoplasia type 2B. *Clin Nucl Med* 1998;23:13–15.

17
Lymphoma

Accurate staging and follow-up of Hodgkin's disease (HD) and non-Hodgkin's lymphoma (NHL) is important in achieving success with modern oncologic therapy. Pretherapy nuclear imaging can assist in staging and serves as a baseline for monitoring response to treatment. Nuclear imaging also can evaluate suspected recurrence and indicate the need for salvage therapy. (AIDS-related lymphoma is discussed in Chapter 7, AIDS.)

SCANS AND PRIMARY CLINICAL INDICATIONS

I. Gallium scan   Page 270
  ● To aid in the initial evaluation and staging of lymphoma
  ● To differentiate post-therapy residual fibrosis from active disease
  ● To detect recurrent lymphoma
  ● To predict disease prognosis

II. Thallium or sestamibi scan   Page 272
  ● To help in the evaluation of non–gallium-avid lymphomas

III. Fluorodeoxyglucose (FDG) imaging   Page 272
  ● All of the above indications

CLINICAL QUESTIONS

Lymphoma

PATIENT INFORMATION

SCANS

I. GALLIUM SCAN

A. Background

Gallium-67-citrate scanning is highly useful in staging, detecting relapse or progression and monitoring and predicting therapeutic response and outcome for HD and NHL. Optimal dosing and SPECT imaging have made gallium an increasingly useful radiotracer in the evaluation of the lymphoma patient, especially when determining residual tumor after treatment.

B. Radiopharmaceuticals

Gallium-67-citrate is a nonspecific marker of tumor and inflammation. It acts as an iron analog and is transported in the blood bound to transferrin. Most lymphomas have transferrin receptors that avidly bind the gallium and facilitate incorporation into the lysosomes of these active tumor cells.

C. How the study is performed

Gallium is injected intravenously (5–10 mCi [185–370 MBq] adult dose) and images are acquired at 2–3 days to allow blood-pool clearance. The use of a higher (8–10 mCi) gallium dose, as well as SPECT imaging, improve diagnostic accuracy. Delayed images may be necessary up to 4–7 days after injection. The imaging may take less than 30 min for planar chest views, or up to 2–3 hr for a comprehensive examination with whole-body SPECT. The patient should be prepared for these possibilities.

D. Patient preparation

Gallium scanning should be avoided within 24 hr after blood transfusions or gadolinium-enhanced MRI scanning, both of which may interfere with gallium biodistribution. Also, it is advisable to wait 3–4 wk after chemotherapy for follow-up imaging (see below). The nuclear medicine physician may prescribe a gentle laxative to assist bowel clearance. The patient may eat, drink and take medications as usual.

E. Understanding the report

Gallium is normally distributed in the liver, spleen, skeletal system, colon and in varying degrees in salivary and lacrimal glands, nasal region, breasts and genitalia. There is faint renal uptake on the 48- to 72-hr images. Mild hilar uptake also may be a normal finding. Minimal lung uptake may be seen up to 48 hr.

The report describes the location and degree of abnormal uptake, which suggests foci of gallium-avid lymphoma (Fig. 1). Correlation often is made to anatomic imaging such as CT scanning. Comparison with prior gallium studies also may be included in the report.

F. Potential problems

1. Normal distribution. Because gallium has normal distribution in certain organs, diseases affecting them will be less conspicuous. The most frequent activity confounding interpretation is that of normal bowel excretion. Normal up-

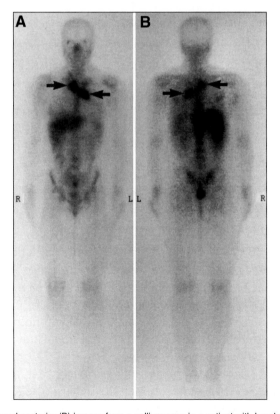

Figure 1. Anterior (A) and posterior (B) images from a gallium scan in a patient with lymphoma show extensive mediastinal uptake (arrows). This study served as a baseline to monitor response to therapy.

take in the pediatric thymus and intense breast uptake in lactating women are expected findings.

2. Nonspecificity. Infection, inflammation, sarcoid and many other cancers besides lymphoma can demonstrate abnormal gallium uptake. Increased uptake can occur at sites of recent surgery, bone-marrow harvesting, fracture, biopsy and intramuscular injections. Severe constipation, bowel inflammation and certain neoplasia can demonstrate abnormal colonic uptake. Liver failure and nephritis can cause increased kidney activity. Thymic hyperplasia with increased uptake is common for 4–10 mo after chemotherapy and radiation therapy. Intense parotid and other salivary gland uptake after local radiation therapy and chemotherapy may be seen. Findings need to be correlated with the clinical examination and the results of other diagnostic tests.

3. False-negative results and biointerference. Chemotherapy (e.g., cisplatin, bleomycin, vincristine) may result in a false-negative study for 3–4 wk after treatment. Small foci of lymphoma as well as a large tumor with inadequate blood flow may result in a false-negative examination. Low-grade NHL may not be gallium-avid. Other potential problems include the alteration of gallium biodistribution caused by the saturation of iron binding sites from iron overload, blood transfusion, chelation therapy and gadolinium administration for MRI.

17

II. THALLIUM OR SESTAMIBI SCAN

Most lymphomas are gallium-avid. Low-grade NHL is less likely to accumulate gallium. If gallium uptake is not present on baseline imaging, scanning with either thallium or sestamibi has been advocated because these radiotracers are often positive with low-grade lymphomas (see Chapter 7, AIDS and Chapter 11, The Skeletal System for more detailed information).

III. FDG IMAGING

FDG scanning with PET is only available at limited locations, but coincidence systems adapted to SPECT gamma cameras and centralized delivery of FDG are making this technology more widely available. This glucose analog localizes to a greater extent in active lymphoma and not in fibrotic or necrotic tissue, differentiating recurrence from treatment effects. The high resolution images provided by FDG scanning can be used for staging of lymphomas, as well as determining response to therapy (Fig. 2), detecting residual and recurrent disease, and determining prognosis. In recent studies, FDG PET staging algorithms have been demonstrated to be more accurate and cost-effective in determining nodal and extra-nodal disease than conventional staging using CT. FDG imaging is more sensitive than bone scanning in identifying skeletal lymphoma lesions; it also can detect bone-marrow involvement, possibly sparing the patient a bone-

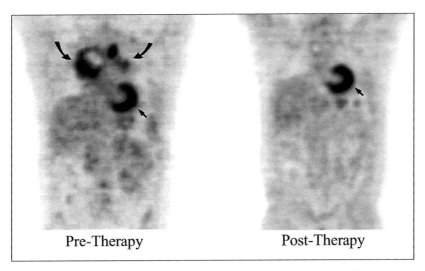

Pre-Therapy   Post-Therapy

Figure 2. FDG PET scans of 19-yr-old man with newly diagnosed HD. Pretherapy scan (left) shows abnormal up-take in mediastinal and bilateral hilar masses (curved arrows) with normal uptake in myocardium (short arrow). The patient received three cycles of chemotherapy. Post-therapy scan (right) shows normal FDG uptake in the my-ocardium (arrow) but no evidence of tumor activity.

marrow biopsy. More studies are required, though, to determine if FDG scan-ning can be used as first-line imaging in place of CT.

Unlike gallium scanning, which requires 2–3 days from injection of gallium to imaging, FDG imaging can be completed in a few hours. FDG eventually may replace gallium scanning, and its reimbursement for the evaluation of lym-phoma has been approved by the United States Health Care Financing Administration. Like gallium, thallium and sestamibi, FDG suffers from a lack of specificity. FDG imaging cannot distinguish one tumor type from another. Uptake also has been described with inflammation, fracture and other benign processes, although this uptake is less intense than the uptake in active lym-phoma (see Chapter 15, Introduction to Cancer and FDG Imaging for more detail).

CLINICAL QUESTIONS

1. Suspected lymphoma: How is initial evaluation and staging done?

Tissue biopsy is necessary to diagnose a suspected lymphoma and determine its histology. Although staging laparotomy was once a mainstay in the initial eval-uation of HD, it is now infrequently used because much of the information that will affect therapeutic decisions can be determined less invasively. CT scanning and percutaneous needle biopsy are the procedures of choice for diagnosing and staging all lymphomas. MRI is used in some centers in place of CT for staging. Bone-marrow biopsy is also used in certain cases.

17

Gallium scanning is able to rapidly survey the entire body and may be useful for problem-solving situations. Yet the major reason to obtain a gallium scan during the initial evaluation is to determine the avidity of the lymphoma for gallium. If the lymphoma is gallium avid, the scan can serve as a baseline for future imaging to monitor response to therapy and to detect early recurrence. In some centers, FDG imaging using PET or coincidence SPECT has largely replaced gallium scanning in the workup of lymphoma.

2. What if the lymphoma is not gallium avid?

Most Hodgkin's lymphomas and NHLs are gallium avid, but low-grade lymphomas may not accumulate gallium. If the initial pretherapy scan fails to show gallium uptake, detecting these low-grade tumors and monitoring response to therapy may be accomplished with thallium or sestamibi scanning or FDG, if available.

3 and 4. Residual mass after therapy on CT scan: Is it active disease or fibrosis? Is salvage therapy required?

CT will demonstrate a residual mass after therapy in nearly 60% of lymphomas despite a complete response. CT cannot differentiate a fibrotic mass from active disease requiring further therapy. Gallium scanning is excellent for resolving this question (76–100% sensitivity and 75–96% specificity). (FDG imaging is also effective in distinguishing viable tumor from post-therapy fibrosis or necrosis.) A pretherapy baseline study must be acquired first to confirm that the tumor is gallium avid. A baseline is especially important if bulky disease is present because it is more likely to leave a residual mass despite successful therapy. Lack of gallium uptake is consistent with fibrosis. Persistent uptake indicates active lymphoma. Thus, gallium scanning can be used to identify those patients who are failing first-line chemotherapy and who may require second-line treatments.

MRI is also being used in some centers, but the accuracy is not as high as with gallium because necrotic tumors may have abnormal signal on MRI, mimicking active disease. Gallium uptake will normalize with successful therapy before MRI signal intensity returns to normal. Often, nuclear imaging and CT or MRI are used in a complementary manner for optimal diagnostic accuracy.

5 and 6. Is nuclear imaging useful in the evaluation for recurrence? Can nuclear imaging help predict prognosis?

Gallium scanning is an accurate predictor of therapeutic outcome. In one study, 94% of patients with a negative gallium scan obtained after two cycles of chemotherapy had a long-term complete response at 31 mo; only 18% of those with a positive gallium scan after two cycles of chemotherapy remained in complete remission at 31 mo. Scanning should be delayed 3–4 wk after chemotherapy (see Potential Problem 3, above).

Gallium uptake also heralds relapse before clinical findings or anatomic imaging are abnormal (95% sensitivity and 89% specificity). A positive gallium scan should be correlated with anatomic modalities such as CT, and the patient should be referred for biopsy or further therapy as clinically warranted. FDG imaging also accurately detects tumor regression and recurrence.

WORTH MENTIONING

1. Radiolabeled antibodies

Iodine-131 and yttrium-90 labeled monoclonal antibodies are being studied for the treatment of NHLs. Preliminary results are promising, and remissions have been obtained in patients in whom conventional therapy has failed.

2. Somatostatin receptor imaging

Somatostatin receptor imaging using Octreoscan also is being studied in the staging and follow-up of HD and NHL.

PATIENT INFORMATION
I. GALLIUM SCAN
A. Test/Procedure

17

Your doctor has ordered a gallium scan to evaluate your lymphoma either to establish the baseline extent of tumor before treatment or to measure the response after therapy.

A small amount of radioactive gallium will be injected into a vein. You will be asked to return in 1–3 days for imaging. During this return visit, you will be positioned next to a special machine called a gamma camera, which does not produce radiation but detects radiation coming from the gallium injected in your body. A series of pictures of your body will then be taken, and you may have to return the next day for delayed pictures. Sometimes pictures over a series of days are needed for proper interpretation. The injection takes only a few min. Each imaging session may take from 30 min to 3 hr.

B. Preparation

You may eat and drink as usual and take your medications. You might be asked to take a gentle laxative to aid in clearance of the radiotracer from your bowel.

C. Radiation and other risks

The amount of radiation used is small and similar to that given by other diagnostic x-ray tests. The effective adult radiation dose to your whole body from this test is about the dose the average person living in the United States receives in 7–14 yr from cosmic rays and naturally occurring background radiation sources. Your radiation dose is about 50–100% of the yearly dose considered safe for doctors and technologists who work with radiation. You can be around other people and use a bathroom normally without risk to others.

D. Pregnancy

If you are pregnant or think you could be pregnant, inform your doctor so that this can be discussed with the nuclear medicine physician.

II. FDG IMAGING
A. Test/Procedure

Your doctor has ordered an FDG PET (coincidence SPECT) scan to evaluate your lymphoma either to establish the baseline extent of tumor before treatment or to measure the response after therapy.

A small amount of radioactive sugar (FDG) will be injected into your vein. After about 45 min, you will be positioned next to a special machine called a PET scanner or coincidence gamma camera, which does not produce radiation but detects radiation coming from the sugar injected in your body. A series of pictures of your body will then be taken. If your brain is to be imaged, the imaging detectors will be brought close to your skull, which may cause claustrophobia, but you can close your eyes. The whole process may take from 1 to 2 hr. It is important that you are able to lie very still for the examination. If you cannot do this, please inform your doctor.

B. Preparation

You will be asked to fast the day of the examination (water is permitted). Please ask your doctor about any medications you are taking. If you are a diabetic, please make sure the PET center knows this, because special instructions may be provided.

C. Radiation and other risks

The amount of radiation used is small and similar to that given by other diagnostic x-ray tests. The effective adult radiation dose to your whole body from this test is about the dose the average person living in the United States receives in 3–7 yr from cosmic rays and naturally occurring background radiation sources. The radiation dose is about 20–40% of the yearly dose considered safe for doctors and technologists who work with radiation. You can be around other people and use a bathroom normally without risk to others.

D. Pregnancy

If you are pregnant or think you could be pregnant, inform your doctor so that this can be discussed with the nuclear medicine physician.

References

1. van Amsterdam JAG, Kluin-Nelemans JC, van Eck-Smit BLF, Pauwels EKJ. Role of Ga-67 scintigraphy in localization of lymphoma. *Ann Hematol* 1996;72:202–207.
2. Front D, Bar-Shalom R, Israel O. The continuing role of gallium 67 scintigraphy in the age of receptor imaging. *Semin Nucl Med* 1997;27:68–74.
3. Bangerter M, Griesshammer M, Binder T, et al. New diagnostic imaging procedures in Hodgkin's disease. *Ann Oncol* 1996;7(suppl 4):S55–S59.
4. Draisma A, Maffioli L, Gasparini M, Savelli G, Pauwels E, Bombardieri E. Gallium-67 as a tumor-seeking agent in lymphomas—a review. *Tumori* 1998;84:434–441.
5. Romer W, Schwaiger M. Positron emission tomography in diagnosis and therapy monitoring of patients with lymphoma. *Clin Positron Imaging* 1998;1:101–110.

17

18
Lung Cancer

Lung cancer causes more deaths in the United States than any other cancer and leads all cancer in mortality in most western countries. The 5-yr survival of patients with lung cancer has not improved during the past decades and overall remains at about 14%. Often, lung cancer presents with a solitary pulmonary nodule (SPN) incidentally diagnosed on a chest x-ray. About a third of SPNs in patients older than 35 yr are malignant.

Chest x-ray, CT and MRI are not accurate in characterizing an SPN as benign or malignant. Sputum cytology, bronchoscopy, percutaneous needle biopsy, mediastinioscopy or open lung biopsy are performed for tissue diagnosis. PET using ^{18}F-fluorodeoxyglucose (FDG) is highly sensitive in identifying lung cancer and is superior to CT in staging the mediastinum.

18

SCANS AND PRIMARY CLINICAL INDICATIONS

I. FDG imaging Page 280
- To diagnose or exclude cancer in SPNs

- To stage lung cancer

- To determine effectiveness of tumorcidal therapy and assess possible recurrence of tumor

II. NeoTect and Octreoscan imaging Page 281
- To assess spread of known small-cell lung cancer

CLINICAL QUESTIONS

PATIENT INFORMATION

SCANS

I. FDG IMAGING

A. Background

Malignant cells have a high rate of glucose utilization under aerobic and anaerobic conditions. FDG images provide semi-quantitative information about glucose metabolism in a suspected tumor. Lung cancers show markedly increased FDG in tumors compared with surrounding normal lung tissue and other benign lesions. The level of FDG localization in a lesion can be semiquantitatively measured using standardized uptake values (SUVs) and correlated with tissue diagnosis (see Chapter 16, Introduction to Cancer and FDG Imaging for additional information).

B. Radiopharmaceuticals

The reader is referred to Chapter 16, Introduction to Cancer and FDG Imaging for information about FDG and how it works.

C. How the scan is performed

Approximately 45–60 min (or longer) after intravenous injection of 6–20 mCi of FDG, imaging is performed on a PET scanner or a coincidence camera (a modified SPECT camera). The interval between injection and imaging is needed

18

for the FDG to accumulate in the tumor and for the background activity to be excreted by the kidneys. Depending on the equipment, the time needed to scan the thorax from the neck to the midabdomen varies from 45 min to 1.5 hr. Before acquiring the emission FDG scan, a transmission scan of the patient's body is typically done so that attenuation correction can be applied to the FDG emission scan.

D. Patient preparation

Except for water, the patient needs to fast for 4–12 hr before the study. Unlabeled serum glucose competes with FDG for entry into tumor cells. If serum glucose is high, the scan may be sub-optimal because relatively low levels of labeled FDG entered the mass. Most centers obtain a blood glucose before administering FDG (see Chapter 16).

E. Understanding the report

The report summarizes the reason for the study, the procedure and the findings. PET studies provide a semiquantitative index of FDG uptake called the SUV, which relates the lesion FDG activity to the injected dose activity. Generally, a lower SUV is associated with benignity, while higher SUVs are associated with malignancy. But, a large lung cancer will have more FDG than a small lesion even though the glucose utilization rate may be the same. There is an indeterminate level of uptake; for lung nodules it is SUV 1.7–2.5

F. Potential problems

1. Dietary compliance. Failure to fast may depress FDG uptake in the tumor.

2. Sensitivity. Coincidence camera imaging is not as sensitive as conventional PET, but the technology is constantly improving. In the lungs, however, its performance is quite good. Lung cancer lesions 1.5 cm or greater are detected with 90% or better sensitivity. The semiquantitative index is helpful in PET, but not yet widely available or standardized for coincidence camera systems.

3. False-positive results. Active inflammatory lesions, such as infections or active granulomas, may be falsely positive; the medical workup would have to be relied upon to reveal active granulomatous disease or infections.

II. NEOTECT AND OCTREOSCAN IMAGING

Technetium-99m-NeoTect is a somatostatin receptor-binding agent. Lung cancer cells are rich in somatostatin receptors. Therefore, this agent localizes in primary lung cancers and some other cancers. Whole-body imaging is easily accomplished, and SPECT images can be obtained. Clinical trials document sen-

18

sitivity of approximately 95% and specificity of approximately 85% for lung cancer lesions >1.0 cm, compared with biopsy.

Indium-111-pentetreotide (Ostreoscan) also binds to somatostatin receptors that are found in abundance on small-cell lung cancers. Similar to neuroendocrine tumor imaging, small-cell lung cancer can be staged using this imaging agent (see Chapter 16, Neuroendocrine Tumors for details about somatostatin receptor imaging).

CLINICAL QUESTIONS

1 and 2. What is the role of the chest x-ray, CT and FDG imaging in patients with an SPN and in staging the mediastinum? When should FDG imaging be used to stage lung cancer?

Based on numerous studies, FDG PET imaging is superior to CT in predicting malignant or benign nature of an SPN. The routine sequence of imaging studies in the workup of patients with suspected lung cancer is chest x-ray followed by CT. A normal chest x-ray rarely is found when lung cancer is present. CT can detect smaller lesions than chest x-ray and sometimes can suggest malignant versus benign status. CT can identify spread to neighboring structures and particularly to lymph nodes in the mediastinum. Based on a lymph node's size (>1.0 cm), CT identifies lymph nodes suspicious for tumor spread, which then require further testing such as sputum cytology, bronchoscopy, percutaneous biopsy, mediastinscopy or open lung biopsy. FDG imaging has sufficiently strong diagnostic power to be cost-effective and clinically useful in this workup progression. Clearly, using PET can reduce the number of thoracotomies performed for nonresectable disease based on evaluation of mediastinal spread. PET also detects extrathoracic metastases, which may be easier sites to biopsy than the lung nodule (Fig. 1).

FDG is clearly important to patient management; those patients whose FDG scans indicate high likelihood of malignancy should undergo thoracotomy, whereas those with an FDG scan that indicates high likelihood of a benign lesion (no uptake or low uptake) can be spared thoracotomy. If a percutaneous biopsy can be performed, it should be done for those patients whose CT or FDG scans indicate that observation rather than surgery is appropriate.

FDG PET is also superior to CT in staging the mediastinum. In determining metastatic involvement of lung cancer, sensitivity of PET based on the studies of 257 patients acquired in 11 centers is 88% and specificity is 91%, whereas CT sensitivity is about 68%. But FDG scans cannot provide the anatomic localization of lymph nodes in the mediastinum as CT can. Thus, both are important for the diagnosis and staging of lung cancer.

FDG imaging can be achieved either by PET or by camera coincidence technologies. PET is superior to coincidence imaging, but both are effective. Coincidence reportedly detects 97% of FDG-avid mediastinal lymph nodes >1.5

A Transaxial

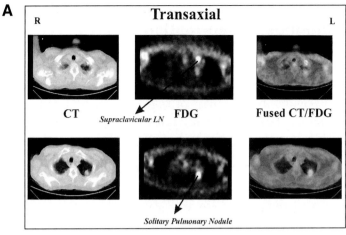

B Coronal

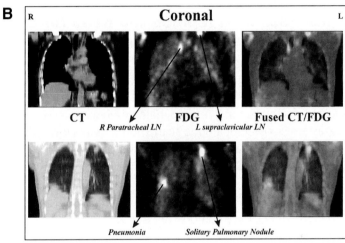

Figure 1. (A) Transaxial tomographic images of CT scan (far left), FDG coincidence scan (middle), and fused CT/FDG images (far right) of upper lung fields (apical slice, top) show an SPN (lower row, arrow) that is hypermetabolic, showing markedly elevated uptake of FDG. Also noted is FDG uptake in a left supraclavicular lymph node (top row, arrow, not apparent on the CT scan), which could be palpated in retrospect. Biopsy of this lymph node revealed squamous cell cancer, sparing the patient a more invasive biopsy of the lung nodule. (B) Coronal tomographic images of CT scan (far left). FDG coincidence scan (middle) and fused CT/FDG images (far right) of an anterior slice (top row) and a posterior slice (bottom row) through the chest. Images show the SPN (posteriorly) in the left apex (bottom row, arrow). Also seen posteriorly is a pneumonic infiltrate in the right lower lobe (bottom row, left arrow). On the anterior slices (top row) a right paratracheal lymph node and the left supraclavicular lymph node (arrows) are seen on FDG and fused CT/FDG images.

cm seen on PET. For PET, sensitivity is 96% (specificity 88%) for detecting cancer in SPNs, based on 588 patient studies reported in 18 publications. Coincidence camera imaging reportedly detects 93% of lung nodules or masses (0.9–4 cm) seen on conventional PET.

Only sparse data for coincidence camera performance have been published as yet. Initial results, without the more recent technological advances including improved count sensitivity and attenuation correction, still reveal sensitivity for detecting cancer in SPNs >1.5 cm of 93%, which far exceeds the capability of CT.

3. Suspected recurrence: Should FDG imaging be used? What prognostic information can it provide?

Recurrent cancers after radiation or chemotherapy avidly accumulate FDG. Consequently, SUVs (i.e., activity taken up in the mass relative to the activity in the dose injected into the patient) in masses containing cancer are higher than SUVs in regions (benign mass or scar tissue) without tumor recurrence.

PET is more accurate than CT in predicting tumor recurrence. Where FDG PET is available, it seems to offer earlier, more accurate detection of tumor recurrence than CT.

The level of tumor FDG (SUV) correlates with prognosis. In a recent study, when the SUV (sometimes called SUR or standard uptake ratio) exceeds 10, median survival is less than 11.4 mo. When SUV is less than 10, median survival is 24.6 mo. SUV is affected by glucose utilization and tumor size.

4. Does the FDG scan replace the need for a bone scan when bone metastases are suspected?

The bone scan is a sensitive test for bone metastases. FDG clearly detects lung cancer metastases, but lung cancer is known to metastasize to distal bones, and the lower extremities are usually omitted from an FDG study because of the excessive time requirements and limited field of view of most PET scanners. If bony metstases are suspected, a bone scan should be performed. Bone scans are appropriate in stage III disease (tumor extension to neighboring structures with or without nodal metastasis) before deciding on curative thoractomy.

5. How cost-effective is FDG PET?

Cost-effectiveness studies have demonstrated that PET plus CT is cost-effective in staging non–small-cell lung cancer. The cost savings are realized by reducing unnecessary curative thoractomies in patients with unresectable disease. The cost-effectiveness analysis is based on comparing two decision strategies: thoracic CT alone versus thoracic CT and thoracic PET. In the management of non–small-cell lung cancer, CT plus PET showed a saving of $1154 per patient without loss of life expectancy compared with the alternate CT alone strategy. Each year, 85,000 patients present with non–small-cell lung cancer in the United States. If all 85,000 were managed using the CT/PET algorithm versus CT alone, the savings would be approximately $98 million per year with no change in life expectancy.

6. What is the role of somatostatin receptor imaging (NeoTect, Octreoscan) in lung cancer?

NeoTect (technetium-labeled somatostatin receptor binding agent) was recently approved by United States Food and Drug Administration for imaging SPNs or masses to confirm or exclude malignancy. In centers where FDG imaging is unavailable, NeoTect SPECT imaging may provide an alternative noninvasive evaluation. NeoTect and Octreoscan (see Chapter 16, Neuroendocrine Tumors) depend on somatostatin receptors rather than tumor or inflammatory cell metabolism of glucose. In addition to lung cancers and neuroendocrine tumors, activated lymphocytes have somatostatin receptors that may cause NeoTect images to be positive. However, the incidence of negative images in granulomas exceeds that of postives.

PATIENT INFORMATION

I. FDG IMAGING
A. Test/Procedure
Your doctor has ordered an FDG scan to determine if you have lung cancer or if the cancer has spread. FDG is a radiopharmaceutical composed of the radioisotope fluorine-18 labeled to a form of sugar (FDG), which is absorbed by tumors. After your blood sugar is checked to see if you have fasted sufficiently for the test, you will receive an intravenous injection of FDG and then have a 45-min waiting period before pictures of your lungs and upper abdomen are taken. It is important for you to be at rest and undistracted by visual (sight) or auditory (hearing) stimuli at the time of the injection. You should not be chewing, swallowing or talking. The whole procedure will take about 1.5–2.5 hr.

B. Preparation
Diet. You need to have fasted for at least 4 hr before the injection of FDG into a vein (usually in your arm).

Medication. There is no restriction on medications.

C. Radiation risks/exposure
The amount of radiation used is small and similar to that given by other diagnostic x-ray tests. The effective adult radiation exposure to your whole body from this test is approximately the dose the average person living in the United States receives in 3–7 yr from cosmic rays and naturally occurring background radiation sources. The radiation dose is about 20–40% of the yearly dose considered safe for doctors and technologists who work with radiation. You can be around other people and use a bathroom normally without risk to others.

D. Pregnancy
If you are pregnant or think you could be pregnant, inform your doctor so that this can be discussed with the nuclear medicine physician.

II. NEOTECT IMAGING
A. Test/Procedure
Your doctor has ordered a NeoTect scan to determine the likelihood that the nodule found on your chest x-ray or CT scan is lung cancer. You will receive

an intravenous injection of NeoTect and then you will have pictures taken by a special camera to detect the radiotracer in your body approximately 2 and 24 hr later.

B. Preparation

There are no dietary or other requirements. If you are well hydrated by drinking plenty of water, your radiation exposure from the test will be minimized due to excretion of the radioactivity in the urine.

C. Radiation risk/exposure

The amount of radiation used is small and similar to that given by other diagnostic x-ray tests. The radiation exposure to your whole body from this test is about the same as the average person living in the United States receives in 5 yr from cosmic rays and naturally occurring background radiation sources. The radiation dose is about 2% of the yearly dose considered safe for doctors and technologists who work with radiation. You can be around other people and use a bathroom normally without risk to others.

D. Pregnancy

If you are pregnant or think you could be pregnant, inform your doctor so that this can be discussed with the nuclear medicine physician.

References

1. Al-Sugir A, Coleman RE. Applications of PET in lung cancer. *Semin Nucl Med* 1998;28:303–319.
2. Valk PE, Pounds TR, Hopkins DM, et al. Staging lung cancer by PET imaging. *Ann Thorac Surg* 1995;60:1573–1582.
3. Gambir SS, Hoh CG, Phelps ME, et al. Decision tree sensitivity analysis for cost-effectiveness of FDG-PET in the staning and management of non-small cell lung carcinoma. *J Nucl Med* 1996;37:1428–1436.
4. Conti PS, Lilien DL, Hawley K, et al. PET and [^{18}F]-FDG in oncology: a clinical update. *Nucl Med Biol* 1996;23:717–735.
5. Shreve PD, Stevenson RS, Deters EC, Kison PV, Gross MD, Wahl RL. Oncologic diagnosis with 2-[fluorine-18] fluoro-2-deoxy-D-glucose imaging: dual-head coincidence gamma camera versus positron emission tomographic scanner. *Radiology* 1998;207:431–437.
6. Coleman RE. PET in lung cancer. *J Nucl Med* 1999;40:814–820.

18

19
Melanoma

The incidence of melanoma, a malignant tumor of melanocytes, has been increasing steadily in recent years. Australia has the highest worldwide incidence of melanoma, with ultraviolet radiation (sun exposure) a recognized major risk factor. In the United States, melanoma causes 6700 deaths per year.

19

a. Lymphoscintigraphy and sentinel node
b. FDG imaging
c. Gallium and other tumor imaging agents

PATIENT INFORMATION

SCANS

I. LYMPHOSCINTIGRAPHY
A. Background

Primary melanoma tumors usually are cutaneous but also may originate in the eye. Staging of cutaneous melanoma is based on tumor thickness (Breslow measurement) and level of invasion (Clark's level), both of which are determined by the pathologist. Resection of the lymph node bed most likely to receive drainage of the tumor often has been performed to identify and remove lymph node metastasis in patients without clinically apparent metastases. Lymphoscintigraphy images have proven the unpredictability of standardized lymphatic drainage patterns. About 10% of trunk melanomas drain to three or more different lymph node beds, which may be in different anatomic locations. The sentinel lymph node is defined as the first lymph node that receives lymph drainage from the tumor site. It is the first node to which a tumor cell would come if it penetrated into lymphatics. Dynamic imaging studies have shown that the sentinel node is not necessarily the node closest to the tumor, nor is it necessarily the hottest node found.

The standard of care for patients without clinically apparent metastases and intermediate stage melanoma (Breslow thickness 0.75–4 mm) has become the sentinel lymph node biopsy. The sentinel lymph node can be identified by lymphoscintigraphy (Fig. 1), with subsequent excision using the intraoperative gamma probe or the blue dye techniques. The blue dye approach uses isosulfan blue dye, injected intradermally at the tumor site in the operating room, followed by a search for blue stained node(s). The blue dye method is challenging for the surgeon and does not provide the road map (as does radionuclide imaging) to identify the anatomic regions containing nodal groups that receive drainage from the tumor site, but blue dye can be used adjunctively with radionuclide imaging and probe. With these approaches, only the nodes at high-

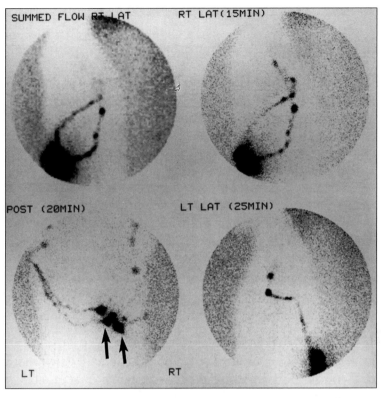

Figure 1. Sentinel lymph node lymphoscintigraphy. Melanoma on back: Lymphoscintigraphy shows drainage to sentinel nodes in both axillae. Four intradermal ^{99m}Tc-filtered sulfur colloid peritumoral injections (arrows) form the activity focus. Discrete channels lead to sentinel lymph nodes in both axillae.

19

est risk for metastasis are resected. Morbidity is significantly reduced compared with that associated with the complete dissection of the nodal bed.

B. Radiopharmaceutical

Technetium-99m-sulfur colloid (filtered or unfiltered) is the most frequently used radiopharmaceutical for lymphoscintigraphy and the only Food and Drug Administration–approved colloid radiopharmaceutical for lymphoscintigraphy in the United States. In Europe ^{99m}Tc-albumin colloid and in Australia ^{99m}Tc-antimony sulfide colloid are used. The main difference between these colloids is particle size.

C. How the test is performed

Within a few hours before scheduled surgery for sentinel lymph node excisional biopsy (often combined with wide excision of the melanoma tumor), lymphoscintigraphy is performed in the nuclear medicine department. Intradermal injections (0.1 ml each) of a summed total dose of approximately 0.5 mCi (1.85 MBq; adult dose) are made surrounding the tumor site at four points, followed immediately by dynamic and static imaging. For trunk lesions it is important to image axillary and cervical as well as inguinal regions. The images demonstrate sentinel lymph node(s) and often the lymphatic vessel(s) draining the tracer from the injections sites. The location of the sentinel node(s) is marked on the skin, and images are sent with the patient to the operating room, where the surgeon uses the gamma detecting surgical probe to assist in finding the sentinel lymph node. The probe is a hand-held wand-like device that is fitted into a sterile glove-sheath for use in the sterile surgical field. As the probe gets closer to the radiation source (the sentinel node) the audible signal increases, alerting the surgeon to the identification of the sentinel node. Using the images, the skin markers and the probe, the surgeon can accurately identify the position of the sentinel node(s) before making an incision. The nodes at risk can be quickly found through a small incision. Operating time and morbidity are substantially reduced.

D. Patient preparation

No dietary or medication restrictions are required for this test.

E. Understanding the report

The report explains the reason for the lymphoscintigraphy, the procedure, the findings and the surgical probe results. The dynamic images often show the lymphatic vessel drainage from the tumor site. One or more sentinel lymph nodes in one or more lymph node beds or anatomic regions also may be imaged.

F. Potential problems

1. Prior surgical intervention. Occasionally, no lymphatic drainage can be seen on images when a deep, wide excisional biopsy preceded sentinel node lymphoscintigraphy. It is thought that deep surgical intervention may so disrupt lymph channels, that the tracer cannot access the lymphatics for transport to lymph nodes.

2. Sentinel versus secondary lymph nodes. Some imaged lymph node(s) will be secondary nodes rather than true sentinel nodes. Secondary nodes accumulate the tracer after it passes through a sentinel node. Usually, the surgeon will excise a secondary node in close proximity to the sentinel node.

II. FDG IMAGING

FDG imaging is highly sensitive in identifying melanoma tumors and their metastases, but it is not as sensitive for detecting micrometastases to sentinel lymph nodes as is histoimmunochemistry pathology. FDG imaging may detect metastases up to 6 mo earlier than conventional anatomic imaging. Coincidence cameras will make FDG imaging more widely available than it has been with conventional PET. If bone metastases are suspected, the bone scan is still recommended as the most sensitive whole-body imaging indicator of bone metastases, even if an FDG study is performed. See Chapter 15, Introduction to Cancer and FDG Imaging, for details on FDG and PET or coincidence camera imaging.

III. GALLIUM IMAGING

Gallium imaging is effective in localizing melanoma tumors and their metastases, particularly in combination with SPECT imaging. See the discussion on gallium imaging in Chapter 17, Lymphoma.

CLINICAL QUESTIONS

1. Biopsy shows malignant melanoma; what is the prognosis?

The Breslow thickness of the tumor measured by the pathologist is the best prognostic indicator for patients with melanoma. Patients with thin lesions (<0.76 mm thick) have 98% 5-yr survivals. Patients with >4 mm thick lesions have 5-yr survivals of about 45%.

2. Biopsy shows malignant melanoma; how is it staged?

Lymphoscintigraphy to identify the sentinel lymph node for excisional biopsy is the standard of care. In patients without clinically apparent metastases and whose primary melanoma is in the intermediate thickness category, 0.76–4.0-mm Breslow thickness, the radionuclide lymphoscintigram is a reliable, accurate and simple method to identify the sentinel node(s) before surgical excision. Using the gamma-detecting probe in the operating room shortens the search for the sentinel node (Fig. 1). This procedure has replaced the elective lymph node dissection (ELND) as the lymph node staging procedure for intermediate thickness melanoma. The experience with ELND was that 20–40% of patients with intermediate thickness tumors had lymph node metastases. Therefore, 60–80% of those patients did not need ELND but were subjected unnecessarily to the expense and morbidity of the procedure. The sentinel node approach selects only those patients with lymph node spread of tumor (indicated by the sentinel lymph node histopathology) to have more invasive lymph node dissection. Thus, the sentinel node staging of melanoma in patients without known metastases has become pivotal in guiding the surgical management of this disease.

3. How can recurrences be detected?

Surgical management of melanoma is excision of the lesion with a margin of approximately 1–3 cm in diameter. Few data support the need for wider exci-

19

sions. Only patients with nodal metastases (by sentinel node biopsy or clinically evident) undergo ELND.

Patients with thicker lesions are at higher risk for recurrence, as are those who have positive lymph nodes at time of diagnosis. These patients typically are closely followed clinically, although there is no consensus on a protocol to screen high-risk patients with FDG or other imaging. Certainly, if an FDG scan shows focal findings in lymph nodes or distant sites, the likelihood of metastatic disease at those sites is high.

Other radiopharmaceuticals available in the United States that are effective in localizing in melanoma tumors and metastases include ^{67}Ga-citrate, thallium, ^{99m}Tc-sestamibi, Octreoscan and NeoTect (as yet unproven). These agents are discussed in other chapters (Chapter 16, Neuroendocrine Tumors; Chapter 17, Lymphoma; Chapter 20, Breast Cancer). Gallium has been widely used in evaluating patients with melanoma. About 75% of melanoma lesions >2 cm are gallium avid. For lesions <2 cm, only about 20% show gallium uptake. Overall sensitivity and specificity have been reported to be 82% and 99%, respectively.

PATIENT INFORMATION

I. LYMPHOSCINTIGRAPHY

A. Test/Procedure

Your doctor has ordered this test to image the sentinel lymph node, which is the first lymph node to receive lymphatic drainage from the tumor site. It is the first lymph node to which a tumor cell would come if it penetrated into a lymph channel from the tumor.

To identify the sentinel lymph node, injections of small amounts of a radioactive material will be made in the skin surrounding the melanoma tumor or the site from which it was removed. Pictures will be taken with a specialized camera.

After we have identified the sentinel node on a picture and marked its location on your skin, in the operating room your surgeon uses a hand-held radiation detecting probe to assist in finding the same sentinel lymph node(s) seen on the picture. The surgeon removes the sentinel lymph node(s) and sends it to the pathologist for examination.

B. Preparation

There are no dietary or medication restrictions.

C. Radiation risks

The only risk of this procedure is a small amount of radiation exposure. The amount used is small and generally is less than that you would receive in a standard diagnostic x-ray test. The radiation exposure to your whole body from this test is about the same as the effective dose a person living in the United States receives in about a week from cosmic and naturally occurring background radiation sources. It is about 1% of the yearly dose safely allowed for doctors and technologists who work with radiation in a hospital. The dose to the skin at the injection site is more, but it will be surgically removed with the tumor. You can be around other people and use a bathroom normally without risk to others.

D. Pregnancy

If you are pregnant or think you could be pregnant, please inform your doctor so that this can be discussed with the nuclear medicine physician.

References

1. Alazraki NP, Eshima D, Eshima LA, et al. Lymphoscintigraphy, the sentinel node concept, and the intraoperative gamma probe in melanoma, breast cancer, and other potential cancers. *Semin Nucl Med.* 1997;27:55–67.
2. Morton DL, Wen DR, Cochman AJ. Management of early stage melanoma by intraoperative lymphatic mapping and selective lymphadenectomy. *Surg Oncol Clin North Am* 1992;1:247–259.
3. Gershenwald JE, Thompson W, Mansfield PF, et al. Multi-institutional melanoma lymphatic mapping experience: the prognostic value of sentinel lymph node status in 612 stage I or II melanoma patients. *J Clin Oncol* 1999;17:976–983.
4. Ross MI, Reintgen DS. Role of lymphatic mapping and sentinel node biopsy in the detection of melanoma nodal metastases. *Eur J Cancer* 1998;34(suppl 3):S7–S11.

19

20
Breast Cancer

The management of patients with breast cancer has changed considerably in recent years with increasing use of less invasive approaches. Radical mastectomy was superceded by simple mastectomy, and lumpectomy frequently is chosen by the patient and doctor as surgical therapy for early cancer. In a continuation of that trend, the sentinel lymph node approach to staging eventually may replace the more invasive axillary lymph node dissection (ALND).

SCANS AND PRIMARY CLINICAL INDICATIONS

CLINICAL QUESTIONS

PATIENT INFORMATION

SCANS

I. MAMMOSCINTIGRAPHY

A. Background

Mammoscintigraphy is adjunctive to mammography and may be particularly helpful for women who are at high risk for breast cancer but whose mammographic examination is suboptimal because of dense breasts, implants or prior surgery. Technetium-99m-sestamibi is the most widely used radiopharmaceutical for mammoscintigraphy, and the only United States Food and Drug Administration (FDA)–approved mammoscintigraphy agent to date.

B. Radiopharmaceuticals

Technetium-99m-sestamibi (Miraluma) accumulates in tumor cells because of transmembrane diffusion driven by electrical potential gradients. The result is high concentration of sestamibi in breast cancer cells compared with surrounding normal breast or fat tissue.

C. How mammoscintigraphy is performed

Sestamibi (20–30 mCi [740–1110 MBq]) is injected intravenously, followed by imaging of the breasts at 10 min, performed in multiple projections. A special table or sponge mattress with cutouts may be used so that the breast hangs down for imaging as the patient is lying prone. The procedure generally takes about 1–1.5 hr.

D. Patient preparation

No dietary or medication restrictions are required.

E. Understanding the report

The report typically describes the reason for the scan and the image findings. Focal areas of radiotracer accumulation may be interpreted as suspicious for or likely to be malignant, whereas diffuse or patchy accumulations of lower levels of activity are more likely to be benign.

Visualizing the tumor on the image is limited primarily by tumor size. In patients with palpable lesions, sensitivity ranges from 83% to 96% (most reports indicate percentages in the low- to mid-90s) and specificity of 90–100%. For nonpalpable lesions, sensitivity decreases to about 55–72%. However, sensitivity and specificity of mammoscintigraphy is not altered by density of the breast tissue, which reduces the ability of mammography to detect small cancers.

F. Potential problems

1. Mammoscintigraphy and screening. Mammoscintigraphy is not sufficiently accurate to replace a biopsy and is too expensive to be a screening tool. Nonetheless, in target populations of high-risk patients who have mammographically compromised studies because of dense breasts, prior surgery, implants or other confounding factors, the mammoscintigraphy study may contribute significantly.

2. Timing of mammoscintigraphy after biopsy/surgery. Nonspecific inflammatory uptake of sestamibi can occur. To minimize this possibility, mammoscintigraphy should be performed no sooner than 10 days after a fine-needle aspiration, 4–6 wk after a breast biopsy and 2–3 mo after breast surgery or radiotherapy.

3. Imaging technique. Special tables and foam mattresses, which allow the breast to be suspended with the patient prone, provide the best positioning for scintillation camera imaging.

II. LYMPHOSCINTIGRAPHY

A. Background

The sentinel lymph node is the first node in a lymph node bed to which a tumor cell would come if it penetrated into lymphatic fluid. Data indicate that if an axillary sentinel node is tumor free, with 97–98% accuracy, there is no tumor spread to any axillary lymph nodes.

Increasingly, published data suggest that the sentinel lymph node approach to staging early breast cancers may become the standard of practice in lieu of ALND. It is not yet the standard of care, in part because there is no true consensus on the best way to identify the sentinel node and localize it in the operating room for excisional biopsy. Nonetheless, using blue dye, radionuclide imaging, intraoperative gamma detecting probe localizations or all of the above, many surgeons are applying the sentinel node approach to staging.

20

B. Radiopharmaceuticals

Technetium-99m-sulfur colloid as a filtered or nonfiltered preparation has been successfully used to image sentinel lymph nodes. In the United States, it is the only FDA-approved colloid agent available for lymphatic mapping. In Europe, ^{99m}Tc-albumin colloid is used, whereas in Australia, a smaller colloid—technetium-antimony sulfide colloid—is used successfully. These labeled colloid particles penetrate from the tissue interstitium into the lymphatics and are transported with lymph fluid to lymph nodes, just as a tumor cell would be.

C. How lymphoscintigraphy is performed

The procedure is performed on the morning of surgery within 2–5 hr of the patient going to the operating room. Some have performed the injections the evening before surgery with success. Imaging is performed to identify sentinel lymph node(s), and lymphatic channels leading to the node(s) can sometimes be identified. The patient's skin can be marked with ink over the sentinel node, with the patient positioned as if on the operating room table. The procedure is usually completed within 1–1.5 hr.

One of two injection sites (or both) are most often used: These are subdermal and peritumoral. If the tumor is nonpalpable, ultrasound guidance may be needed. The injection is followed by finger massage to facilitate uptake of the tracer into the lymphatics and by imaging for up to 1 hr. The skin is marked with ink as the patient lies under the camera to indicate to the surgeon the location of the sentinel lymph nodes.

In the operating room, the surgeon uses the hand-held gamma detecting probe to find the radiotracer-labeled sentinel lymph node(s) seen on the images. The probe's audio signal and count detection meter guide the surgeon's search for the node(s).

For nonpalpable tumors, wire localization is performed, usually with ultrasound guidance, before sending the patient to the operating room (to assist the surgeon in finding the tumor during surgery). The radionuclide is injected after the wire has been placed, followed by imaging. Subdermal injection is preferred to minimize leakage of radiotracer through skin puncture sites made for wire placement.

D. Patient preparation

No preparations are required for this procedure. If it is performed immediately before surgery, the preparations for surgery apply.

E. Understanding the report

The report describes the procedure and the findings on the images. Lymphatic drainage of the breast is most frequently to the axilla, but internal mammary drainage is also evident in 20–30% of cases. In inner-quadrant tumors, lymphatic drainage may be exclusively to internal mammary nodes Supraclavicular and infraclavicular nodes are also occasionally seen. Extra-axillary drainage has been more often reported with peritumoral injections of the radiocolloid than with subdermal injections.

F. Potential problems

1. Importance of breast positioning. During imaging the breast tissue may need to be shifted medially and inferiorly to optimize visualization of axillary nodes and laterally for visualizing internal mammary nodes. The soft-tissue attenuation easily can hide the small amount of radiotracer uptake into a sentinel lymph node; large breasts tend to be more problematic. Frontal and lateral imaging helps in this regard. If the tumor is near the axilla, the injected dose can obscure visualization of the sentinel node.

2. Optimum methods. The optimum injection site (subdermal versus peritumoral) has not yet been established. Some physicians use both for each patient. The optimum volume of injection has not been established. The optimum particle size has not been defined, although success is reported with several preparations.

CLINICAL QUESTIONS

1. Once a diagnosis of early breast cancer is made, how is it staged?

The staging procedure for breast cancer is axillary lymph node dissection. The presence and number of tumor-positive lymph nodes removed in an ALND is used to assess prognosis and select adjuvant therapy. As public awareness of breast cancer has increased, along with concomitant acceptance of mammography and self-examination by women, mean tumor size at the time of diagnosis has decreased. Up to 30% may be <1 cm. Thus, ALND has yielded decreasing incidence of axillary node metastases (10–18% for tumors <1 cm), which has led to some consideration of selecting patients for ALND based on tumor size.

Axillary lymph node dissection is an invasive procedure with significant morbidity; even 20 yr after surgery, about 40–45% of women suffer from lymphedema. Among women who have undergone radical mastectomy, up to 60% have lymphedema; about 30% of those treated with modified radical mastectomy or breast conserving surgery with axillary dissection have lymphedema. For women who also are treated with radiation to the axilla, the incidence of lymphedema increases. Lymphedema is unsightly, it is a psychologically distressing and constant reminder of the cancer, and it causes limited range of shoulder motion and limited use of the arm, painful seromas and paresthesias, all of which are common sequelae of axillary dissection. Thus, the sentinel node approach to staging early breast cancer in lieu of the ALND has enormous appeal to patients and caregivers.

Other nuclear imaging procedures that have the potential to contribute to noninvasive staging include the sestamibi mammoscintigram and fluorodeoxyglucose (FDG) imaging. Mammoscintigraphy images may reveal a focus of axillary lymph node activity, which may represent a metastasis. Unfortunately, the accuracy of this test to detect metastases to lymph nodes is limited.

When the primary tumor is >2 cm, axillary lymph node involvement is detected by PET using FDG with 94% sensitivity. It appears that micrometastases in smaller lymph nodes are likely missed by PET (sensitivity, 33%) when the primary breast cancer is <2 cm.

Thus, the sentinel lymph node approach to staging early breast cancer is undoubtedly the most accurate of the lesser invasive methods relative to ALND. Micrometastases are perhaps even better identified with the sentinel node than the ALND, because multiple sections of the node and histoimmunochemical stains (not done when as many as 10–25 nodes from axillary dissection are submitted at once to the pathologist) are easily done for only one, two or three sentinel node(s) and significantly increase the detection of micrometastases. Studies indicate that 16% of primary tumors <1 cm are associated with micrometastases in sentinel lymph nodes; 33% of tumors 1–2 cm are associated with sentinel node micrometastases; 41% of tumors 2–5 cm are associated with sentinel node micrometastases; 75% of tumors >5 cm are associated with lymph node

20

metastases. If the sentinel node is tumor-positive, the surgeon may opt to do an axillary dissection for therapeutic and informational purposes.

2. Do women with small tumors (<2 cm) need axillary staging?

Because of wide use of mammographic screening and self-examinations, more women present with small tumors (<2 cm) than ever before. Some physicians have suggested that because axillary lymph nodes usually were free of metastases in patients with small tumors, axillary dissection should be abandoned when the tumor is <1–2 cm. The recent data from sentinel lymph node excisional biopsies and histoimmunochemical pathology examinations showed the incidence of micrometastases or macrometastases to be significant (16%) for small tumors (0.1–1.0 cm). Figure 1 shows a sentinel node in the axilla and a chain of three nodes in the internal mammary region, the most inferior of which is a sentinel node, as it was the first node to receive tracer in the chain.

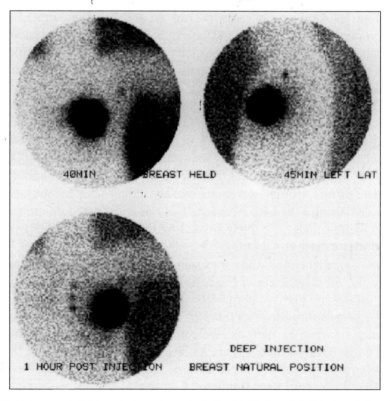

Figure 1. The large, round, dark focus is the peritumoral injection into the breast. A distinct sentinel node is seen in the axilla on the anterior (top left) and lateral (top right) views, as the breast is moved medially to clear the axilla. The bottom image shows a chain of three internal mammary nodes, the most inferior of which is the sentinel node, as it filled first.

WORTH MENTIONING

1. Other radiopharmaceuticals

Other radiopharmaceuticals that may be used to image breast cancer include FDG, ^{99m}Tc-tetrofosmin (see Chapter 1, Cardiovascular Diseases), ^{99m}Tc-methylene diphosphonate (MDP)—a widely used bone scan agent (see Chapter 11, The Skeletal System), ^{111}In-pentetreotide (somatostatin analog receptor imaging binding agent; see Chapter 16, Neuroendocrine Tumors) and monoclonal antibodies such as anticarcinoembryonic antigen antibody labeled to ^{99m}Tc. Tetrofosmin and MDP (imaged at 5–10 min after intravenous injection) are reported to give excellent results in imaging primary breast cancers with 90% overall accuracy. Tetrofosmin behaves similarly to sestamibi, but clinical reports in breast cancer are not as numerous as the published literature for sestamibi.

2. Monitoring response to therapy

Initial data suggest FDG can monitor chemotherapy response in patients. Metabolic changes in breast cancer can be detected after 8 days of initiating therapy, before tumor shrinkage. Studies have shown early (6–13 days from initiating chemotherapy) decrease in FDG tumor uptake, which correlates with response to therapy.

3. Sestamibi and the p-glycoprotein multidrug resistance gene

Sestamibi is a substrate of p-glycoprotein, which is found in cells that overexpress the multidrug resistance gene (*MDR1*). These tumor cells pump out a variety of products, including sestamibi. Thus, wash-out of sestamibi from the tumor by association with the *MDR1* gene may have prognostic and therapeutic implications that remain to be characterized.

20

PATIENT INFORMATION

I. MAMMOSCINTIGRAPHY

A. Test/Procedure

Your doctor has ordered mammoscintigraphy (also called scintimammography) to evaluate a region of suspicion in your breast for possible cancer or because you are at high risk for breast cancer and other evaluations (mammograms, ultrasound) are not adequate. After an intravenous injection of the radiotracer (technetium sestamibi or equivalent other agent), pictures will be taken of your breasts using a special camera that detects the radioactive tracer in your breast tissue.

B. Preparation

There are no dietary or medication restrictions for this test.

C. Radiation risk

The only risk of this procedure is a small amount of radiation exposure. The amount used is generally about the same as that given by diagnostic x-ray tests. The radiation exposure to your whole body from this test is about the same as the dose the average person living in the United States receives during 10–15 years from cosmic rays and naturally occurring background radiation sources. The radiation dose is about 50–100% of the yearly dose considered safe for doctors and technologists who work with radiation. You can be around other people and use a bathroom normally without risk to others.

D. Pregnancy

If you are pregnant or think you could be pregnant, inform your doctor so that this can be discussed with the nuclear medicine physician.

II. LYMPHOSCINTIGRAPHY
A. Test/Procedure

Your doctor has ordered this test because you have breast cancer. This test is to identify the sentinel lymph node, which is the first lymph node to receive lymphatic drainage from the tumor. It is the first lymph node to which a tumor cell would come if it penetrated into a lymph channel from your breast tumor.

After we have identifed the sentinel node on a picture and marked its location on your skin, in the operating room, your surgeon will use a hand-held radiation-detecting probe to assist in finding the same sentinel lymph node(s) seen on the picture.

B. Preparation

There are no dietary or medication restrictions for this procedure.

C. Radiation risk

The only risk of this procedure is a small amount of radiation exposure. The amount used is very small and generally is less than that given by diagnostic x-ray tests. The radiation exposure to your whole body from this test is about the same as the dose a person living in the United States receives in about 1 wk from cosmic rays and naturally occurring background radiation sources. It is about 1% of the yearly dose considered safe for doctors and technologists who work with radiation. The dose at the injection site is more, but that tissue will likely be surgically removed. You can be around other people and use a bathroom normally without risk to others.

D. Pregnancy

If you are pregnant or think you could be pregnant, inform your doctor so that this can be discussed with the nuclear medicine physician.

References

1. Khalkhali I, Villanueva-Meyer J, Edell SL, et al. Impact of breast density on the diagnostic accuracy of Tc-99m sestamibi breast imaging in the detection of breast cancer [abstract]. *J Nucl Med* 1996;288:74P.

2. Khalkhali I, Cutrone JA, Mena IG, et al. Scintimammography: the complementary role of Tc-99m sestamibi prone breast imaging for the diagnosis of breast carcinoma. *Radiology* 1995;196:421–426.

3. Jackson VP, Hendrick RE, Feig SA, Kopans DB. Imaging of the radiographically dense breast. *Radiology* 1993;188;297–301.

4. Taillefer R. The role of ^{99m}Tc-sestamibi and other conventional radiopharmaceuticals in breast cancer diagnosis. *Semin Nucl Med* 1999;29:16–40.

5. Alazraki NP, Halkar RK. Using the sentinel node concept to stage breast cancer. In: Taillefer R, Waxman AD, Khalkali I, Biersack HJ, eds. *Radionuclide Imaging of the Breast.* New York, NY: Marcel Dekker Inc.; 1998.

6. Ganz PA. The quality of life after breast cancer: solving the problem of lymphedema. *N Engl J Med* 1999;340:383–385.

7. Veronesi U, Paganelli G, Galimberti V, et al. Sentinel-node biopsy to avoid axillary dissection in breast cancer with clinically negative lymph nodes. *Lancet* 1997;349:1864–1867.

8. Cox CE. Guidelines for sentinel node biopsy and lymphatic mapping of patients with breast cancer. *Ann Surg* 1998;227:645–653.

9. Alazraki NP, Eshima D, Eshima LA, et al. Lymphoscintigraphy, the sentinel node concept and intraoperative gamma probe in melanoma, breast cancer, and other potential cancers. *Semin Nucl Med* 1997;27:55–67.

20

21
Colorectal Cancer

Colorectal cancer is the fourth most common cancer in the United States and the second most common cause of cancer death. In 1997, there were an estimated 131,300 new cases and 54,900 deaths. The treatment of localized colorectal cancer is surgery, but 15–20% of patients present with simultaneous distant metastases, and 30–40% of patients treated by potentially curative resection relapse. The most common sites of metastases are the liver, the peritoneal cavity, the pelvis, the retroperitoneum and the lungs. Early detection and surgical excision of isolated recurrences, particularly in the liver or lung, may lead to a cure in up to 25% of patients. The size and number of hepatic metastases affect the prognosis; furthermore, the presence of extrahepatic metastases is a relative contraindication to surgical resection of hepatic metastases. Consequently, accurate noninvasive detection of metastases plays a critical role in selecting patients who would benefit from surgery and avoids unnecessary surgery in patients for whom chemotherapy would be more appropriate.

21

SCANS AND PRIMARY CLINICAL INDICATIONS

I. Fluorodeoxyglucose (FDG) imaging   Page 306

- To clarify an equivocal lesion on CT/MRI

- To detect hepatic and extrahepatic metastases

- To distinguish tumor from postoperative and postradiation changes

CLINICAL QUESTIONS

PATIENT INFORMATION

I. FDG imaging (See Chapter 15, Introduction to Cancer and FDG Imaging)

SCANS

I. FDG IMAGING
A. Background

Recurrent tumors of the colon and rectum are not well imaged by conventional modalities. CT is often unable to distinguish tumor from postoperative or postradiation therapy changes. FDG PET provides a sensitive test for detecting extrahepatic metastases from colorectal cancer and appears to have an even higher accuracy than CT or CT portography in detecting hepatic metastases (Fig. 1). (See Background at the beginning of Chapter 18, Lung Cancer, for more information on FDG.)

B–F. Radiopharmaceuticals, how the study is performed, patient preparation, understanding the report and potential problems

See Chapter 16, Neuroendocrine Tumors, B–F.

II. ONCOSCINT IMAGING
A. Background

OncoScint is more sensitive than CT/MRI for evaluating the extrahepatic abdomen and pelvis (Fig. 2). In particular, OncoScint may detect tumor in normal sized lymph nodes and distinguish postoperative and postradiation changes from tumor. OncoScint is also more sensitive than CT in detecting recurrent disease presenting as diffuse carcinomatosis. Because OncoScint accumulates in normal he-

21

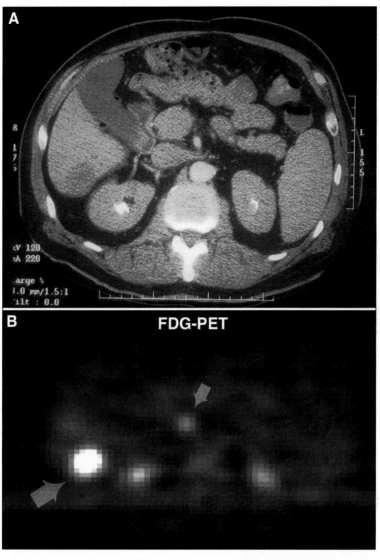

Figure 1. (A) A CT scan in a patient with rising CEA after surgical resection of a colon carcinoma shows a single hepatic metastasis. (B) An FDG PET study confirmed the hepatic metastasis (large arrow) but showed an additional nodal metastasis in the porta hepatis that was not detected by CT (small arrow). The remaining two focal areas of activity represent FDG in the renal collecting system.

patocytes, it is much less sensitive than CT for detecting hepatic metastases. In a recent study of patients with recurrent disease, CT and OncoScint in combination had a sensitivity of 88%, significantly greater than CT or OncoScint alone. OncoScint appears to be superior to FDG in detecting diffuse carcinomatosis.

B. Radiopharmaceuticals

Indium-111-satumomab pentetide (OncoScint CR/OV, CYT-103) is a B72.3 murine IgG monoclonal antibody directed against a high molecular weight glycoprotein, TAG-72, which is expressed in the majority of colorectal and more

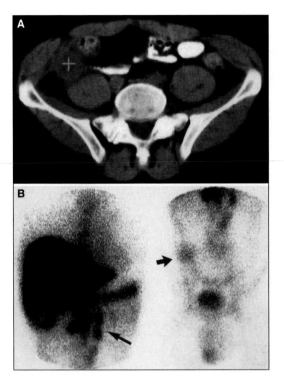

Figure 2. A 47-yr-old man had a right hemicolectomy and appendectomy for a perforated appendiceal carcinoma; significant local inflammation was noted at surgery. The patient subsequently presented with a rising CEA. (A) CT scan shows a right lower quadrant mass (marker has been placed over the mass) interpreted as tumor recurrence versus fibrosis. The remainder of the CT scan was normal. (B). The 72-hr planar OncoScint images show abnormal uptake in the region of the right lower quadrant mass identified on CT (short arrow); this abnormality persisted on delayed images, whereas colon activity cleared (not shown). There was also intense uptake in the mid- and lower abdomen (long arrow) indicative of extensive disease. Planned surgery was cancelled, and the patient was placed on chemotherapy. (Reprinted with permission from Markowitz A, Saleemi K, Freeman LM. Role of In-111 CYT-103 (OncoScint) immunoscintigraphy in the evaluation of patients with recurrent colorectal cancer. *Clin Nucl Med* 1993;18:685–700.)

than 90–95% of common epithelial ovarian cancers. The radiotracer also localizes in normal liver, spleen and bone marrow.

C. How the study is performed

The patient receives an intravenous injection of 1 mg of antibody labeled with 5 mCi (185 MBq) of ^{111}In. Imaging typically is performed at 72 hr and often is repeated at 96 or 120 hr to confirm abnormalities or to distinguish between normal activity in the bowel and tumor.

D. Patient preparation

The study should not be performed within 6 wk of abdominal surgery because of uptake due to nonspecific postsurgical inflammatory changes. The nuclear medicine department often will give the patient a cathartic before imaging. No other patient preparation is required. The patient should understand that two imaging sessions may be required to distinguish between tumor or bowel activity. Prior CT/MRI scans should be made available to the nuclear medicine physician if these are not available at his or her institution.

E. Understanding the report

The report will indicate the presence or absence of any evidence for recurrent or metastatic disease and will localize the sites of abnormality as accurately as possible.

F. Potential problems

1. False-negative and false-positive results. A negative scan does not exclude disease. The specificities of CT and OncoScint appear to be identical, about 75–80%; their combined sensitivity exceeds that of either test alone.

2. Human antimouse antibody (HAMA) formation. Approximately 55% of patients receiving OncoScint will develop HAMA although in one third of patients, HAMA levels become undetectable by 6 mo. Elevated HAMA may prevent a repeat study and may prevent the patient from receiving any other murine monoclonal antibody. HAMA may interfere with two-site murine antibody-based immunoassays for CEA and CA 125 and often results in spuriously high values. If HAMA may be present, the laboratory should be notified so that appropriate measures can be taken to prevent HAMA interference.

3. Repeat OncoScint scans? OncoScint scans may be repeated if there is a continuing question regarding recurrent disease. Because of the possibility of HAMA formation (see 2, above), HAMA testing should be performed and can be arranged by the nuclear medicine physician through Cytogen Corp., the supplier of OncoScint. If HAMA values are <50 ng/ml, imaging is rarely affected; HAMA levels between 50 and 400 ng/ml may be associated with an altered biodistribution that could reduce the sensitivity of the scan. If the serum HAMA level is >440 ng/ml, repeat imaging studies should not be performed because of too great a loss in sensitivity.

III. CEA-SCAN IMAGING

A. Background

Initial data suggest that the accuracy of CEA-Scan for assessing resectability may be greater than that of CT alone, both in patients undergoing evaluation for curative abdominopelvic resection of colorectal cancer and in the subset of patients with suspected or proven liver metastases. For patients with recurrent disease, the additional use of CEA-Scan with CT potentially doubles the number of patients who could be saved the cost, morbidity and mortality of unnecessary abdominopelvic surgery.

B. Radiopharmaceuticals

CEA-Scan (^{99m}Tc-arcitumomab) is a ^{99m}Tc-labeled murine monoclonal antibody Fab′ fragment that is reactive with CEA, a tumor-associated antigen that is expressed by a variety of cancers as well as certain inflammatory states such as Crohn's disease. The sensitivity and specificity of the scan do not depend on the levels of circulating antigen; CEA is present in >95% of all colorectal cancers, regardless of the serum CEA levels.

C. How the study is performed

The patient receives an intravenous infusion of 20–30 mCi (740–1110 MBq) of ^{99m}Tc-CEA-Scan over 30 min; planar and SPECT images are obtained 2–5 hr

21

later. Initial images typically are obtained 2 hr after injection, when gut activity is minimal; at 2 hr, however, tumor-to-background ratios are suboptimal, and delayed images also are obtained when the lesion-to-background ratio is optimized. On later 4- to 5-hr images, gut activity may present a problem in interpretation. Total imaging time ranges from 1 to 3 hr; total time in the nuclear medicine department is approximately 5 hr.

D. Patient preparation

1. Allergy to murine-derived products. CEA-Scan should not be administered to patients who are known to be hypersensitive to murine-derived products.

2. Hydration and catheterization. The patient should be well hydrated to minimize artifacts resulting from bladder filling. Catheterization immediately before imaging is recommended for the patient with suspected disease within the pelvis or for any patient who is unable to empty the bladder.

E. Understanding the report

See FDG imaging, understanding the report, above.

F. Potential problems

1. False-negative results. A negative scan does not exclude disease.

2. HAMA formation. HAMA formation after CEA-Scan is approximately 1% and is rarely a problem after CEA-Scan administration.

CLINICAL QUESTIONS

1. In presumed solitary colorectal cancer is nuclear imaging indicated?

CT is the standard imaging procedure for patients with suspected primary colorectal cancer; in addition to searching for metastatic disease, CT provides excellent anatomic definition that may be useful in surgical planning. The use of nuclear imaging of patients deemed resectable by CT imaging may not be cost-effective, and additional supporting data need to be obtained if these tests are to be recommended as a routine procedure. Nuclear imaging may be valuable in selected cases, particularly if equivocal lesions are demonstrated by CT scanning or if the presence or absence of metastatic disease will alter the surgical management. However, even if the patient has multiple, synchronous unresectable metastases, the management of primary colorectal cancer usually includes palliative resection of the primary tumor to prevent bowel obstruction.

2. How should high-risk colorectal cancer patients be monitored after resection of the primary tumor?

To detect recurrence, postsurgery patients often are followed-up by measurement of serum levels of CEA; however, the sensitivity of the test is only about

60%. As many as one third of patients with recurrent colorectal cancers do not have elevated CEA levels. FDG PET imaging is more sensitive than CEA monitoring in detecting recurrent disease, but the clinical role, cost-effectiveness and timing of periodic imaging in screening asymptomatic but relatively high-risk patients (Dukes' B2 and C tumors) with no CEA elevation needs further evaluation before specific recommendations can be made. If CEA is elevated, see Clinical Question 3, below.

3. Is the patient with elevated CEA after surgery for colorectal cancer still a surgical candidate?

Early detection and prompt treatment of recurrences may lead to a cure in up to 25% of patients. CT and MRI have limited sensitivity for evaluating the extrahepatic abdomen, for detecting recurrent tumors in normal-sized lymph nodes and for distinguishing postoperative and postradiation changes from tumor. Nuclear imaging substantially increases the accuracy of staging these patients (Figs. 1 and 2). There have been no large comparisons of FDG PET, OncoScint and CEA-Scan; however, the available data suggest that FDG PET with attenuation correction will provide superior lesion detection, sensitivity and specificity. FDG PET is not available in many centers but OncoScint and CEA-Scan are widely available, can be imaged with standard SPECT instrumentation and, when combined with CT, result in improved sensitivity compared with CT alone. OncoScint may be superior to FDG PET in detecting diffuse carcinomatosis. CEA-Scan is superior to OncoScint in detecting hepatic metastases.

4. Does the questionable recurrence of a lesion on CT/MRI represent colorectal cancer or postoperative/ postradiation changes?

Nuclear imaging often can resolve questionable lesions noted by CT/MRI or in patients with a nondiagnostic fine-needle aspiration biopsy. The choice of imaging procedures depends on the availability of FDG, the type of camera equipment available and local expertise. A positive scan, especially with CT or MRI co-registration, may be very helpful in identifying the optimal site for biopsy.

21

References

1. Jessup JM, Markowitz AJ, Guillem JG, et al. Colorectal cancer. *CA Cancer J Clin* 1996;47:70–128.
2. Delbeke D. Oncological applications of FDG PET imaging: brain tumors, colorectal cancer, lymphoma and melanoma. *J Nucl Med* 1999;40:591–603.
3. Hughes K, Pinsky CM, Petrelli NJ, et al. Use of carcinoembryonic antigen radioimmunodetection and computed tomography for predicting the resectability of recurrent colorectal cancer. *Ann Surg* 1997;226:621–631.

4. Rigo P, Paulus P, Kaschten BJ, et al. Oncological applications of positron emission tomography with fluorine-18-flurodeoxyglucose. *Eur J Nucl Med* 1996;23:1641–1674.
5. Dominguez JM, Wolff BG, Nelson H, et al. In-111-CYT-103 scanning in recurrent colorectal cancer—does it affect standard management? *Dis Colon Rectum* 1996;39:514–519.
6. Markowitz A, Saleemi K, Freeman LM. Role of In-111 CYT-103 (OncoScint) immunoscintigraphy in the evaluation of patients with recurrent colorectal cancer. *Clin Nucl Med* 1993;18:685–700.

21

22
Ovarian Cancer

Approximately 1 in 70 women will develop an ovarian malignancy. Lymphatic spread to the pelvic and paraaortic lymph nodes is also common, particularly in advanced disease. The initial treatment is surgery followed by chemotherapy with or without radiation. Accurate staging and the amount of residual disease influence the selection of therapy and survival.

Detection of recurrent disease is based on elevation of serum markers such as CA 125 or carcinoembryonic antigen, imaging procedures (chest x-ray, CT, MRI) and surgery (laparotomy, laparoscopy). However, the serum marker CA 125 has a high false-negative rate and does not predict extent or location of disease. CT and MRI are limited in the detection of small tumor deposits, tumor in normal sized nodes and diffuse miliary disease and in distinguishing scar/adhesions from recurrent tumor. Exploratory surgery does not detect extra-abdominal tumors, is expensive, has an increased complication rate and yields false-negative results in 20–50% of patients. For patients with recurrent disease, nuclear imaging offers more accurate staging than conventional imaging procedures, can better direct therapy, can reduce the need for invasive staging procedures and can reduce the costs of patient management.

22

SCANS AND PRIMARY CLINICAL INDICATIONS

CLINICAL QUESTIONS

SCANS

I. FDG IMAGING
A. Background

Most ovarian malignancies arise from the ovarian epithelium, a single layer of cells on the surface of the ovary. Epithelial ovarian cancers commonly disseminate by exfoliation. The cancer cells migrate with the peritoneal fluid and may implant throughout the abdomen and pelvis. Lymphatic spread to the pelvic and paraaortic lymph nodes is also common, particularly in advanced disease. The initial treatment is surgery followed by chemotherapy with or without radiation. The disease is often advanced at the time of diagnosis, and the overall 5-yr survival rate is only 39%. Accurate staging and the amount of residual disease influence the selection of therapy and survival. (See Chapter 15, Introduction to Cancer and FDG Imaging, for the background regarding FDG.)

B–F. Radiopharmaceuticals, how the scan is performed, patient preparation, understanding the report and potential problems

See Chapter 18, Lung Cancer.

22

II. ONCOSCINT IMAGING
A. Background

See FDG, Background, above. OncoScint CR/OV (satumomab penetide) is an ^{111}In-labeled whole antibody that targets a tumor associated glycoprotein (TAG-72) that is expressed by up to 97% of epithelial ovarian carcinomas.

B–F. Radiopharmaceuticals, how the scan is performed, patient preparation, understanding the report and potential problems

See Chapter 21, Colorectal Cancer.

CLINICAL QUESTIONS

1. Is nuclear imaging indicated in a patient with pelvic mass and suspected ovarian carcinoma?

Ultrasonography and CT are standard imaging procedures in this setting. In addition to searching for metastatic disease, CT provides excellent anatomic definition that may be useful in surgical planning. The sensitivity of OncoScint in this setting is quite high (95%), but the specificity is low (50%); the TAG-72 antigen also may be expressed by benign ovarian tumors. For these reasons, OncoScint should not be used to determine whether a newly discovered ovarian mass is benign or malignant.

FDG imaging appears promising and can detect sites of disease missed by CT; however, FDG also can accumulate in sites of inflammation, and the cost-effectiveness of routine FDG imaging in the initial staging has not been established. FDG imaging may be valuable in selected cases, particularly if equivocal lesions are demonstrated by CT scanning, and the presence or absence of metastatic disease will alter the surgical approach.

2. Does a questionable metastasis on CT/MRI represent ovarian carcinoma?

Nuclear imaging can be useful in evaluating a site of questionable disease. FDG is superior to OncoScint in detecting hepatic metastases and appears to be superior in the rest of the abdomen, although FDG bladder activity may obscure lesions in the central pelvis. OncoScint is a valuable alternative to FDG for evaluating extrahepatic disease and diffuse miliary spread.

3. Should a second-look laparotomy be performed for clinical staging and possible tumor resection in a patient with no evidence of recurrence after 1 yr?

Clinical metastases will develop in approximately one third of patients during the first year after surgical resection. For this reason, many clinicians advocate a second-look laparotomy for clinical staging and possible tumor resection at 1 yr. Replacing the second-look laparotomy with FDG PET imaging followed by laparoscopy when FDG PET imaging shows lesions suspicious for metastatic disease appears to reduce unnecessary invasive staging procedures and reduces total health care costs.

4. Is a patient with known local recurrence a surgical candidate?

FDG or OncoScint imaging can be especially valuable if the presence of additional metastatic sites will alter the proposed therapy (see Clinical Question 5, below).

5. Do elevated tumor markers after surgery for ovarian carcinoma represent recurrent disease?

FDG PET appears to be more sensitive and more specific than CT in detecting recurrent disease, particularly for lesions 1 cm or larger. As experience increases and FDG imaging becomes more widely available, FDG imaging is expected to have an increasingly important role in the management of patients with ovarian cancer. OncoScint combined with CT imaging is significantly more sensitive than CT alone, and Oncocint may be more sensitive than FDG for detecting carcinomatosis.

References

1. Coleman RE. Clinical PET in oncology. *Clin Positron Imaging* 1998;1:15–30.
2. Rigo P, Paulus P, Kaschten BJ, et al. Oncological applications of positron emission tomography with fluorine-18-flurodeoxyglucose. *Eur J Nucl Med* 1996;23:1641–1674.
3. Surwitt EA, Childers JM, Krag DN, et al. Clinical assessment of In-111-CYT-103 (OncoScint) immunoscintigraphy in ovarian cancer. *Gynecol Oncol* 1993;48:285–292.
4. Casey MJ, Gupta NC, Muths CK. Experience with positron emission tomography (PET) scans in patients with ovarian cancer. *Gynecol Oncol* 1994;53:331–338.
5. Smith GT, Hubner KF, McDonald T, Thie JA. Cost analysis of FDG PET for managing patients with ovarian carcinoma. *Clin Positron Imaging* 1999;2:63–70.

22

23
Prostate Cancer

Prostate cancer is the most frequently diagnosed cancer in men in the United States and accounts for 40% of new cancer cases. Approximately 80% of these patients will be candidates for curative therapy. Regardless of the treatment option (radical prostatectomy, interstitial implants [brachytherapy], external beam irradiation), as many as half of these patients will not be cured by local therapy.

SCANS AND PRIMARY CLINICAL INDICATIONS

I. Capromab pendetide (ProstaScint) scan

Page 318

- To determine if curative therapy is a treatment option when newly diagnosed prostate cancer patients present with a high risk for metastatic disease

- To determine if salvage radiotherapy is a treatment option when a patient presents with a rising prostate-specific antigen (PSA) after radical prostatectomy or brachytherapy

II. Bone scan (see Chapter 11, The Skeletal System)

- To determine if skeletal metastases are present when a patient with newly diagnosed prostate cancer presents with a PSA > 10 ng/ml

- To determine if salvage radiotherapy is a treatment option when a patient presents with a rising PSA after radical prostatectomy or brachytherapy

23

CLINICAL QUESTIONS

PATIENT INFORMATION

SCANS

I. CAPROMAB PENDETIDE (PROSTASCINT) SCAN

A. Background

Patients with prostate cancer that has metastasized to lymph nodes or bones are no longer candidates for therapeutic options such as radical prostatectomy or interstitial implants. The likelihood of metastases can be estimated from the PSA, clinical stage and the Gleason score (an index of the aggressiveness of the tumor based on histologic features of the biopsy). CT and MRI are limited in their ability to detect early lymph-node metastases because lymph nodes <1 cm in diameter are considered normal.

Detection of metastases with ProstaScint does not depend solely on lymph node size; detection depends primarily on the amount of labeled antibody localizing in the tumor. In a recent multicenter trial, the sensitivity, specificity and accuracy of CT/MRI in detecting extraprostatic carcinoma was 20%, 68% and 48%, respectively, compared with 75%, 86% and 81%, respectively, for ProstaScint, even though the trial was completed before the optimal imaging techniques for ProstaScint were defined.

B. Radiopharmaceutical

Indium-111-capromab pendetide (ProstaScint) is a murine IgG1 monoclonal antibody that targets a prostate specific transmembrane glycoprotein (prostate-specific membrane antigen [PSMA]) that is expressed on prostate epithelial cells, some marrow cells and colonic crypt cells. The antibody does not target PSA or prostate acid phosphatase. Lymph-node metastases often have a higher PSMA expression than the primary prostate cancer, and poorly differentiated tumors usually have higher PSMA expression than well-differentiated tumors. Unlike

PSA, the expression of PSMA is not suppressed by androgen deprivation or androgen blockade.

C. How the study is performed

Patients receive an intravenous injection of approximately 5 mCi (185 MBq) of the ^{111}In-labeled antibody and typically return at 96 hr for planar imaging of the torso and SPECT imaging of the pelvis. The antibody immediately distributes within the blood pool, and blood-pool activity will persist through 96–120 hr. Because many lymph nodes are adjacent to blood vessels, a mild irregularity or dilatation of the blood vessel may be confused with lymph-node activity. To minimize this problem and improve diagnostic accuracy, a SPECT image of the blood pool is routinely obtained. In some centers, the blood pool scan is performed immediately after injection of the antibody; in other centers, red blood cells are labeled with ^{99m}Tc when the patient returns for the 96-hr monoclonal antibody scan. The ^{99m}Tc blood-pool and ^{111}In monoclonal-antibody images are then obtained sequentially or simultaneously during an imaging session that lasts 1–2 hr, depending on the specific protocol. If bowel activity is present, the patient may be given a bowel preparation and asked to return the following day for additional imaging.

D. Patient preparation

There is no specific patient preparation required before injection of the antibody. The patient will be given a bowel preparation to take before the diagnostic imaging session at 96 hr. Some centers catheterize the patient at the time of imaging to minimize bladder activity.

E. Understanding the report

The report often articulates the reason for the scan and may include relevant clinical data such as PSA, Gleason score and clinical stage of the disease. The report will state if there is activity in the prostatic fossa, if there is evidence for nodal metastases in the pelvis or metastases outside the pelvis and will describe the location of any suspected metastases as precisely as possible.

23

F. Potential problems

1. Human antimouse antibody (HAMA) formation. HAMA formation occurs in 8% of patients after a single ProstaScint infusion (0.5 mg of antibody) and in 19% of patients after second infusion. The presence of HAMA may increase the risk of an allergic reaction or alter the distribution of the antibody. HAMA testing can be arranged by the laboratory performing the examination if the patient has previously received a murine monoclonal antibody injection. If patients have never received an intravenous injection of a murine monoclonal antibody, routine HAMA testing is not indicated.

2. Test availability. The United States Food and Drug Administration has approved ProstaScint to be used only by physicians who have had specific training in the performance and interpretation of ProstaScint scans. It is not practical to provide training for staff at every institution with nuclear imaging capability; consequently, the test is not available at every institution, but it is widely available throughout the United States.

CLINICAL QUESTIONS

1 and 2. When is the newly diagnosed patient a candidate for definitive therapy? Does a patient with increased risk factors have pelvic lymph-node metastases?

The risk of metastases in men with newly diagnosed prostate cancer can be estimated from the clinical stage, Gleason score and PSA. A common algorithm for estimating risk has been published by Partin et al. Patients at low risk for metastatic disease are candidates for definitive therapy. Patients at high risk for metastatic disease may undergo a pelvic lymph node dissection; if metastases are detected, the patient usually is spared the expense and morbidity of definitive therapy and generally is managed with hormonal therapy. When patients are at increased risk for metastatic disease, ProstaScint and bone scans are increasingly used to search for nodal and extranodal metastases, particularly if the patient is a poor surgical candidate. If nodal metastases are detected outside the prostate bed, the patient may be a candidate for extended field radiotherapy. If distant metastases are detected, the patient can be spared the expense and morbidity of definitive therapy (Fig. 1).

3 and 4. Should a bone scan be obtained to search for bony metastases? Can a ProstaScint scan replace a bone scan for detection of bony metastases?

Patients with a PSA < 10 ng/ml are unlikely to have bony metastases detected by bone scan. A bone scan is recommended for newly diagnosed prostate cancer patients presenting with bone pain or a PSA $\geq$ 10–20 ng/ml; a high-grade Gleason score also increases the risk of bony metastases. Nevertheless, many urologists continue to perform a baseline bone scan in patients with a PSA < 10 ng/ml to document benign abnormalities such as degenerative joint disease or previous fractures before definitive surgical or radiation therapy treatment, especially in patients who are at greater risk for subsequent bony metastases. A ProstaScint scan cannot replace the bone scan because the bone scan is much more sensitive for bony metastases.

23

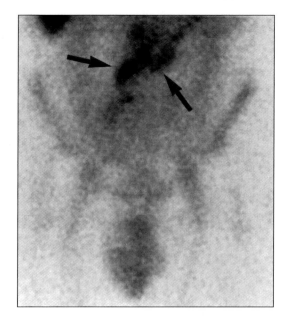

Figure 1. A 56-yr-old patient was referred for a ProstaScint scan because of a rising PSA after radical prostatectomy. Planar images of the pelvis show abnormal actvity corresponding to iliac and periaortic nodes (arrows). The tip of the liver is also visible. Normal uptake is seen in the pelvic marrow, iliac arteries, colon and scrotum.

5. Is a patient with a rising PSA after radical prostatectomy or brachytherapy a candidate for salvage radiation therapy?

The value of salvage radiotherapy in men with an elevated PSA after radical prostatectomy is still controversial. A bone scan should be obtained to exclude bony metastases. Even with a negative bone scan, a major problem in evaluating the effectiveness of radiation therapy has been the fact that there was no accurate way to determine if the cancer was potentially curable (confined to the prostatic fossa) or if it was incurable (spread beyond the pelvis and planned radiation field). Criteria that favored a good response to salvage radiotherapy included disease confined to the prostatic fossa (positive surgical margin on the pathology report), Gleason grade ≤ 3, negative seminal vesicles, PSA doubling time > 6 mo, PSA nadir of zero after surgery and PSA recurrence delayed for at least 2.5 yr after the radical prostatectomy. In the absence of these criteria, the response to salvage radiation therapy could be as low as 20%.

Initial reports show that salvage radiotherapy is much more likely to result in a sustained reduction in PSA when the ProstaScint scan shows disease confined to the prostatic fossa or pelvic nodes. If the scan indicates the presence of metastases that cannot be encompassed in the radiation field, radiation therapy is unlikely to be of benefit and hormonal therapy is more appropriate (Fig. 1). Depending on the scan and clinical presentation, additional testing may be performed to confirm the presence of disease not amenable to radiation therapy.

23

WORTH MENTIONING

1. Fluorodeoxyglucose (FDG) imaging

Fluorine-18 FDG imaging is useful in detecting many primary and metastatic cancers. As of 2000, FDG imaging is not indicated in the routine management of prostate cancer, and its potential application to prostate cancer is still under evaluation (see Chapter 15 for a discussion of FDG imaging). Preliminary data suggest that prostate cancers that accumulate FDG are more aggressive than prostate cancers that are not detected by FDG imaging.

PATIENT INFORMATION

I. PROSTASCINT SCAN
A. Test/Procedure

Your doctor has ordered a ProstaScint scan to determine if prostate carcinoma has spread to the lymph nodes or other sites outside the prostate gland. You will receive an intravenous injection of a radioactive antibody that targets prostate cancer cells. The antibody circulates in the blood, and you will be instructed to return about 3–4 days later to be scanned. You will likely be given a preparation to cleanse your bowel before the scan.

Many lymph nodes are adjacent to blood vessels; consequently, a mild irregularity or dilatation of the blood vessel may be confused with lymph node activity. To minimize this problem, a scan of the blood pool is also obtained. An ounce of blood is withdrawn, labeled with a different radioactive tracer and reinjected. Comparison of the blood-pool scan with the antibody scan improves the diagnostic accuracy. A blood-pool scan can be obtained immediately after the antibody is injected, but it is usually obtained at the time you return for your antibody scan. The imaging session lasts 1.5–3 hr, depending on the specific protocol. The imaging session requires you to lie motionless on a table while a camera moves over you or rotates around you. If bowel activity is present, you may be given another bowel preparation and asked to return the following day for additional imaging. Occasionally a catheter may be needed to drain your bladder.

B. Preparation

Diet. There are no dietary restrictions.

Medications. There are no medication restrictions. Prescription medications do not interfere with the test.

C. Radiation and other risks

The radiation dose is comparable to x-ray studies using contrast such as a barium enema. The radiation dose to the whole body is about half the dose allowed a radiologist or nuclear medicine technologist in 1 yr. The radioactive tracer is eliminated in your urine and feces; it also decays rapidly. Even if no radioactive tracer were eliminated in your urine or feces, less than 5% of the injected dose would remain in your body after 2 wk because of natural decay of the tracer. There is no risk to the people around you.

References

1. Hinkle GH, Burgers J, Neal CE, et al. Multicenter radioimmunoscintigraphic evaluation of patients with prostate carcinoma using indium-111 capromab pendetide. *Cancer* 1998;83:739–747.
2. Kahn D, Williams RD, Haseman MK, et al. Radioimmunoscintigraphy with In-111-labeled capromab pendetide predicts prostate cancer response to salvage radiotherapy after failed radical prostatectomy. *J Clin Oncol* 1998;16:284–289.
3. Burgers JK, Hinkle GH, Haseman MK. Monoclonal antibody imaging of recurrent and metastatic prostate cancer. *Semin Urol* 1995;13:103–112.
4. Partin AW, Subong ENP, Walsh PC, et al. Combination of prostate-specific antigen, clinical stage, and Gleason score to predict pathological stage of localized prostate cancer. A multi-institutional update. *JAMA* 1997;277:1445–1451.
5. Oesterling JE. Using PSA to eliminate the staging radionuclide bone scan: significant economic implications. *Urol Clin North Am* 1993;20:705–711.
6. Lawton CA, Grignon D, Newhouse JH, et al. Oncodiagnosis panel: 1997: prostate carcinoma. *RadioGraphics* 1999;19:185–203.
7. Polascik TJ, Manyak MJ, Haseman MK, et al. Comparison of clinical staging algorithms and [111]indium-capromab pendetide immunoscintigraphy in the prediction of lymph node involvement in high risk prostate carcinoma patients. *Cancer* 1999;85:1586–1592.

23

24
Thyroid Cancer

Patients with papillary and follicular thyroid carcinomas (differentiated thyroid cancers) have a favorable prognosis. The overall survival rate at 10 yr for middle aged adults is 80–95%; however, patients who are not treated with ^{131}I have a cumulative tumor recurrence rate at 30 yr that approaches 40%. The risk of recurrence is higher in patients with tumors ≥ 1.0 cm, poorly differentiated follicular subtypes, Hürthle-cell carcinomas, tumor invasion of the thyroid capsule, vascular invasion, lymph-node metastases, distant metastases and age at presentation <16 yr or >45 yr.

Papillary carcinomas are often multicentric (up to 80% in some series) and bilateral in approximately one third of cases. The tumor spreads via regional lymphatics within the thyroid to adjacent lymph nodes and occasionally to the lungs. Follicular carcinoma is less likely to be multicentric, but it may metastasize to lungs or bones via hematogenous spread.

24

SCANS, THERAPY AND PRIMARY CLINICAL INDICATIONS

I. Post-thyroidectomy ^{131}I or ^{123}I scan Page 326

- To confirm the presence of a thyroid remnant and determine the ablation dose of ^{131}I

- To detect local and distant metastases

CLINICAL QUESTIONS

PATIENT INFORMATION

24

SCANS AND THERAPY

I. POST-THYROIDECTOMY ^{131}I OR ^{123}I SCAN

A. Background

The primary treatment for thyroid carcinoma is a total thyroidectomy. The purpose of the postsurgical ^{131}I scan is to determine if subsequent radioiodine therapy is appropriate. Scans are obtained for two reasons: First, to detect a post-surgical thyroid remnant and determine the ablation dose and, second, to detect thyroid cancer metastases.

1. To confirm the presence of a postsurgical thyroid remnant. An ^{131}I scan often is obtained approximately 6 wk after a total or near-total thyroidectomy for thyroid cancer to confirm the presence of a thyroid remnant and determine what percent of the administered dose concentrates in the remnant. Some specialists use the percent uptake to determine the ablation dose of ^{131}I; in the unlikely event that the scan shows no evidence of a thyroid remnant, ablation doses of ^{131}I rarely are given.

A secondary goal of the ^{131}I scan is to search for metastatic disease. If metastases are detected, the patient usually is given a larger therapeutic dose of ^{131}I. To avoid stunning (see Clinical Question 3, below), the first post-thyroidectomy scan is sometimes obtained with ^{123}I instead of ^{131}I because ^{123}I does not have a beta emission. The ^{123}I scan can confirm the presence of a thyroid remnant, and the 24-hr uptake can be measured to help determine the ^{131}I ablative dose; however, the usual dose of ^{123}I for thyroid scanning (see Chapter 9, The Thyroid) is not as effective in detecting small metastases as ^{131}I.

2. The radioiodine scan to search for metastatic thyroid cancer. Protocols may vary among institutions. In general, thyroid hormone is stopped, the patient's thyroid-stimulating hormone (TSH) is documented to exceed 30–50 μU/ml, the serum thyroglobulin is measured and a diagnostic whole-body scan with ^{131}I is obtained. If metastases are detected or if substantial residual activity is present in the thyroid bed, a therapeutic dose of ^{131}I is given. To avoid stunning, some experts administer 5–6 mCi of ^{123}I instead of ^{131}I, but there is not as much experience in the use of ^{123}I for whole-body scanning.

B. Radiopharmaceuticals

1. Iodine-131. Iodine-131-sodium iodide is used for the pretherapy scan. Other radiopharmaceuticals may be used to search for metastatic thyroid cancer, but unless the cancer accumulates iodine, therapy will not be effective. Iodine-131 is a beta- and gamma-emitting isotope of iodine. Extra-thyroidal iodide is transported rapidly across the membrane of the follicular cell where it is oxidized, bound to tyrosine (organified) and subsequently incorporated into thyroid hormone. The relatively high-energy photon of ^{131}I can be imaged with conventional gamma cameras; its beta particle has an average path length of 0.8 mm in tissue, and it deposits all of its energy near its source. The beta particle of ^{131}I is responsible for 90% of the radiation dose to tissue.

24

2. Iodine-123. Iodine-123-sodium iodide is sometimes used to confirm the presence of a thyroid remnant because it has no beta emission and avoids the problems of stunning (see Clinical Question 3).

C. How the study is performed

1. Iodine-131. The adult patient swallows a capsule containing approximately 2–5 mCi (74–185 MBq) of ^{131}I-sodium iodide; many physicians prefer the lower dose to minimize stunning. After receiving the radioiodine, the patient goes home and returns 48–72 hr later for a whole-body scan. The uptake in the thyroid bed often is measured at the time of the scan, and the percent uptake may be a factor in planning treatment. The scan takes approximately 1 hr.

2. Iodine-123. The patient swallows capsules containing 0.5–5.0 mCi (18.5–185 MBq) of ^{123}I-sodium iodide and returns for scanning at 24 hr. Depending on the protocol, the scan and uptake measurement may take up to 1 hr.

D. Patient preparation

1. Explain the goal of the scan to the patient. The goal of the diagnostic ^{131}I or ^{123}I scan is to determine if ^{131}I therapy needs to be administered. If the scan shows evidence of metastatic disease or significant activity remaining in the thyroid bed, the patient should proceed to ^{131}I therapy. To plan appropriately, the patient needs to be aware that a diagnostic scan may lead immediately to therapy, which may require hospitalization.

2. Hypothyroid state. A disadvantage of ^{131}I therapy has been the requirement that patients be hypothyroid at the time of the scan and subsequent therapy. Thyroid hormone may suppress differentiated thyroid cancers, and tumor suppression will result in reduced or absent ^{131}I uptake. An appropriate hypothyroid state often is confirmed by a TSH level that exceeds 30 μU/ml before therapy. Patients on thyroxine suppression need to stop the thyroxine for approximately 6 wk before therapy to reach a hypothyroid state. Alternatively, triiodothyronine (T3) can be substituted for thyroxine and then stopped for 2 wk to minimize the duration of the hypothyroid state. Many physicians document that the TSH is elevated before proceeding to a scan (see Clinical Question 7).

3. Low-iodine diet. Patients often are given a low-iodine diet for 1–2 wk before therapy and placed on a low-iodine diet in the hospital. A low-iodine diet shrinks the iodide pool in the body, increases the percentage of ^{131}I in the iodide pool and potentially increases the uptake of radioiodide by the thyroid remnant or tumor. A simplified low-iodine diet (see Clinical Question 1) is provided by Lakshmanan et al.

4. No food for 4 hr before radioiodine administration. The patient may drink water but should not eat for 4 hr before radioiodine administration because food may delay absorption of the radioiodine.

5. Intravenous contrast. Patients should not be scheduled for treatment if they have had intravenous contrast within the preceding 4–6 wk. The iodine in the contrast will increase the iodide pool and decrease the uptake of ^{131}I by the thyroid remnant or tumor.

6. Exogenous iodine in diet or medications. Amiodarone and mineral/vitamin supplements containing iodine will increase the iodide pool and decrease the uptake of ^{131}I by the thyroid remnant or tumor. The patient should be asked about vitamin or mineral supplements and asked to discontinue any supplements containing iodine for several weeks before therapy.

7. Pregnancy. Pregnancy must be excluded.

8. Laxatives. Occasionally patients are given a mild laxative the day before the scan to minimize gut activity.

E. Understanding the report

The report describes the presence or absence of activity in the thyroid bed, the presence or absence of distant metastases and, if ablative therapy is contemplated, may include the percent uptake in the neck at 72 hr. Activity within the thyroid bed is common after surgery and usually represents a thyroid remnant, although the possibility of residual tumor cannot be excluded.

F. Potential problems

1. Hypothyroidism. The patient may find it difficult to tolerate the hypothyroid state. Hypothyroidism can be minimized by switching the patient from thyroxine to triiodothyronine for 4–6 wk, stopping the triiodothyronine for 2 wk and then checking the TSH (see Clinical Question 11).

2. Intravenous contrast or exogenous iodine. See 5 and 6 under Patient Preparation.

II. THALLIUM, SESTAMIBI AND FDG SCANS

A. Background

Thallium, sestamibi and FDG are accumulated by many thyroid cancers and may detect medullary carcinomas, Hürthle cell carcinomas and differentiated and anaplastic thyroid carcinomas that fail to concentrate radioiodine. These agents may be useful in detecting metastatic thyroid cancer and guiding external beam radiation therapy, but they do not emit beta radiation and cannot be used for therapy, nor can they be used to predict the response to ^{131}I therapy. They have an advantage in that no specific patient preparation is required, and the patient may remain on suppressive doses of thyroid hormone. Thallium, sestamibi and FDG scans are most often obtained in the clinical setting of a rising thyroglobulin and a negative radioiodine scan.

24

B–E. Radiopharmaceuticals, how the study is performed, patient preparation and understanding the report

Thyroid carcinomas including poorly differentiated and anaplastic thyroid carcinomas often accumulate these radiopharmaceuticals. Images are obtained 15–30 min after thallium (3–5 mCi [101–185 MBq]) or sestamibi (10–20 mCi [370–740 MBq]) injection and 60 min after FDG injection (10–15 mCi [370–555 MBq]). Depending of the imaging protocol, imaging will require 45–90 min. No special preparation is required.

F. Potential problems

1. Normal biodistribution. The normal biodistribution of thallium and sestamibi could obscure disease in the abdomen, pelvis and heart.

2. Response to ^{131}I therapy. Uptake of these tracers in a tumor site cannot be used to predict the response to ^{131}I therapy.

III. ^{131}I THERAPY
A. Background

Iodine-131 is used to ablate thyroid remnants after total or near-total thyroidectomy to destroy any tumor cells remaining in the remnant and to facilitate monitoring for recurrence with subsequent radioiodine scans and thyroglobulin measurements. Iodine-131 also is used to treat distant metastases. Because of the risks of injury to the superior and recurrent laryngeal nerves and the parathyroid glands, it is rare for a surgeon to perform a total thyroidectomy; in 90–100% of patients, there is some thyroid tissue remaining. Papillary thyroid carcinoma is multicentric in 20–80% of patients (the wide range reported in the literature is probably related to the diligence with which the pathologists searched for tumor foci). Because papillary carcinoma, and to a lesser extent follicular carcinoma, can be multifocal, a thyroid remnant after surgery may still contain thyroid cancer. Total or near-total thyroidectomy results in a lower recurrence rate and is a prerequisite to optimize ^{131}I therapy.

The radiation dose to the tumor depends on the amount of ^{131}I accumulated by the tumor and length of time the ^{131}I remains in the tumor. If a metastasis or thyroid remnant accumulates as little as 0.15% of the administered dose per gram of tumor, 100 mCi of ^{131}I can still deliver 8000–10,000 rads to the tumor, a radiation dose sufficient to destroy about 80% of thyroid cancers. The optimal dosage of ^{131}I required to ablate the thyroid remnant is debated but ranges from 30 to 100 mCi (1110 to 3700 MBq) with many therapists tending toward the higher dosage. Some therapists calculate a dose of ^{131}I based on an estimate of the remnant or tumor size, the uptake and the residence time of the ^{131}I in the tumor/remnant. Treatment of patients with a papillary carcinoma > 1.5 cm with a combination of thyroidectomy, ^{131}I ablation and thyroid hormone suppression results in a lower recurrence rate than surgery alone, surgery plus external radiation or surgery plus thyroid hormone.

Total or near-total thyroidectomy followed by ^{131}I ablation of the thyroid remnant facilitates the use of serum thyroglobulin to monitor recurrence of thyroid cancer. Once the thyroid is completely ablated, the serum thyroglobulin level with endogenous TSH stimulation becomes a highly sensitive and specific marker for thyroid cancer because the only source of thyroglobulin in the body is thyroid cancer. Endogenous or exogenous TSH stimulation may be needed to detect a rise in thyroglobulin and maximize the sensitivity of tumor detection. The absence of measurable thyroglobulin does not mean that there are no metastases; the metastases may be nonfunctional or may produce too little thyroglobulin to be detected. Furthermore, some patients have antithyroglobulin antibodies, which will interfere with the measurement. For these reasons, a diagnostic radioiodine scan often is obtained at the time of the first post-therapy thyroglobulin measurement.

B. Radiopharmaceutical

Iodine-131 emits a gamma photon that can be imaged and a beta particle that provides the radiation to ablate thyroid remnants and iodine-avid thyroid cancers. When ^{131}I is trapped and organified by normal thyroid tissue or by differentiated thyroid cancers, it decays inside the cell and emits a beta particle, which disrupts the nearby cellular DNA, prevents further cell division and leads to cell death.

C. How the therapy is performed

The patient swallows capsules containing the prescribed dose of ^{131}I, and if hospitalization is required, the patient remains isolated in a hospital room until the level of ^{131}I in the body falls below 30 mCi or 1110 MBq (see discussion of regulations below). Visitors may be allowed in the patient's room for very limited periods of time, depending on the radiation levels. Thyroxine is resumed at the time of discharge or 2–3 days after ^{131}I administration.

Depending on the state, it may not be necessary to hospitalize the patient. In the past, Nuclear Regulatory Commission regulations required hospitalization if a patient received greater than 30 mCi (1110 MBq) of ^{131}I; moreover, the patient had to remain in the hospital until the total amount of ^{131}I in the body dropped below a prescribed level. The Commission recently has revised its regulations and allows physicians to release patients with higher levels of ^{131}I if the treating physician can ascertain that there will not be any significant radiation exposure to the general public and patient's family. Some states, called agreement states, may not allow physicians this option, and physicians may not be comfortable with or want to assume the increased liability of releasing a patient who may not adhere to radiation safety precautions. Other countries have different regulations governing the release of patients after ^{131}I therapy.

24

Patients often return for a whole-body imaging session 3–10 days after ^{131}I therapy because the sensitivity for the detection of metastatic disease is increased after the higher doses administered for ablation or therapy.

D. Patient preparation

The patient preparation is the same as for the radioiodine diagnostic scan (See above).

E. Understanding the report

The report summarizes the indication for therapy, indicates that informed consent was obtained and states the dosage of ^{131}I given. If a whole-body scan is obtained 3–10 days after ^{131}I administration, that report will describe the presence or absence of activity within the thyroid bed and the presence or absence of metastatic disease.

F. Potential problems

See Patient Preparation and Potential Problems under the post-thyroidectomy ^{131}I or ^{123}I scan, above, and Clinical Question 10, below.

CLINICAL QUESTIONS

1. Should a low-iodine diet be prescribed before ^{131}I therapy?

A low-iodine diet should be prescribed for 1–2 wk before radioactive iodine therapy. The rationale for a low-iodine diet is to shrink the extrathyroidal iodide pool so that the administered radioactive iodide will occupy a greater percentage of the pool and uptake into the thyroid remnant or tumor will be correspondingly enhanced. Iodized salt, sea salt, milk, other dairy products, eggs, seafood, kelp or seaweed, seaweed derivatives such as algin (which often is used as a stabilizer in processed food), foods containing red dye no. 3 (red or pink cereals, candies or vitamins) and many restaurant foods are high in iodine. A more detailed low-iodine diet is provided in the reference by Lakshmanan et al.

24

2. Should a radioiodine scan be obtained after a thyroidectomy for thyroid cancer?

The role of the postsurgery scan, ^{131}I ablation of the thyroid remnant and ^{131}I therapy for metastases is well established. In patients with tumors $\geq$ 1.0 cm or any of the other risk factors described in the introduction, a strong argument can be made for a total thyroidectomy followed by ^{131}I ablation of the thyroid remnant to remove or destroy any remaining thyroid tissue including multicentric or bilateral foci of tumor. In a recent study, ^{131}I therapy was the single most powerful prognostic indicator for disease-free survival. Not only does ^{131}I therapy followed by thyroid hormone reduce tumor recurrence, this approach also reduces mortality and can offset the augmented risks incurred by delayed therapy, age > 45 yr at the time of diagnosis, tumors > 1.5 cm, multicentricity, local invasion or regional metastases. Total ablation of the thyroid also facilitates follow-up with radioiodine scans and thyroglobulin measurements to detect recurrence. Post-therapy care should include suppression of TSH with thyroxine and follow-up with serum thyroglobulin determinations and whole-body radioiodine scans.

3. What is stunning, and how can it be minimized?

The typical dose of ^{131}I to detect residual thyroid tissue in the neck or to scan for metastatic disease ranges from 2 to 5 mCi (74–185 MBq) with most therapists tending toward the lower dose. The radiation from these diagnostic doses may "stun" the residual thyroid or thyroid cancer, reducing the uptake of ^{131}I after a therapy dose a few days later. Stunning can be minimized by reducing the diagnostic dose. Anecdotal evidence suggests that stunning also can be minimized by treating immediately at the completion of the diagnostic scan (48–72 hr) rather than rescheduling the therapeutic dose 4–7 days after the diagnostic dose. If a patient cannot be treated immediately, however, some data suggest that a delay of 10–14 days may allow some recovery from stunning, but the patient must remain hypothyroid during this delay.

To minimize stunning in the post-surgical patient, some physicians omit the diagnostic scan and simply administer an ablative dose once the patient is determined to be hypothyroid. There are four potential disadvantages to this approach:

1) If no remnant is detected, an ablative dose may not be indicated
2) A higher therapeutic dose is usually administered if metastases are detected on the diagnostic scan
3) The presence of a 5–10% uptake in a thyroid remnant may suggest the need for a more complete thyroidectomy rather than ^{131}I therapy
4) The uptake may be used to help calculate the therapeutic dose

An ^{123}I diagnostic scan with 0.5–5.0 mCi (18.5–185 MBq) avoids stunning and can be substituted for the ^{131}I diagnostic scan to evaluate the thyroid remnant after a thyroidectomy. One potential limitation of this approach is the relatively short 13-hr half-life of ^{123}I compared with the 8-day half-life of [131]I. Some experts argue that the sensitivity for detecting distant metastases is optimal 48–72 hr after radioiodine administration. Because of the short half-life of ^{123}I, the sensitivity for detecting distant metastases may be reduced although this problem can be countered by administering a higher dose of [123]I. A recent study, however, suggests that the sensitivity of ^{123}I and ^{131}I are similar in the initial evaluation of the patient immediately after throidectomy. Disadvantages of ^{123}I include increased cost and less experience as a whole-body scanning agent for metastatic disease.

24

4. Should a postsurgical thyroid remnant be ablated with ^{131}I?

Over the long term, near total thyroidectomy followed by ^{131}I therapy plus thyroid hormone confers a distinct outcome advantage in patients with initial tumors $\geq$ 1.0 cm. This approach reduces tumor recurrence and mortality sufficiently to offset the increased risks associated with age $<$ 40 yr at the time of diagnosis, tumor size $\geq$ 1.0 cm, multicentric foci and local invasion or regional metastases. If the patient does not have any of the risk factors listed above, some experts do not obtain a scan and simply suppress the residual thyroid with thyroid hormone.

5. What are the risks of ^{131}I therapy?

Cytopenia. A mild transient cytopenia may occur in patients receiving relatively high doses of radioiodine (approximately 200 mCi) to treat metastatic disease.

Nausea and vomiting. Nausea and occasional emesis may occur 4–24 hr after radioiodine administration. This is transient and generally resolves by 36–48 hr. The patient should be treated with antiemetics at the first sign of nausea. Some physicians prescribe antiemetics prophylactically, especially in patients who may be at higher risk for this complication (patients receiving 150–200 mCi of ^{131}I, children and small adults).

Sialadenitis. The salivary glands also concentrate iodide; consequently, sialadenitis may occur in 10–30% of patients receiving about 200 mCi of ^{131}I. This complication can be minimized by having the patient suck lemon drops or other hard candy (see reference by Robbins et al.) and by good hydration to stimulate the flow of saliva.

Cystitis. Radiation cystitis is a possible complication but can be avoided by having the patient drink fluids liberally and void every 1–2 hr during the first 24–48 hr. Frequent voiding also minimizes the whole-body and gonadal radiation exposure.

Oligospermia. The therapeutic doses of radioiodine used to treat thyroid cancer may result in clinically significant oligospermia. The effect appears to be minimal after 100 mCi or less, appears to be dose dependent and is usually reversible. High-risk patients who are likely to undergo multiple high-dose therapies should consider long-term storage of semen before treatment. The dose to the testes can be reduced by good hydration, frequent voiding and laxatives to ensure 1–2 stools per day for 2–4 days after therapy.

Female fertility. Although transient amenorrhea may occur in the first year after ^{131}I therapy, there appears to be no significant difference in the fertility rate, birth rate and premature delivery rate among women with differentiated thyroid cancer treated with ^{131}I and women treated with surgery and hormone suppression.

24

Dysgeusia. Some studies report that taste dysfunction may occur in up to 48% of patients from 1 to 5 days after therapy. Taste dysfunction may be perceived as a loss of taste or taste distortion (metallic or chemical taste). It is transient in the majority of patients but may persist up to a year or longer.

Leukemia. There is probably no increased risk of leukemia among patients receiving no more than 200 mCi of radioiodine per treatment in whom treatments are spaced by at least 6–12 mo and in whom the total dose does not exceed 800 mCi. When cumulative doses exceed 1000 mCi, the incidence of leukemia may increase.

Pulmonary fibrosis. Pulmonary fibrosis has been reported to occur in patients with diffuse pulmonary metastases who have been treated with ^{131}I in doses that exceed 250 mCi. The complication can be minimized by limiting the amount of ^{131}I accumulated in the lungs to 80 mCi. The percentage of administered ^{131}I that will accumulate in the lungs can be determined by a pretherapy diagnostic scan.

6. Should ^{131}I therapy be given after a lobectomy for a supposedly benign tumor that later proved to be a thyroid carcinoma?

The preferred treatment is to excise the remaining lobe and then ablate any remnant with ^{131}I. If a large amount of residual thyroid tissue remains, it is difficult to ablate the remaining tissue with ^{131}I, use thyroglobulin measurements to monitor recurrence or effectively treat functioning metastases.

7. Is ^{131}I therapy of value in the treatment of medullary thyroid cancer?

Iodine-131 often is administered to ablate any remaining thyroid tissue after a thyroidectomy for medullary thyroid carcinoma. Medullary carcinoma of the thyroid comprises about 10% of all thyroid malignancies and is often hereditary. Although the progenitor calcitonin producing parafollicular C-cells do not concentrate radioactive iodide, the hereditary forms of the disease may be multicentric, and ^{131}I ablation has been associated with a fall in plasma calcitonin levels, probably because of destruction of malignant parafollicular C-cells adjacent to normal thyroid tissue in the remnant. The role of ^{131}I-metaiodobenzylguanidine (MIBG) in the diagnosis and treatment of medullary thyroid cancer is briefly discussed in Chapter 16, Clinical Question 6.

8. Is ^{131}I therapy of value when a patient has a rising thyroglobulin but a negative radioiodine scan?

Iodine-131 is the most effective therapy for metastatic differentiated carcinoma of the thyroid. The diagnostic scan may not detect metastatic thyroid cancer for several reasons: (a) the tumor volume or the concentration of ^{131}I is too low to be detected with the relatively low 2 mCi (74 MBq) scanning doses but can be detected and treated with the higher 100–200 mCi (3700–7400 MBq) doses often administered for therapy; (b) the tumor has dedifferentiated enough so that it no longer concentrates ^{131}I; or (c) the patient is still taking exogenous thyroid hormone, has recently had a contrast study or is consuming foods or supplements high in iodine.

Once option (c) is excluded by careful history, many physicians will treat the patient with a rising thyroglobulin but a negative diagnostic scan because ^{131}I can be an effective therapy for small or micrometastases that were not visualized on the diagnostic scan (see Worth Mentioning).

A metastasis or thyroid remnant that accumulates as little as 0.15% of the injected dose per gram of tumor can receive a radiation dose of 8000–10,000 rads after administration of 100 mCi of [131]I. A post-therapy scan and post-therapy measurements of the serum thyroglobulin are important aids to monitor the response to therapy.

9. Is ^{131}I therapy of value in the treatment of anaplastic thyroid cancer?

Anaplastic thyroid cancers do not concentrate ^{131}I; consequently, ^{131}I therapy is not efficacious. If there is a question regarding the anaplastic nature of metastatic thyroid cancer, a diagnostic radioiodine scan should be obtained. Regardless of tumor histology, if the scan demonstrates tumor uptake of radioiodine, ^{131}I therapy is likely to be beneficial.

10. Should a routine radioiodine scan be obtained after ^{131}I therapy?

Imaging 3–10 days after ^{131}I therapy can detect small or poorly functioning metastases that are missed on the diagnostic scan. In many centers, post-therapy scans are routine because there is no increased risk associated with the additional images (Fig. 1).

11. Should recombinant human thyrotropin be administered instead of making the patient hypothyroid before a radioiodine scan or therapy?

To optimize a diagnostic radioiodine scan or ^{131}I therapy, the TSH must be elevated. This traditionally has been accomplished by discontinuing exogenous thyroid hormone until the patient becomes hypothyroid (see Patient Preparation, above). Recombinant human thyrotropin is commercially available and provides an expensive alternative to the traditional approach; however, the patient avoids the symptoms associated with the hypothyroid state. Preliminary data suggest that whole-body radioiodine scans after administration of recombinant thyrotropin in a patient who continues taking thyroid hormone may not be as sensitive in detecting metastatic disease as withdrawing thyroid hormone

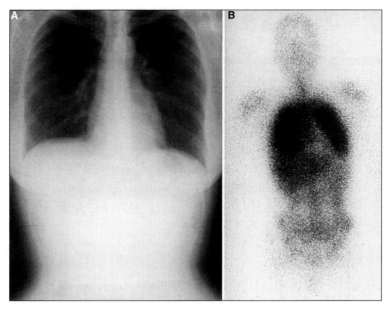

Figure 1. A 44-yr-old nutritionist underwent thyroidectomy for papillary thyroid carcinoma. The thyroid remnant was ablated with 100 mCi (3700 MBq) of ^{131}I. (A) The chest radiograph was normal. (B) A post-therapy scan obtained approximately a week after ^{131}I administration showed diffuse pulmonary metastases. Minimal uptake was noted in the thyroid bed. The liver was visualized because of circulating proteins iodinated by the thyroid remnant or the tumor; the liver activity does not represent diffuse hepatic metastases.

and allowing the endogenous TSH to rise. Recombinant thyrotropin is particularly appropriate for patients who refuse to become hypothyroid. Currently (2000), recombinant thyrotropin is FDA approved as a preparation for a diagnostic radioiodine scan and to enhance the sensitivity of a thyroglobulin measurement but not as preparation for ^{131}I therapy.

12. When should a patient be rescanned after an ablation dose or ^{131}I therapy?

If the post-^{131}I therapy scan shows only a thyroid remnant and no local or distant metastases, the patient is placed on thyroid hormone. A follow-up scan and thyroglobulin measurement are typically obtained 6–12 mo after ablation of the thyroid remnant, and the patient is re-examined every 9–12 mo until he/she has been rendered tumor free, as determined by the serum thyroglobulin assay and radioiodine scan. Further follow-up is individualized. Some physicians repeat the diagnostic scan and thyroglobulin measurement at 1- to 3-yr intervals, especially in patients with high-risk tumors. Evaluation often is continued every 2–5 yr for 20 yr, and some specialists recommend surveillance for life because of the potential for late recurrences. The combination of the diagnostic scan and serum thyroglobulin measurement improves detection of recurrent disease.

24

WORTH MENTIONING

1. Lithium in combination with ^{131}I therapy

A suboptimal therapeutic response after ^{131}I therapy may occur if the ^{131}I has a short residence time in the tumor; ^{131}I has a half-life of about 8 days, and a short residence time will decrease the potential radiation dose to the tumor. Lithium inhibits thyroid hormone secretion and ^{131}I release from the thyroid gland without affecting ^{131}I uptake. For this reason, lithium has been proposed as an adjuvant to ^{131}I therapy. Retarding the release of ^{131}I from the tumor will augment the radiation delivered to the tumor for any given dose of [131]I. Additional studies regarding lithium and ^{131}I therapy will probably be appearing in the literature.

2. ^{111}In-OctreoScan

Indium-111-OctreoScan binds to somatostatin receptors (see Chapter 16, Neuroendocrine Tumors). High doses of ^{111}In-OctreoScan or a beta-emitting isotope attached to an OctreoScan-type ligand with a high affinity for somatostatin receptors are under investigation for the treatment of neuroendocrine tumors, including medullary carcinoma.

3. ^{131}I-MIBG therapy for metastatic medullary thyroid cancer

Iodine-131-MIBG has been used to treat metastatic medullary carcinoma of the thyroid in patients whose metastases have been documented to concentrate MIBG after a diagnostic scan using ^{123}I or ^{131}I-MIBG. Iodine-131-MIBG therapy is discussed in more detail in Chapter 16, Neuroendocrine Tumors, Clinical Questions 5 and 6.

4. [131]I therapy combined with the surgical probe

When a patient has palpable neck disease, some institutions administer a therapeutic dose of ^{131}I and then send the patient to surgery 4–5 days later. With the use of the surgical probe, the surgeon can more easily locate and excise the sites of bulky tumor; any metastatic sites not removed are treated with [131]I.

5. [123]I scan to predict the response to ^{131}I therapy

When patients present with a rising thyroglobulin but a negative ^{131}I scan, ^{131}I therapy may still be of value (see Clinical Question 8). Preliminary results suggest that a 5-mCi (185-MBq) [123]I scan will predict the results of ^{131}I therapy. If no metastatic site is identified on the 5-mCi (185-MBq) [123]I scan, there will be no tumor identified on the post ^{131}I therapy scan and no decline in thyroglobulin; consequently, unnecessary ^{131}I therapy can be avoided.

24

PATIENT INFORMATION

I. POST-THYROIDECTOMY ^{131}I OR ^{123}I SCAN

The post-thyroidectomy ^{131}I or ^{123}I scan is often a prelude to therapy; for this reason, the purpose of the scan and the implications of the results should be discussed with your physician. A standardized patient information summary is not provided because physicians may differ in the choice of the diagnostic isotope (^{131}I versus ^{123}I) and in patient preparation, particularly in regard to withdrawing thyroid hormone versus the administration of recombinant TSH.

II. THALLIUM, SESTAMIBI AND FDG SCANS

Patient information for thallium and sestamibi scans is comparable with that provided in Chapter 3 except that the scanning procedure to search for malignancy will include whole-body imaging. Patient information for an FDG scan is provided in Chapter 15.

References

1. Schlumberger MJ. Papillary and follicular thyroid carcinoma. *N Engl J Med* 1998;338: 297–306.
2. Mazzaferri EL. An overview of the management of papillary and follicular thyroid carcinoma. *Thyroid* 1999;9:421–427.
3. Singer PA, Cooper DS, Daniels GH, et al. Treatment guidelines for patients with thyroid nodules and well-differentiated thyroid cancer. *Arch Intern Med* 1996;156:2165–2172.
4. Samaan NA, Schultz PN, Hickey RC, et al. Well-differentiated thyroid carcinoma and the results of various modalities of treatment. A retrospective review of 1599 patients. *J Clin Endocrinol Metab* 1992;75:714–720.
5. Dadparvar S, Krishna L, Brady LW, et al. The role of iodine-131 and thallium-201 imaging and serum thyroglobulin in the management of differentiaed thyroid carcinoma. *Cancer* 1993;71:3767–3773.
6. Utiger RD. Follow-up of patients with thyroid carcinoma. *N Engl J Med* 1997;337:928–930.
7. Lakshmanan M, Schaffer A, Robbins J, et al. A simplified low iodine diet in ^{131}I scanning and therapy of thyroid cancer. *Clin Nucl Med* 1988;13:866–868.
8. Reynolds JC, Robbins J. The changing role of radioiodine in the management of differentiated thyroid cancer. *Semin Nucl Med* 1997;27:152–164.
9. Sweeney DC, Johnston GS. Radioiodine therapy for thyroid cancer. *Endocrinol Metab Clin North Am* 1995;24:803–839.
10. Ladenson PW, et al. Comparison of administration of recombinant human thyrotropin with withdrawal of thyroid hormone for radioactive iodine scanning in patients with thyroid carcinoma. *N Engl J Med* 1997;337:888–896.
11. Robbins J, Merino MJ, Boice JD, et al. Thyroid cancer: a lethal endocrine neoplasm. *Ann Intern Med* 1991;115:133–147.
12. Park HM, Park YH, Zhou XH. Detection of thyroid remnant/metastasis without stunning: an ongoing dilemma. *Thyroid* 1997;7:277–280.
13. Britton KE, Foley RR, Siddiqi A, et al. I-123 imaging for the prediction of I-131 therapy for recurrent differentiated thyroid cancer, RDTC, when I-131 tracer is negative but raised thyroglobulin, Tg [abstract]. *Eur J Nucl Med* 1999;26:1013.

24

25 Polycythemia Vera and Essential Thrombocythemia

Polycythemia vera (PV) is a stem-cell clonal disease characterized by an increased total red cell mass often associated with splenomegaly, leukocytosis and thrombocytosis. PV needs to be distinguished from secondary causes of polycythemia caused by living at high altitude, chronic pulmonary disease, smoking, massive obesity, cyanotic heart disease, certain hemoglobinopathies and erythopoeitin-producing tumors. PV also needs to be differentiated from pseudopolycythemia, in which there is an increase in hematocrit caused by a contracted plasma volume.

The diagnosis of PV is based on an elevated red cell volume, normal arterial saturation and either splenomegaly or two of the following: thrombocytosis, leukocytosis, an elevated neutrophil alkaline phosphatase, an elevated vitamin B_{12} or an elevated unconjugated B_{12} binding capacity. In difficult cases, in vitro cultures of erythroid progenitors and measurement of erythropoetin levels can contribute to the diagnosis; erythropoetin is elevated in secondary polycythemia and suppressed in primary polycythemia.

Essential thrombocythemia or essential thrombocytosis is an idiopathic myeloproliferative disorder characterized by a persistent elevation of circulating platelets. Patients may present with recurrent spontaneous bleeding or thrombotic episodes; their platelet counts commonly exceed 1,000,000/μl. It is important to note that most patients presenting with platelets in excess of 1,000,000/μl have reactive, not primary, thrombocytosis. Reactive thrombocythemia can occur secondary to infection, splenectomy, malignancy, trauma, noninfectious inflammation, iron deficiency or blood loss, and these conditions need to be excluded before instituting myelosuppressive therapy.

25

PROCEDURES AND PRIMARY CLINICAL INDICATIONS

CLINICAL QUESTIONS

PROCEDURES

I. RED CELL VOLUME

A. Background

The primary indication for a measurement of red cell volume is suspected PV. There is an increased risk of PV in men when the hematocrit exceeds 0.50 and in women when the hematocrit exceeds 0.45. Patients with suspected PV usually are referred for a measurement of the red cell volume or red cell mass. The test actually measures red cell volume; however, the specific gravity of red cells is almost the same as that of water, and the red cell volume typically is equated with the red cell mass. PV needs to be distinguished from pseudopolycythemia, which is also known as Gaisböck's syndrome, stress polycythemia, relative polycythemia and spurious polycythemia. In pseudopolycythemia, the red cell mass is normal but the plasma volume is contracted and the hematocrit is consequently elevated. When clinically requested, the plasma volume was measured using ^{125}I-albumin, but this drug is not available in the United States (2000); the procedure was similar to that described for red cell volume.

25

B and C. Radiopharmaceutical and how the procedure is performed

Approximately 20 ml of blood are withdrawn. The red cells are separated and labeled with 0.5 μCi (18.5 KBq) of chromium-51 (^{51}Cr) and a known quantity is injected back into the patient. After equilibration for 15–20 min, a sample of blood is withdrawn, and the red cell volume is determined using the indicator dilution technique (the more dilute the tracer concentration, the larger the measured volume).

D. Patient preparation

No specific preparation is required. A phlebotomy before the test should be avoided because this will lower the red cell volume. The patient should avoid any other radionuclide tests just before measurement of red cell volume because residual radioactivity in the blood may lead to spurious results.

E. Understanding the report

The report will provide the red cell volume as well as reference values. The International Committee for Standardization in Hematology recommends reference values for red cell volume of 25–35 ml/kg in men and 20–30 ml/kg in women and 40 ml/kg for plasma volume for both sexes. Other normal values based on height, weight and sex may be reported. Because blood volume correlates best with lean body mass, an elevated red cell volume could be interpreted as normal in an obese individual. Some institutions adjust the red cell volume for lean body mass.

F. Potential problems

1. Measurement of plasma volume. Usually a measure of red cell volume is sufficient to diagnose or exclude polycythemia. If the red cell volume is normal and the hematocrit is elevated, the plasma volume is assumed to be reduced. The plasma volume can be estimated indirectly from the red cell volume and the venous hematocrit. This calculation assumes that the ratio of the whole-body hematocrit to the venous hematocrit is approximately 0.91. This assumption is valid in healthy individuals, but this ratio can fluctuate widely (0.7–1.2) in patients, and estimates of plasma volume based on this calculation can be quite spurious.

2. Obesity. Expression of the results as milliliter per kilogram may underestimate the degree of polycythemia in obese individuals.

3. Phlebotomy. A patient with PV may have a normal red cell volume if the measurement is made after the patient has been phlebotomized.

4. Iron deficiency. Patients with PV may have a normal red cell volume if they have a concurrent iron deficiency.

25

II. SODIUM PHOSPHATE ^{32}P THERAPY

A. Background

In patients with PV, symptoms are associated with an increased blood volume and increased viscosity. More than 35% of patients give a history of a hemorrhagic or thrombotic episode during the course of the disease. Untreated patients survive an average of 2 yr. See Introduction for additional information.

B–F. Radiopharmaceutical, how the procedure is performed, patient preparation, understanding the report and potential problems

Sodium phosphate ^{32}P is a beta emitter; there is no gamma emission. Phosphorous-32 is excreted in the urine but as long as the patient is continent, ^{32}P therapy presents no radiation risk to the public. The typical dose of ^{32}P ranges from 3 to 5 mCi (111–185 MBq), and it is administered intravenously in an outpatient setting. There is no special patient preparation. Phosphorous-32 therapy is not associated with acute adverse effects and can be repeated if an adequate response is not obtained or if the patient relapses. There is probably an increased risk of leukemia and there may be an increased risk of nonhematological malignancies, but the degree of risk is debated (See Clinical Question 3).

CLINICAL QUESTIONS

1. Is the red cell volume elevated? Does the patient have PV?

The measured red cell volume is compared with the expected red cell volume derived from normal populations matched for sex, weight or body surface area. The red cell volume correlates best with lean body mass, and the expected red cell volumes may be overestimated in obese individuals. An elevated red cell volume supports the diagnosis of PV.

2. Should a patient with PV be treated with ^{32}P?

The course of PV and the optimal therapy are still debated. Treatment consists of phlebotomy and myelosuppressive therapy. Regardless of the eventual therapeutic approach, phlebotomy should be used initially to reduce the red cell mass. Phlebotomy can be performed repeatedly and has been used to manage individuals with mild disease, young patients and those with polycythemia of uncertain cause. Recent data, however, suggest that phlebotomy may not be acceptable as permanent treatment because of poor clinical tolerance and the frequency of vascular complications. In a prospective trial conducted by the Polycythemia Vera Study Group, phlebotomy alone was associated with an increased risk of death in the first 4 yr because of hemorrhage or thrombosis, whereas ^{32}P therapy was associated with an increased risk of lymphocytic leukemia and other nonhematologic malignancies. Phlebotomy and ^{32}P therapy were both superior to treatment with chlorambucil. The chemotherapeutic agent most commonly used for marrow suppression in patients with PV is hydroxyurea for which the risk of leukemia remains debatable.

In most cases, ^{32}P therapy provides long, trouble-free remissions and successfully reduces the morbidity associated with the disease. The initial dose ranges from 3 to 5 mCi (111–185 MBq). No form of therapy is clearly better in

25

terms of patient survival, but management of patients with ^{32}P is simpler and may be particularly appropriate in elderly patients. Remissions may last 6–24 mo. Phosphorus-32 therapy can be repeated if a relapse occurs.

3. Should a patient with essential thrombocythemia be treated with sodium phosphate?

Treatment options include hydroxyurea, anagrelide and sodium phosphate ^{32}P. Phosphorus-32 is probably associated with an increased risk of secondary malignancy; however, because of its ease and patient tolerance, ^{32}P is a viable treatment option and should be considered particularly in poorly compliant patients or in patients older than age 50 yr.

4. What is the risk of ^{32}P therapy?

There is no acute toxicity from ^{32}P therapy. The risk of acute leukemia with phlebotomy alone is about 1%; with ^{32}P therapy, the risk varies from 2% to 15% at 10 yr. The large discrepancy between studies reporting 2% and studies reporting 15% is probably related to cumulative dose of ^{32}P, the stage of the disease and other forms of therapy that the patient may have received.

References

1. Lamy T, Devillers A, Bernard M, et al. Inapparent polycythemia vera: an unrecognized diagnosis. *Am J Med* 1997;102:14–20.
2. International Committee for Standardization in Haematology. Recommended methods for measurement of red-cell and plasma volume. *J Nucl Med* 1980;21:793–800.
3. Najean Y, Dresch C, Rain J. The very-long-term course of polycythemia: a complement to the previously published data of the Polycythaemia Vera Study Group. *Br J Haematol* 1994;86:233–235.
4. Berk PD, Goldberg JD, Donovan PB, et al. Therapeutic recommendations in polycythemia vera based on Polycythemia Vera Study Group protocols. *Semin Hematol* 1986;23:132–143.
5. Murphy S, Iland H, Rosenthal D, Laszlo J. Essential thrombocythemia. an interim report from the Polycythemia Vera Study Group. *Semin Hematol* 1986;23:177–182.
6. Buss DH, Cashell AW, O'Connor ML, et al. Occurrence, etiology and clinical significance of extreme thrombocytosis: a study of 280 cases. *Am J Med* 1994;96:247–253.

25

26
Intracavitary Therapy

Malignant pleural and peritoneal effusions can present as difficult problems in the management of the cancer patient. Discomfort and respiratory distress due to fluid in the chest and abdomen can be among the most distressing symptoms encountered as a result of malignant disease. Instillation of chromic phosphate ^{32}P (a colloidal suspension of radioactive phosphorus) provides a therapeutic alternative in the management of the patient with a malignant effusion. Phosphorus-32 chromic phosphate also has been used as an adjunct to cytoreductive surgery and chemotherapy in patients with ovarian cancer.

INTRACAVITARY THERAPY AND PRIMARY CLINICAL INDICATIONS

CLINICAL QUESTIONS

26

THERAPY

I. TREATMENT OF MALIGNANT ASCITES

A. Background

Malignant ascites most commonly results from ovarian, renal cell or gastrointestinal tract tumors. Seeding of the peritoneum results in serosal irritation with increased fluid production and decreased fluid removal secondary to obstructed lymphatics. Ascites can be a major source of morbidity, causing severe dyspnea, coughing, and hiccoughing secondary to diaphragmatic irritation. Treatment with ^{32}P chromic phosphate results in a cessation or significant decrease in ascites in 50–80% of patients. Most of the patients who respond will do so soon after treatment; however, the maximum response usually requires 3 mo. The clinical response is enhanced if there is adequate dispersion of the radioactive colloid throughout the peritoneal cavity.

The imaging agent, ^{99m}Tc-sulfur colloid, can be injected before intracavitary instillation of the ^{32}P-chromic phosphate to exclude loculation and ensure adequate colloid dispersion (see Potential Problems, below).

B. Radiopharmaceutical

Phosphorous-32 chromic phosphate is a colloidal suspension with ^{32}P incorporated into the colloid. Phosphorus-32 has a half-life of 14.3 days, an average beta range in tissue of 3.2 mm and a maximum range of 8.0 mm. The average dose ranges from 10 to 20 mCi (370–740 MBq) of ^{32}P-chromic phosphate. The distribution of chromic phosphate ^{32}P is largely fixed within 24 hr with less than 10% of the dose remaining in the intracavitary fluid. Dose calculations based on a uniform distribution of ^{32}P in a capillary layer covering the intraperitoneal surface give an estimated surface dose of about 30–60 Gy (3000–6000 rads) for typical administered doses. This therapy is most effective if tumor implants are small. Large, bulky tumor masses will not be penetrated by the beta emission of ^{32}P. There is no gamma emission, and the patient does not present a radiation risk to the public.

C. How the procedure is performed

A catheter is placed in the abdominal cavity for ^{32}P-chromic phosphate infusion (see Potential Problems, below).

D. Patient preparation

No specific preparation is required other than catheter placement for the chromic phosphate ^{32}P infusion.

E. Understanding the report

The report describes the adequacy of tracer dispersal if ^{99m}Tc-sufur colloid was infused for imaging and gives the dose of chromic phosphate ^{32}P administered as well as the volume of co-administered fluid.

26

F. Potential problems

1. Loculation. Administration of ^{32}P-chromic phosphate into a loculated space reduces its therapeutic effectiveness and substantially increases the risk of complications. Adequate dispersal can be ensured by first infusing a solution containing 1–3 mCi of ^{99m}Tc-sulfur colloid in 250–1000 ml of saline. The distribution of ^{99m}Tc-sulfur colloid can be determined by imaging the 140 keV gamma photon of ^{99m}Tc; there is no beta emission and no risk to the patient if the instilled ^{99m}Tc-sulfur colloid is contained within a loculated space. If loculation is detected by imaging, the catheter can be repositioned or reinserted. Once adequate dispersion is established with ^{99m}Tc-sulfur colloid imaging, the ^{32}P-chromic phosphate is premixed in 250–1000 ml of saline and infused. Premixing ^{32}P-chromic phosphate with the saline results in a more uniform distribution.

2. Complications. Complications are minor and usually temporary but they may include nausea, abdominal pain, vomiting, diarrhea and low-grade fever.

II. TREATMENT OF MALIGNANT PLEURAL EFFUSION

A. Background

Malignant pleural effusions commonly result from breast, lung or ovarian cancer or lymphoma. They can produce profound respiratory symptoms and if left untreated may progress to fibrothorax.

B–E. Radiopharmaceutical, how the procedure is performed, patient preparation and understanding the report

See those under treatment of malignant ascites, above.

F. Potential problems

Loculation. Pretherapeutic infusion of ^{99m}Tc-sulfur colloid for imaging will identify or exclude loculation (see Potential Problems under treatment of ascites, above). The study can also exclude the possibility of a bronchopleural fistula.

III. ADJUVANT THERAPY FOR OVARIAN CARCINOMA

A. Background

Each year, approximately 20,000 American women are diagnosed with ovarian carcinoma, with 90% of the tumors occurring in patients between the ages of 40 and 65 yr. Because the initial disease is usually asymptomatic, tumors often are advanced at the time of diagnosis, and the large majority of patients require adjuvant therapy. Patients with a high-grade stage 1 tumor, ascites, tumor ex-

26

crescencies on the ovarian surface or tumor rupture during surgery are at risk for abdominal recurrence. Multiagent chemotherapy has become the adjuvant therapy of choice after surgery; however, radiation therapy alone or in conjunction with chemotherapy is also under investigation.

Intra-abdominal ^{32}P-chromic phosphate is an appealing option for adjuvant therapy because of its low toxicity and the potential for the ^{32}P colloid to match the primary spread pattern of ovarian carcinoma within the abdominal cavity; metastatic deposits directly adjacent to sites of ^{32}P localization receive therapeutic radiation from the beta particle during ^{32}P decay. A number of studies report encouraging results, but they are limited by the inclusion of patients with various tumor grades and stages, prior therapies, different doses of ^{32}P-chromic phosphate, differences in timing and instillation technique, and lack of well-controlled randomized trials.

B–F. Radiopharmaceutical, how the procedure is performed, patient preparation, understanding the report and potential problems

See those under treatment of malignant ascites and malignant pleural effusion, above.

CLINICAL QUESTIONS

1. Which patients with malignant ascites should receive intracavitary therapy?

Systemic chemotherapy is typically used for treatment of the underlying malignancy, but the decrease in ascitic volume may be limited. Paracentesis also is often ineffective because effusions usually reaccumulate rapidly, and repeated paracentesis depletes the protein reserves of patients who often are already debilitated. If the ascites is causing significant morbidity, is not responding to conventional therapy and the patient has a life expectancy exceeding several months, treatment with ^{32}P-chromic phosphate should be considered.

2. Which patients with a malignant pleural effusion should receive intracavitary therapy?

Malignant effusions in patients with breast cancer or lymphoma as well as acellular effusions often respond to systemic chemotherapy. For malignant effusions that do not respond, intrapleural instillation of a sclerosing agent such as tetracycline, doxycycline or an antineoplastic agent is usually the treatment of choice. These cause a painful chemical irritation, which results in obliteration of the pleural space. Talc powder also has been used, but it is quite painful and may require general anesthesia during administration. If sclerosing agents are unsuccessful or contraindicated, instillation of ^{32}P-chromic phosphate suspension may be useful. Phosphorous-32-chromic phosphate therapy is painless, and partial or complete responses can be obtained in about 50–60% of patients.

WORTH MENTIONING

1. Low-dose ^{32}P-chromic phosphate in conjunction with platinum analog chemotherapy for the treatment of ovarian carcinoma

The platinum analogs cisplatin and carboplatin appear to exert their primary effect by the formation of lethal platinum-induced cross links between DNA bases. These cross links may sensitize the cells to radiation damage. Consequently, the radiation from low-dose intraperitoneal treatments of ^{32}P-chromic phosphate may act synergistically with platinum analog chemotherapy to provide an advantage in the treatment of disseminated intraperitoneal ovarian cancer.

2. Radioimmunotherapy of ovarian carcinoma

Intracavitary ^{32}P-chromic phosphate therapy is nonselective; the ^{32}P colloid deposits randomly on the peritoneal surfaces. Radioimmunotherapy offers a more targeted approach. The monoclonal antibody *HMFG*1, for example, recognizes a glycoprotein tumor associated antigen encoded by the gene *muc-1*, which is overexpressed on at least 97% of ovarian adenocarcinomas. Intraperitoneal administration of *HMFG*1 labeled with a beta-emitting isotope offers the potential of eradicating microscopic residual disease. Preliminary results using this approach are encouraging.

References

1. Young RC, Walton LA, Ellenberg SS, et al. Adjuvant therapy in stage I and stage II epithelial ovarian cancer. *N Engl J Med* 1990;322:1021–1027.
2. Spanos WJ, Day T, Jose B, et al. Use of P-32 in stage III epithelial carcinoma of the ovary. *Gynecol Oncol* 1994;54:35–39.
3. Pattillo RA, Collier BD, Abdel-Dayam H, et al. Phosphorus-32-chromic phosphate for ovarian cancer: I. Fractionated low-dose intraperitoneal treatments in conjunction with platinum analog chemotherapy. *J Nucl Med* 1995;36:29–36.
4. Taylor A, Baily NA, Halpern SE, Ashburn WL. Case report: loculation as a contraindication to intracavitary P-32 chromic phosphate therapy. *J Nucl Med* 1975;16:318–319.
5. Cubberly D, Datz FL, Taylor A. Value of preinjection tracer before P-32 treatment of effusion: unexpected bronchopleural fistula. *AJR Am J Roentgenol* 1982;139:166–167.
6. Nicholson S, Gooden CSR, Hird V, et al. Radioimmunotherapy after chemotherapy compared to chemotherapy alone in the treatment of advanced ovarian cancer: a matched analysis. *Oncol Rep* 1998;5:223–226.

26

27
Bone Pain Palliation

Bone metastases can develop in any patient with cancer. The most common cancers metastasizing to bone are breast, prostate and lung. If these cancers are not cured, skeletal metastases will develop and most patients will have progressive bone pain. As many as 50% of these patients report inadequate pain control. The initial treatment is non-narcotic analgesics, which often progresses to opiates. Opiate analgesia may be complicated by somnolence, mood changes, nausea and constipation, and additional drugs may be required to treat these symptoms. External radiation therapy can provide significant palliation, but additional sites often become symptomatic while the primary site is being treated; furthermore, bone marrow toxicity may limit the number of sites that can be treated. Radionuclide therapy (unsealed source therapy) involves the intravenous administration of therapeutic bone-seeking radiopharmaceuticals that deliver a high local dose of radiation directly to the sites of bony metastases. There are now compelling data to show that radionuclide therapy is equally effective in inducing pain relief as external beam therapy, although the onset of pain relief is slower. More importantly, radionuclide therapy irradiates all the painful sites with a single treatment, suppresses the development of new painful sites, reduces the need for subsequent external beam therapy and appears to decrease total patient care costs.

27

THERAPY AND PRIMARY CLINICAL INDICATIONS

Clinical Questions

PATIENT INFORMATION

THERAPY

I. RADIONUCLIDE THERAPY FOR BONE PAIN PALLIATION

A. Background

Radionuclide therapy (unsealed source therapy) involves the single intravenous administration of a bone-seeking radiopharmaceutical that delivers a high local radiation dose directly to the sites of bony metastases. There is no acute toxicity, and the drugs typically are administered in an outpatient setting. The response rate is 60–80% with approximately 20% of patients becoming pain free. Although these agents are effective in palliating bone pain and may result in a fall in tumor markers such as prostate-specific antigen (PSA), there is no evidence that they prolong survival. Furthermore, they only target bony metastases; there is no effect on soft-tissue metastases. Radionuclide therapy can be combined with local beam therapy or hormonal therapy. Toxic effects are mild and are generally limited to platelet depression, which tends to slowly return toward baseline levels over 8–24 wk.

B. Radiopharmaceuticals

1. Strontium-89 (Metastron). Strontium-89 is a beta emitter with a physical half-life of 50.5 days. The typical therapy dose ranges from 3 to 4 mCi (111–148 MBq). Strontium is accumulated in metabolically active bone because of its chemical similarity to calcium. The distribution of strontium in bone is equivalent to that of standard bone imaging agents, and, like them, it is accumulated preferentially at bony sites of tumor invasion. There is prolonged retention of strontium at tumor sites with some activity remaining up to 100 days after injection. After strontium administration, platelets decrease an average of about 30–50% with the nadir occurring about 4–6 wk post-therapy; platelets recover slowly and rise toward pretreatment levels in 12–24 wk. Most of the strontium that is not accumulated in bone is eliminated in the urine over 1–2 days. A few patients will have an acute exacerbation of their pain a few days after strontium administration. This exacerbation is known as a flare and typically lasts 1–2 days; anecdotally, these patients appear to be more likely to have a favorable clinical response. In responders, pain relief typically begins from 1–3 wk after administration and lasts an average of 3–6 mo (range, 2–12 mo).

2. Samarium-153-ethylenediaminetetramethylenephosphonic acid (EDTMP). Samarium-153 (lexidronam, Quadramet) contains ^{153}Sm, which is a beta and gamma emitter with a half-life 46.3 hr; because of the gamma emission, the distribution of ^{153}Sm-EDTMP can be imaged (Fig. 1). The therapy dose is approximately 1 mCi (37 MBq)/kg. Its distribution is equivalent to that of routine bone imaging agents and, like strontium, it accumulates preferentially at the site of tumor invasion of bone. Approximately 35% of the dose is excreted in the first 24 hr, with most of the excretion occurring in the first 6 hr; if metastases are widespread, retention can approach 100%. Patients should be well hydrated and void at least every 1–2 hr during the first 8 hr after injection to minimize the dose to the kidneys and bladder. After ^{153}Sm-EDTMP therapy, platelets may fall to 30–50% of baseline values; the nadir occurs at 3–5 wk after injection, and platelets tend to return to pretreatment levels by 8–10 wk. Patients may have a transient increase in bone pain (flare reaction), which is usually mild and occurs within 72 hr after injection. In responders, pain relief usually occurs within 1–2 wk and lasts an average of 2.6 mo (range, 1–8.8 mo).

3. Rhenium-186-etidronate and ^{117m}Sn diethylenetriamine pentaacetic acid. These drugs are investigational agents in the United States, but they may become available in the future. The response rates are likely to be similar to the two approved agents. There may be differences in onset of action, duration of response and marrow toxicity. Controlled, double-blind studies may be required to answer these questions.

C. How the procedure is performed

27

The drugs are infused through an intravenous line over a few minutes. The typical therapy dose of ^{89}Sr ranges from 3 to 4 mCi (111–148 MBq), and the typical dose of ^{153}Sm-EDTMP is 1 mCi (37 MBq) per kg. There is no acute toxicity, and the patient may leave as soon as the infusion is complete.

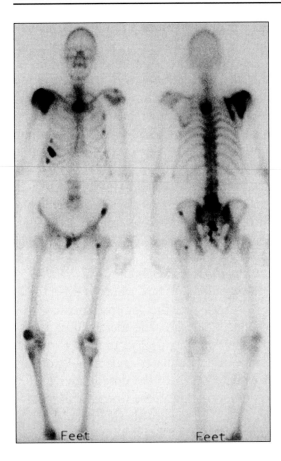

Figure 1. A patient with metastatic prostate cancer was referred for ^{153}Sm-EDTMP therapy. Because of multiple sites of disease and the need for opioid analgesia, the patient was treated with 1 mCi (37 MBq)/kg and returned 24 hr later for whole-body imaging. The distribution is equivalent to the distribution obtained with the standard bone scan, which can be seen in Chapter 11, Figure 2.

D. Patient preparation

1. Pregnancy. Pregnancy needs to be excluded immediately before therapy in women of childbearing age.

2. Bone scan. A recent bone scan needs to be obtained to ensure that the sites of the patient's pain correspond to areas of abnormal uptake on the bone scan. If the bone scan is normal, the patient's pain may not be due to metastatic disease; if it is due to metastasis, the normal bone scan indicates that the metastatic site will not accumulate the therapeutic tracer, and the patient is unlikely to benefit from therapy.

3. Pretherapy laboratory tests. A complete blood count, platelet count, creatinine and a test for subclinical disseminated intravascular coagulopathy (DIC) should be obtained within a week of therapy. In general, granulocytes should exceed 2000/μl, and platelets should exceed 60,000 and preferably 100,000/μl. Patients should not receive radionuclide therapy until 6–8 wk after treatment with long-acting myelosuppressive chemotherapy (nitrosoureas) or 4 wk after

27

hemibody irradiation or other forms of myelosuppressive chemotherapy. Similarly, myelosuppressive therapy or hemibody radiation should not be given for 6–12 wk after radionuclide therapy because of the potential for severe leukopenia or thrombocytopenia. Patients with DIC are probably at increased risk of severe thrombocytopenia after therapy.

4. Calcium supplements. Calcium may reduce the effectiveness of the therapy, and calcium supplements should be discontinued for 2 wk before treatment.

5. Bisphosphonates. Etidronate or other bisphosphonates may interfere with therapy (see Potential Problems, below).

E. Understanding the report
The report lists the radiopharmaceutical and dose administered; it also may contain recommendations for follow-up monitoring of possible marrow toxicity.

F. Potential problems
1. Impending spinal cord compression or impending pathologic fracture. Radionuclide therapy may be administered for pain relief, but it is not adequate treatment for either of these conditions.

2. Short life expectancy. Pain relief may not occur for 1–3 wk after therapy, depending on the drug used. The delay in onset of pain relief may preclude this form of therapy in patients with a very short life expectancy.

3. Hypercalcemia. Unless accompanied by renal failure, hypercalcemia is not a contraindication.

4. Renal failure. The therapeutic radiopharmaceuticals are eliminated in the urine. Patients with renal failure may need a reduction in the administered dose. Dialysis does not preclude therapy, but the radiation safety officer will need to be consulted before therapy is scheduled.

5. The patient is taking etidronate or other bisphosphonates. These drugs may interfere with uptake in the bone and at the metastatic sites. The therapist should be consulted; it may be necessary to obtain a bone scan. If the bone scan shows good uptake at the metastatic sites, comparable uptake can be expected with any of the therapeutic radiopharmaceuticals and treatment can proceed.

6. Incontinence. Most of the therapeutic radionuclides that are not accumulated in bone are eliminated in the urine over the first 1–2 days. Most incontinent patients given special instructions for radiation safety can be managed at home with a condom catheter or indwelling bladder catheter, but management of incontinent patients should be discussed with the nuclear medicine physician before treatment.

27

CLINICAL QUESTIONS

1. Should a patient with painful bony metastases receive radionuclide therapy?

Treatment usually is reserved for patients who have failed hormonal or chemotherapy. In these patients, the primary indication is severe bone pain because of metastatic disease that requires narcotic analgesia or limits mobility; some physicians treat patients with multiple metastases demonstrated on bone scan even if the pain is not yet requiring narcotic analgesia. Available data suggest that radionuclide therapy alone is an effective approach. Studies comparing radionuclide therapy to external beam therapy have shown comparable rates of response, although the response rate is quicker after external beam therapy. Radionuclide therapy, however, treats all bony metastatic sites with a single dose, lessens the likelihood that nonpainful bony metastases will become painful and reduces the need for subsequent external beam therapy. The response rate is 60–80%, with about 20% of patients becoming pain free. The risks are quite small; the main toxicity is a subclinical thrombocytopenia, which tends to return to the baseline level in 8–24 wk. Some clinicians treat patients with multiple metastases and one or two sites of severe pain with radionuclide therapy in combination with external beam radiotherapy.

2. Should a patient with nonpainful bony metastases receive radionuclide therapy?

In theory, this approach may have advantages because radionuclide therapy suppresses the development of new painful sites and reduces the need for subsequent external beam therapy in patients with painful bony metastases. However, the advantage of radionuclide therapy in patients who have widespread bony metastases but no bone pain has not been documented.

3. What are the alternatives to radionuclide therapy for painful bony metastases?

Hormone therapy. Bony metastases from breast or prostate cancer often will respond to hormonal manipulations. Patients with breast cancer may respond to drugs such as tamoxifen, whereas patients with prostate cancer may respond to bilateral orchiectomy, estrogens, antiandrogens or total androgen blockade. Eventually, hormonal therapy fails, and other forms of pain palliation need to be implemented.

Chemotherapy. Many cancers will respond to chemotherapy, and chemotherapy is often an initial or second-line approach. Platelet depression will be exacerbated if hemibody or radionuclide therapy are combined with cytotoxic chemotherapy.

Analgesics. Pain may be controlled with increasing doses of opiate analgesia. Potential complications include opiate-induced nausea, constipation or somnolence, which can negatively impact quality of life.

27

External beam radiotherapy. Local external beam radiotherapy is the treatment of choice for a single, severely painful bony metastasis that is refractory to hormonal therapy or chemotherapy. It consists of a beam of x-rays directed at a specific tumor site; toxicity is minimal. Radionuclide therapy is more appropriate for multiple sites of pain. The two therapies can be combined when a patient has one or two sites of especially severe pain but multiple sites of metastatic disease and bone pain. This appears to be a cost-effective approach and can reduce lifetime health service costs.

Hemibody radiotherapy. Wide field radiotherapy may be used as palliative therapy to treat patients with multiple sites of pain. It may be administered as upper or lower hemibody therapy or it may be administered sequentially to the upper and lower body. Toxicity may include thrombocytopenia, pancytopenia, pneumonitis and gastroenteritis.

4. What are the contraindications to radionuclide therapy?

Bone pain that is not due to metastatic disease. A bone scan is recommended before radionuclide therapy to make sure that the sites of the patient's pain correspond to sites of metastatic disease. The radiopharmaceuticals used in radionuclide therapy have the same distribution as seen on the bone scan; uptake at the metastatic sites on the bone scan will ensure that the radiopharmaceutical will be delivered to the painful site.

Pregnancy. Pregnancy is a contraindication to radionuclide therapy.

DIC. There is probably an increased risk of severe thrombocytopenia after treatment of patients with underlying DIC.

Marrow suppression. Platelets should exceed 60,000 and preferentially 100,000/μl. Granulocytes should exceed 2000/μl. In patients with severe marrow suppression, the risk of bleeding and the requirement for platelet transfusions is substantially increased. There also may be an increased risk of granulocyte depression and infection.

Etidronate therapy. See Potential Problems, above.

Terminal patient. If the patient's life expectancy does not exceed several weeks, he or she is unlikely to survive long enough to benefit from radionuclide therapy. This is particularly true if the patient is treated with strontium.

5. Can a patient with lytic metastases be treated?

27

The critical factor in determining which patients may respond to radionuclide therapy is a bone scan showing abnormal uptake corresponding to the sites of pain, not the presence of lytic or blastic lesions on an x-ray (Fig. 2). Lytic lesions can be treated provided that the lytic sites are shown to have abnormally increased uptake on a bone scan.

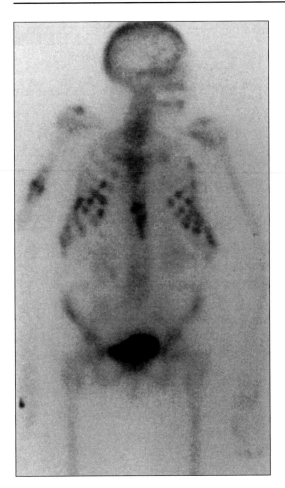

Figure 2. A 62-yr-old woman with multiple myeloma presented with severe anterior rib pain only modestly controlled with narcotic analgesia. A chest radiograph showed multiple lucent lesions throughout the bones of the chest consistent with myeloma. She had been treated with chemotherapy and involved field radiotherapy. A bone scan shows multiple areas of abnormal uptake in the anterior ribs corresponding to the sites of the patient's pain. The patient had a pathologic fracture of the right humerus. Based on the pain and the bone scan, the patient was treated with ^{89}Sr with a subsequent reduction in her pain and pain medications. (Reprinted with permission from Edwards GK, Santoro J, Taylor A. Use of bone scintigraphy to select patients with multiple myeloma for treatment with strontium-89. *J Nucl Med* 1994;35:1992–1993.)

6. Can a patient be treated more than once?

If a patient responds to radionuclide therapy and the pain recurs, the patient may be retreated ≥3 mo after the initial therapy. The response rate to retreatment ranges from 50 to 70%.

WORTH MENTIONING

1. Combination therapy

Studies are under way that combine radionuclide therapy with radiosensitizers such as doxorubicin (adriamycin) in an attempt to improve pain palliation and increase survival.

2. Multiple dose therapy

Preliminary results suggest that five repeated therapies of 30 mCi (1110 MBq) of [153]Sm-EDTMP each at 3-mo intervals may normalize the PSA and induce a remission of bone lesions in addition to providing a palliative effect.

27

PATIENT INFORMATION

I. RADIONUCLIDE THERAPY FOR BONE PAIN PALLIATION

A. Procedure

You have been referred for radionuclide therapy because you have bone pain due to cancer that has spread to the bones. Treatment consists of a single injection. An intravenous line will be placed in an arm vein, and you will receive an infusion of a radioactive drug. The actual infusion of the drug will take no more than 10 min. The radioactive drug preferentially goes to areas where tumor is invading bone. The principal radiation travels only a fraction of an inch and irradiates the tumor where it is invading bone. Sixty to 80% of patients will have a reduction in pain or a decrease in the use of pain medication, and about 20% of patients will become pain free. If treatment is successful but the pain recurs, there is the possibility of additional treatments. The treatment will not make you ill and you will be able to leave after the drug is injected.

B. Preparation

Diet. You should drink a lot of fluids before you come for your therapy. There are no special dietary requirements.

Medications. If you are taking calcium or calcium-containing vitamins, you should stop taking these supplements for 2 wk before therapy. If you are taking etidronate or other bisphosphonates for osteoporosis or to treat your cancer, let your doctor know before you come for your therapy. These medications may interfere with the uptake of the radioactive drug in the bone around the tumor.

C. Radiation and other risks

There will be some radiation to your bone marrow resulting in a decrease in your platelets and white cells, which may result in an increased risk of bleeding or infection. This is rarely a problem, but your platelets and white cells will need to be monitored by blood tests for 6–12 wk after your therapy.

Some of the radioactive drug will be excreted in your urine. You should sit down to urinate and double flush the toilet for 2–7 days depending on which drug you receive (check with your doctor when you have your therapy). Always wash your hands after using the toilet. If any urine gets on your clothes or bedding, wash them separately with an extra rinse cycle. If you are incontinent, check with your doctor before scheduling the therapy.

27

D. Pregnancy

If you are pregnant or think you may be pregnant, inform your doctor before scheduling treatment.

References

1. Laing H, Ackery DM, Bayly RJ, et al. Strontium-89 chloride for pain palliation in prostatic skeletal malignancy. *Br J Radiol* 1991;64:816–822.
2. Porter AT, McEwan AJB, Powe JE, et al. Results of a randomized phase-III trial to evaluate the efficacy of strontium-89 adjuvant to local field external beam irradiation to the management of endocrine resistant metastatic prostate cancer. *Intl J Radiat Oncol Biol Phys* 1993;25:805–813.
3. Bolger JJ, Dearnaley DP, Kirk D, et al. Strontium-89 (Metastron) versus external beam radiotherapy in patients with painful bone metastases secondary to prostatic cancer: preliminary report of a multicenter trial. *Semin Oncol* 1993;20:32–33.
4. Quilty PM, Kirk D, Bolger JJ, et al. A comparison of the palliative effects of strontium-89 and external beam radiotherapy in metastatic prostate cancer. *Radiother Oncol* 1994;31:33–40.
5. McEwan AJB, Amyotte GA, McGowan DG, et al. A retrospective analysis of the cost effectiveness of treatment with Metastron (^{89}Sr-chloride) in patients with prostate cancer metastatic to bone. *Nucl Med Comm* 1994;15:499–504.
6. Tu S, Delpassand ES, Jones D, et al. Strontium-89 combined with doxorubicin in the treatment of patients with androgen-independent prostate cancer. *Urol Oncol* 1996;2:191–197.
7. Silberstein E. Dosage and response in radiopharmaceutical therapy of painful osseous metastases. *J Nucl Med* 1996;37:249–252.
8. McEwan AJB. Unsealed source therapy of painful bone metastases: an update. *Semin Nucl Med* 1997;27:165–182.
9. Malmberg I, Persson U, Ask A, et al. Painful bone metastases in hormone-refractory prostate cancer: economic costs of strontium-89 and/or external radiotherapy. *Urology* 1997;50:747–753.
10. Papatheofanis FJ. Short-term reduction in pain medication costs following systemic radionuclide therapy in prostate cancer patients. *Veteran Health System J* 1998;3:63–66.
11. Edwards GK, Santoro J, Taylor A. Use of bone scintigraphy to select patients with multiple myeloma for treatment with strontium-89. *J Nucl Med* 1994;35:1992–1993.

28 Radiation, Radiopharmaceuticals and Imaging Devices

Medical diagnostic imaging often uses ionizing radiation in the form of x-rays and gamma-rays. Ionizing radiation includes beta-particles, which are the most common form of internally administered radiation used for therapy. Beta-particles contribute to the radiation dose in some medical imaging procedures, but beta-particles are not useful for imaging because they travel distances of only a few millimeters in tissue. Nonionizing imaging techniques include MRI and ultrasound. This chapter briefly describes the types of ionizing radiation and units of radiation exposure. It also includes a discussion of naturally occurring background radiation and the risks of somatic injury, cancer and genetic damage after radiation exposure. The chapter concludes with a brief discussion of radiopharmaceuticals and imaging equipment used in nuclear medicine.

Radiation: Units, exposure and risk

28

1. What are curies, becquerels, roentgens, rads, rems, grays and sieverts?

The activity of a radioactive substance is measured in terms of the rate at which the nuclei of its radioactive atoms disintegrate. The units of activity include the curie (Ci), defined as 3.7×10^{10} disintegrations per second (dps) and the newer metric unit, the becquerel (Bq), which is defined as one disintegration per second. The becquerel has been adopted as the standard international (Systeme Internationale, SI) unit to express the administered dose of a radionuclide, although the curie is still the most commonly used unit in the United States. Other SI units include the gray and the sievert (see below). The activities administered to patients are usually in the range of millicuries (1 mCi = 3.7×10^7 dps), microcuries (1 µCi = 3.7×10^4 dps) or megabecquerels (1 MBq = 10^6 dps).

The basic unit of radiation exposure is the roentgen (R). It refers to the amount of ionization produced by a beam of x-rays or gamma-rays in air and is used to specify radiation levels in the environment. Exposure levels are measured with radiation detection devices such as Geiger counters. The amount of

28

radiation energy absorbed by irradiated tissue is called the radiation dose and is specified in rads or grays. A dose of 1 rad is defined as 100 ergs of energy absorbed per gram of tissue; 1 gray is defined as 1 joule of energy per kilogram of tissue and is equal to 100 rads.

The biologic effect of radiation depends not only on the number of ergs per gram of tissue but also on the linear energy transfer of the radiation (the density of ionizations produced by the radiation). For a given path length, alpha-particles and neutrons produce 10–20 times more ionizations than x-rays, gamma-rays or even beta-particles and have a much greater biologic effect. To account for the different biologic effects resulting from different types of radiation, the radiation dose in rads or grays is multiplied by a radiation weighting factor to obtain a new measurement called the equivalent dose, which relates the dose in rads or grays to the biologic risk. The equivalent dose is specified in rems (roentgen-equivalent-man) or sieverts. For x-rays, gamma-rays and beta-particles, the weighting factor is 1; consequently, for diagnostic ionizing radiation, roentgens, rads and rems turn out to be numerically equivalent, although they actually represent different quantities. One roentgen results in an absorbed dose of 1 rad, which is equivalent to 1 rem in tissue. Because the values are numerically equivalent, the radiation dose is sometimes expressed in millirads instead of millirems. Similarly, grays and sieverts (Sv) are numerically equivalent; 1 Sv is equal to 100 rems. The radiation dose from diagnostic nuclear medicine procedures is generally quite low and is expressed in millirems (1/1000 rem; mrem), millisieverts (mSv) or microsieverts (μSv).

2. What is the radiation dose to the nuclear medicine patient?

Once administered to the patient, radiopharmaceuticals do not distribute uniformly throughout the body; they are designed to target specific organs, tumors or pathways and avoid others. Consequently, the whole body does not receive a uniform radiation dose after a radiopharmaceutical administration. Different tissues receive different exposures depending on the amount of the radiopharmaceutical going to a particular tissue and how long it remains there. After administration of a renal radiopharmaceutical (5 mCi of ^{99m}Tc-mercaptoactyl-triglycine [MAG3]), the radiation exposure to the red marrow, for example, is approximately 9 mrem, whereas tissues such as the bladder may receive doses as high as 850 mrem depending on the volume of urine in the bladder and the frequency of voiding.

The radiation dose often is expressed as the total body dose, the total energy absorbed in the body divided by the mass of the total body. A limitation of the total body dose approach is that it does not distinguish between a radiation dose delivered to a relatively radiosensitive tissue such as the marrow and the same radiation dose delivered to a relatively radioresistant tissue such as the brain. The concept of "effective radiation dose" has been developed to define a single quantity that could express the overall potential deleterious effect of radiation

28

exposures. This concept allows the risk of the different radiation doses to different tissues throughout the body to be expressed in a single measurement. The effective radiation dose equivalent is the whole body radiation dose that would have to be given to produce a risk equivalent to the sum of the risks from the individual radiation doses to the various organs. The radiation dose described in the patient information forms refers to the effective radiation dose. The effective dose from diagnostic nuclear medicine procedures is typically in the range of 100–1000 mrem (1–10 mSv) with an average of about 330 mrem (3.3 mSv). For comparison, background radiation is estimated to be approximately 300 mrem (3.0 mSv) per year.

The term "dose" is also used to refer to the dosage or amount of a radioactive tracer administered to a patient. It is important to distinguish between the use of the term "dose" to describe the administered activity (millicuries or megabecquerels) and the absorbed radiation dose (rems, sieverts); failure to recognize this distinction may lead to confusion.

3 and 4. What is the radiation exposure from background radiation? What is the radiation exposure from a transcontinental flight?

An understanding of naturally occurring environmental radiation is useful in placing medical radiation in perspective. Radiation from cosmic rays and naturally occurring radioactive atoms results in a continuous low-level radiation exposure. Background radiation increases with altitude and varies with location depending on the abundance of natural radioactive elements in rocks or soil. Background radiation from cosmic rays, for example, is about 50 mrem/yr in mile-high Denver, but it is only 25 mrem/yr at sea level. Perhaps the greatest variability in background radiation is due to indoor radon, which exposes the bronchial epithelium to alpha-particle radiation.

Another source of natural radioactivity is the human body itself, which contains radioactive potassium-40 (^{40}K) and carbon-14 (^{14}C). Radioactive lead-210 (^{210}Pb) and polonium-210 (^{210}Po) have been observed in cigarette smoke; these tracers emit alpha-particles, have been found in the bronchial epithelium of cigarette smokers and may contribute to the increased risk of lung cancer observed in smokers. Modern air travel also increases the exposure of the public to radiation; a typical transcontinental flight exposes each passenger to a radiation dose of approximately 0.5 mrem/hr. For comparison, naturally occurring background radiation in the United States results in an estimated average annual dose equivalent of about 300 mrem (3.0 mSv).

5. What are the effects of high doses of radiation (nuclear weapons, radiation accidents)?

The effects of high doses of radiation are the changes associated in the popular mind with radiation: hair loss, skin burns, loss of oral and intestinal mucosal integrity, depletion of stem cells, aspermia, agranulocytosis, sepsis, generalized de-bility and death. The eventual survival time and mode of death after whole-body exposure depend on the dose level. At very high doses of 10,000–15,000 rad (100–150 Gy), death occurs in a few hours and appears to result from neurologic and cardiovascular breakdown (central nervous system or CNS syndrome) although the exact cause of death is unclear. At dose levels of 500–1200 rad (5–12 Gy), death occurs within a few days and results from destruction of the gastrointestinal mucosa (GI syndrome). At lower dose levels of 250–500 rad (2.5–5.0 Gy), death occurs several weeks after exposure, due to effects on bone marrow (hematopoietic syndrome). In the GI and hematopoietic syndromes, the principal cause of death is the depletion of the stem cells of the gut epithelium and marrow.

6 and 7. How is the risk of low-level radiation determined? What is the risk of cancer from low-level radiation?

Radiation effects on human beings may be classified as *somatic,* affecting the irradiated person, or *genetic,* affecting progeny. The acute somatic effects of high-dose radiation have been described in Question 5; delayed somatic effects include cancer. Since the earliest use of x-rays, radiation production of tumors has been noted. Carcinogenesis has been postulated to require an initiator and a promoter. The usually long latent period of one to four decades between radiation exposure and the appearance of a tumor suggests radiation does not create malignant cells per se, but functions as an initiator.

The most extensive data that permit a quantitative assessment of risk from radiation as a function of dose come from the Japanese survivors of Hiroshima and Nagasaki and from the therapeutic irradiation of patients with ankylosing spondylitis. A significant increase in the incidence of leukemia was found in the Japanese survivors, which peaked about 10 yr after exposure and then declined. An elevated incidence of other cancers, including lung, breast and thyroid cancers, has been detected, but these cancers appear to have much longer latent periods than leukemia. In spondylitic patients, an increased incidence of leukemia was found, which was comparable to that seen in the Japanese study. However, a sharp distinction must be made between the long-term effects produced by massive amounts of radiation (nuclear bombs, radiation for cancer therapy) and the long-term effects produced by low levels of diagnostic radiation, which may differ in dose levels and dose rates by factors of thousands or more.

It is not possible to directly determine the incidence rate of cancer or severe hereditary disorders from very low radiation doses. Carcinogenic and mutagenic changes produced by radiation are indistinguishable from those occurring spontaneously. Furthermore, the increase in radiation exposure from diagnostic studies over background radiation is so small that any resulting increases in cancer are difficult if not impossible to demonstrate by epidemiologic methods. The naturally occurring incidence of cancer is just too high compared with any slight increase that might occur from an additional low dose of diagnostic radiation superimposed on background radiation.

28

Data from the Japanese survivors of Hiroshima and Nagasaki show that the risk becomes significant at the 95% confidence level only for doses in excess of 20,000 mrem (200 mSv). The problem is how to extrapolate the documented risk from high-dose radiation delivered at a high-dose rate to low dose radiation delivered at a low-dose rate. This is an area of debate. Proponents of a hypothesis called "hormesis" argue that low-dose radiation is actually beneficial. Others argue for a threshold effect; up to a certain dose level (the threshold), there is no increased risk. Others argue that the known risk from high-dose radiation (Hiroshima, Nagasaki) can be extrapolated by mathematical modeling to determine the risk from low-dose radiation. The primary mathematical models that have been examined are the linear, linear-quadratic and the quadratic. The linear model implies that the total population risk of 100 rem given to 10,000 individuals is the same as 1 rem given to 1,000,000 individuals. For purposes of radiation protection, the no-threshold, linear model is applied because it is the most conservative; however, for risk estimates, the best data appear to support a linear-quadratic model. At low doses the effect is linear but the effect is much less than the effect observed at high doses; the total population risk of 100 rem given to 10,000 individuals is substantially higher than 1 rem given to 1,000,000 individuals.

In conclusion, the risk of cancer from low-dose levels remains hypothetical and is based on extrapolations from data for persons exposed to higher-dose levels and high dose rates. Using the linear-quadratic model, the International Commission on Radiation Protection (ICRP) has estimated that an effective dose of 500 mrem (5 mSv), which is typical for many nuclear medicine procedures, would result in 1 additional fatal cancer among 4000 exposed individuals. The risk is 1 in 2000 among those younger than 15 yr and 1 in 8000 among those older than 70 yr. The risk of dying from cancer in the United States is 25%. Using the ICRP estimates that extrapolate from high radiation doses and high-dose rates, the risk of a 35-yr-old person dying from cancer would increase from approximately 25% to 25.03% following a nuclear medicine examination.

8. What are the genetic effects of low-dose radiation?

The descendants of the Japanese survivors of Hiroshima and Nagasaki are the largest population available for estimating the genetic hazards of radiation exposure. No increase has been observed in the incidence of prenatal or neonatal deaths or the frequency of malformations. Even if an increase in genetic hazards had been observed, there would still be the problem of extrapolating the genetic effects from high-dose, high-dose-rate irradiation to low-dose irradiation delivered at a low-dose rate. However, complete data from Japan are not yet available. The number of people exposed was small by genetic standards, and insufficient time has passed for the appearance of recessive mutations which may require several generations for expression.

9. What are the radiation exposure guidelines for radiation workers, the general public and patients?

Using the available data regarding carcinogenic and genetic effects, even though they are incomplete, the National Council of Radiation Protection has issued

28

permissible dose standards for individuals who work with radiation. The maximum total effective dose equivalent is 5 rem/yr (50 mSv/yr). Nuclear medicine patients can be released if the total effective dose equivalent to any one individual member of the general public is not likely to exceed 500 mrem (5 mSv); however, nuclear medicine facilities are required to give patients written guidelines to minimize the radiation dose to other individuals if the total effective dose equivalent is likely to exceed 100 mrem (1 mSv). Guidelines regarding the maximum total effective dose have not been issued for patients; as a general rule, diagnostic testing should be conducted with the smallest radiation dose practical and designed to achieve the most favorable risk-benefit ratio. Radiation should be used only when indicated for diagnostic purposes; this particularly applies to children and patients who may be pregnant. However, there should be no hesitation in using radiation when the diagnostic procedure can yield information essential to the management of a patient (see Question 11). In many clinical settings, the risk of not performing the diagnostic study will substantially exceed the risk of the study itself.

10. Can studies using ionizing radiation be performed in pregnant women?

Doses of irradiation during pregnancy that approach the level of 10–15 rem (0.1–0.15 Sv) to a fetus may result in an increased incidence of fetal malformations, fetal death, or persistent damage of genetic material, depending on the stage of pregnancy during which the radiation is delivered. The fetal dose from nuclear medicine procedures typically ranges from 0.1 to 1.0 rem. The fetus is particularly susceptible to congenital defects during the first trimester of pregnancy. Studies that must be done in pregnant women should be performed with careful attention to techniques that reduce the potential risk to the fetus. If the radiopharmaceutical is excreted by the kidneys, for example, forcing fluids and frequent bladder emptying will minimize the radiation exposure to the embryo or fetus. Radiolabeled material that crosses the placental barrier should usually be avoided. Consultation with the diagnostic specialist using these imaging tools may help distinguish between an indicated and an unwarranted study; furthermore, consultation also can assist in the design, timing and format of the study to minimize the risk to the fetus (see Chapter 13, Women's Health, Clinical Question 11 and Chapter 2, Pulmonary System and Thromboembolism, Clinical Question 7 for additional discussion of the use of ionizing radiation in pregnant or nursing mothers).

11. How can the risk of ionizing radiation be minimized for potentially pregnant women?

If a woman is potentially pregnant, special consideration should be given to the relatively high radiosensitivity of the fetus, particularly during the first trimester. Thus, it is important to ask if the patient suspects that she may be pregnant and to ask when she had her last menstrual period. If she responds

28

that she could be pregnant, the procedure should be postponed, if possible, until pregnancy can be confirmed or ruled out. If the patient does not think she is pregnant, fetal risk can be minimized by limiting the radiation exposure to the first 10 days of the menstrual cycle before ovulation and potential conception. This precaution becomes more important if radiologic examination of the abdomen or pelvis (CT, intravenous urogram, barium enema, lumbar spine series) is planned or if the radiopharmaceutical concentrates in the abdomen, pelvis or bladder.

12. Is there any risk to a patient's family or colleagues after a nuclear medicine test using a diagnostic radiopharmaceutical?

The person likely to receive the highest radiation dose from a patient who has been given a diagnostic radiopharmaceutical is a child sitting in the lap of the patient. Even in the worst case, the dose to the child is unlikely to exceed 100 mrem (1 mSv) and falls within accepted guidelines (see Question 9). It is helpful to remember that radiation exposure falls off with the square of the distance from the source; the radiation exposure to a family member can be substantially reduced if the family member simply sits across the room from the patient. In summary, the radiation exposure to friends, family members or the general public is not a concern; it is highly unlikely that any person will receive a radiation dose even approaching the 500 mrem (5 mSv) limit specified for any member of the general public. For comparison purposes, background radiation exposure is about 300 mrem/yr (3.0 mSv/yr).

13. What is a radiopharmaceutical?

A radiopharmaceutical is a radioactive drug that is designed to image or measure a particular structure or process. The ability of radiopharmaceuticals to function as indicators of specific physiologic processes often provides an important measure of disease that might not be apparent based on anatomic or structural changes alone. A radiopharmaceutical consists of a gamma-ray, x-ray or beta-emitting radionuclide that often is combined with a nonradioactive component to better tailor it for concentration by a particular organ or physiologic process. Unlike standard drugs such as those used for the treatment of infections or hypertension, radiopharmaceuticals are administered in tracer quantities; consequently, they typically elicit no physiological or pharmacologic response and do not affect the process being imaged or measured.

Radiopharmaceuticals used for imaging emit electromagnetic radiation such as x-rays and gamma-rays, whereas radiopharmaceuticals used in therapy emit particulate radiation such as beta-particles.

A prominent difference between x-rays and beta-particles lies in their ability to penetrate matter. Beta-particles travel only a few millimeters in soft tissue before expending all of their energy, whereas x-rays and gamma-rays distribute their energy more diffusely and can transverse many centimeters of tissue.

28

14. What is technetium-99m?

Technetium-99m (^{99m}Tc), for which 99 is the atomic weight and m stands for metastable), serves as the principal radionuclide for many radiopharmaceuticals. Technetium-99m, often abbreviated as technetium, is used widely in nuclear medicine procedures because it is readily available, has a short 6-hr half-life and has an ideal gamma energy for standard imaging equipment (140 keV). Furthermore, ^{99m}Tc does not emit particulate radiation such as beta particles, and radiopharmaceuticals containing ^{99m}Tc result in minimal radiation to the patient.

15. What is a PET radiopharmaceutical?

Positron-emitting radionuclides of carbon-11 (^{11}C), oxygen-15 (^{15}O) and nitrogen-13 (^{13}N) can be incorporated into a variety of biologic tracers and substrates, which can be used to image receptor sites and other physiologic and metabolic processes. Positrons (positive electrons) are emitted from radioactive nuclei with an excess of protons. Positrons travel only a few millimeters in tissue before colliding with a negative electron; this encounter results in the annihilation of both particles, with the creation of two 511 keV photons that travel at 180 degrees in opposite directions (see Question 19). The half-lives of many of these positron-emitting radionuclides are in the range of a few minutes, necessitating on-site cyclotron production facilities. Fluorine-18 (^{18}F), however, is one positron emitter with a longer half-life of 110 min. Fluorine-18 can be made in an off-site production facility, used to label deoxyglucose, which can then be shipped to the user; ^{18}F-fluorodeoxyglucose is the most common PET radiopharmaceutical (see Chapter 15, Introduction to Cancer and FDG Imaging). Generator systems are available to produce rubidium-82 (^{82}Rb) for myocardial imaging studies and gallium-68 (^{68}Ga) for labeling purposes. These generator systems also can make positron imaging possible without an on-site cyclotron.

16. What is the risk of an allergic reaction to a radiopharmaceutical?

The chemical quantities of a radionuclide or a radiopharmaceutical injected into a patient are generally quite small. For example, the amount of iodide used in a thyroid uptake study is thousands of times less than the iodide present in ordinary iodized table salt consumed at a meal. Radiopharmaceuticals almost never provoke the type of hypersensitivity reactions that can occur after administration of the contrast media used in x-ray studies.

17. What is a gamma (scintillation) camera?

Most common nuclear medicine studies image the distribution of a radiopharmaceutical in the body with a gamma (scintillation) camera. The gamma camera consists of a collimator, crystal, an array of photomultiplier tubes, system electronics and a computer. The collimator is typically a single slab of lead or

28

tungsten containing many small holes; only photons traveling parallel to the collimator holes can reach the crystal located behind the collimator. The crystal absorbs the photons and emits the absorbed energy as a flash or shortly spaced series of flashes of light—scintillations—proportional in brightness to the energy absorbed. An array of photomultiplier tubes converts the light flashes from the crystal into an electronic signal that can be used to determine the energy of the photon and the location of its interaction with the crystal. The signal is subsequently digitized and stored in a computer for image production, processing, analysis and display. The photon detection components of a gamma camera (collimator, crystal, photomultiplier tubes and initial electronics) often are referred to as a detector. Gamma camera systems may contain one, two or three detectors and often are designed for SPECT imaging (see Question 18). Systems with two or more detectors can be used to acquire two or more images simultaneously and reduce the imaging time.

18. What is a SPECT imaging system?

SPECT uses a standard gamma camera but houses it in a special gantry that can rotate around the patient. Images are acquired at multiple angles, usually encompassing 180 or 360 degrees around the body. These multiple angle data sets are subsequently used to produce computer reconstructed tomographic images that can be displayed as coronal, sagittal and transverse slices. SPECT imaging provides greater contrast as well as better anatomic delineation than is generally possible with planar imaging. The ability to quantitate tracer distribution is not as good with SPECT as with PET (see below) because of problems of collimation and attenuation, which are inherent in the detection of single photons. An area of SPECT research is the improvement of the resolution and quantitative capacity of SPECT imaging systems.

19. What is a PET imaging system?

PET is one of the fastest-growing areas in nuclear medicine. PET imaging systems dramatically expand the capacity to image in vivo physiology and biochemistry because they can image the high-energy photons of positron-emitting tracers such as ^{18}F, ^{11}C, ^{13}N and ^{15}O, tracers that are easily incorporated into biologically active molecules and key substrates of metabolism. There are two types of PET imaging systems: dedicated PET imaging systems that only image positron-emitting radiopharmaceuticals and hybrid systems that image both PET radiopharmaceuticals and traditional single-photon emitters such as ^{99m}Tc (see Question 20).

Positrons (positive electrons) travel only a few millimeters in tissue before colliding with a negative electron. This encounter results in the annihilation of both particles, with the creation of two 511 keV photons, which travel at 180 degrees in opposite directions. Most modern dedicated PET systems consist of dozens to several hundred detectors that are arranged in a circular or polygonal configuration. The system only registers a count if two detectors that are

28

180 degrees apart detect a photon at the same time (a coincidence event). The coincidence circuitry and a reconstruction algorithm are used to identify the site of a positron emission; collimators are not required. The collection of multiple counts coupled with filters, reconstruction algorithms and other computer-controlled image manipulation techniques provide reconstructed cross-sectional images. Dedicated PET systems often incorporate techniques to correct for tissue attenuation and can provide accurate quantitative data describing radiopharmaceutical distribution.

20. What is a coincidence camera imaging system?

Dedicated PET imaging systems are not designed to image single-photon emitting radiopharmaceuticals, which account for the large majority of nuclear medicine procedures. Similarly, standard gamma cameras are not designed to image the high-energy 511 keV photons of PET radiopharmaceuticals, although cardiac viability studies can be performed using detectors with thick crystals and specially designed collimators (see Chapter 1, Cardiovascular Diseases). The use of PET radiopharmaceuticals, particularly ^{18}F-fluorodeoxyglucose is increasing, and many institutions seek to image with ^{18}F but do not have the volume of procedures to justify investing in a dedicated PET system. Coincidence camera systems are designed to image single-photon and positron-emitting radiopharmaceuticals.

The typical coincidence camera system is a hybrid SPECT system with two detectors that can be used to image standard radiopharmaceuticals. The two detectors also can be positioned on opposite sides of the body to image positron-emitting radiopharmaceuticals using coincidence circuitry (see Question 19), and they can rotate around the body allowing the production of tomographic images. Currently, coincidence camera systems cannot match the image quality and quantitative measurements of a dedicated PET system, in part because the two flat detectors of a coincidence camera system have a much lower count rate than can be obtained with the circular array detectors in a dedicated PET system. In addition, today's coincidence systems lack methods of accurate and reliable attenuation correction. As research progresses, the count rate and image quality of the coincidence systems for imaging PET radiopharmaceuticals will improve.

References

1. Cohen BL, Lee IS. A catalog of risks. *Health Phys* 1979;36:707–722.
2. Cormack J, Towson JEC, Flower M. Radiation protection and dosimetry in clinical practice. In: Murray IPC, Ell PJ, eds. *Nuclear medicine in clinical diagnosis and treatment,* Edinburgh: Churchill Livingstone; 1994:1367–1388.
3. Gibbs SJ. Radiobiology. In: Sandler MP, Coleman RE, Wackers JFT, Patton JA, Gottschalk A, Hoffer PB, eds. *Diagnostic nuclear medicine,* 3rd ed. Baltimore: Williams and Wilkins; 1996:309–327.

28

29
Comparative Costs of Diagnostic Procedures

The actual cost for any medical procedure depends upon the definition of "cost." Is the cost defined as the charge to the patient, the cost to the patient's insurance carrier, health maintenance organization (HMO) or the combined charge? Do different insurance carriers or HMOs have different contracts with the facility and different costs? Is cost defined as the actual dollars spent for the total resources that were required to perform the procedure? If so, how was overhead for space, lights, cleaning and equipment amortization determined? What has been allowed in the cost to defray procedures performed on patients who cannot or do not pay?

One way to attempt to compare "costs" for diagnostic procedures is to use the payment allowed by Medicare, which is based on a relative resource methodology. Each November, Medicare publishes a *Medicare B Locality Fee Schedule.* The fees allowed are the sum of several components: physician work, malpractice costs, practice expense costs and a geographic factor that adjusts for the locality in which one practices such as rural or urban. Most radiology and all nuclear medicine procedure payments by Medicare consist of two parts: physician and technical. When a radiologic procedure is performed in a private office, for example, the physician is paid the sum of the physician and technical allowed fees, or the so-called global fee. In a hospital, however, the radiologist would be paid only the physician component of the total or global allowed fee.

The following Comparative Cost table is based on the total or global fees allowed for medical procedures

29

by Medicare in an urban area in the northeast United States in 1999. This Comparative Cost table was constructed using commonly accepted coding practices. The *Medicare B Locality Fee Schedule* uses *Current Procedural Terminology Fourth Edition* (CPT4) which is a systematic listing and coding of procedures and services performed by physicians and is a product of the American Medical Association. Each procedure is identified with a five-digit code. This coding system is recognized and used by all medical insurance companies and payers in this country. Medicare uses an additional coding system to code drugs and radiopharmaceuticals, medical products, and some procedures that it may wish to particularly monitor, for example, PET imaging for lung cancer. The table does not include any special fees that may be charged by a facility for room use such as during a biopsy, endoscopy or catheterization, nor does it include contrast media costs because, in many parts of the country, these are rolled into the CT/MRI procedure costs.

In the table, radiopharmaceutical costs are in parentheses after each listed nuclear medicine procedure. Medicare pays the invoice cost for the radiopharmaceutical, a charge that may vary from one facility to the next. But more importantly, the choice of a radiopharmaceutical, or accessory agent such as dipyridamole or adenosine for stress cardiac testing, is dependent upon the particular clinical circumstance. For example, the cost for radiopharmaceuticals for tumor imaging varies from less than $100 for ^{67}Ga-citrate to nearly $1000 for ^{111}In-pentetreotide (OctreoScan). We have elected to use the Florida "allowed" radiopharmaceutical cost list, which was published in their Medical B Newsletter (#159, 6/26/98) for most of the procedures. For those radiopharmaceuticals that are not on that list, we used invoice data provided by several large institutions. It should be emphasized that the actual cost to a facility may be greater or less than the figures provided; the data provide a cost comparison based on Medicare payments. The procedures listed below follow the order of the chapters.

Comparative Cost of Diagnostic Procedures (1999)

Indication	Procedure	Medicare B Payment (Global Fee)	
		Procedure	Radiopharmaceutical
Coronary artery disease	Stress/rest exercise SPECT	$ 555	(55–90)
	Stress ECG	$ 132	
	Dobutamine echocardiogram	$ 142	(15)
	Coronary angiography	$1955	
Congestive heart failure	Radionuclide ejection fraction	$ 275	(30–94)
	Echocardiogram ejection fraction	$ 246	
Pulmonary embolism	V/P scan	$ 285	(75)
	CT chest with contrast, spiral	$ 351	
	Pulmonary angiogram	$ 897	
Renovascular hypertension	Kidney scan w/ACE inhibitor	$ 248	(35–94)
	Renal ultrasound with duplex Doppler	$ 387	

29

Comparative Cost of Diagnostic Procedures (1999)

Indication	Procedure	Medicare B Payment (Global Fee) Procedure	Radiopharmaceutical
Renovascular hyper. cont.	Angiogram of kidneys	$ 956	
	CT with contrast	$ 417	
	Magnetic resonance angiography	$ 513	
	Captopril-stimulated plasma renin	$ 61	
Pyelonephritis	Kidney SPECT scan with DMSA	$ 274	(73)
	CT with contrast	$ 417	
	Renal ultrasound	$ 119	
Urinary reflux	Radionuclide cystourography	$ 116	(35)
	Contrast cystourography	$ 119	
Hepatic hemangioma	RBC SPECT scan	$ 280	(94)
	CT Liver with/without contrast	$ 417	
	MRI abdomen	$ 538	
	Liver ultrasound	$ 89	
Acute cholecystitis	Hepatobiliary scan	$ 193	(34)
	Abdominal ultrasound	$ 123	
	CT with contrast	$ 344	
Gastroparesis	Gastric emptying scan	$ 209	(15)
	Upper GI series	$ 96	
	Endoscopy	$ 180	(plus procedure room/medications)
Gastrointestinal bleeding	RBC scan	$ 280	(94)
	Selective mesenteric angiogram	$1445	
	Colonoscopy	$ 279	(plus procedure room/medications)
Osteomyelitis, foot	Three-phase bone scan	$ 247	(23)
	WBC scan	$ 176	(458)
	^{67}Ga scan	$ 176	(48)
	X-ray	$ 31	
	MRI	$ 531	
Fever of unknown origin	Whole-body gallium scan	$ 306	(48)
	Whole-body WBC scan	$ 306	(196)
	CT chest with contrast	$ 351	
	CT abdomen with contrast	$ 344	
Brain tumor recurrence	MRI of brain with/without contrast	$1132	
	CT with/without contrast	$ 352	
	SPECT brain scan with ^{201}Tl	$ 323	(75)
	PET brain scan with ^{18}F-FDG	(not priced by Medicare)	
Brain death	EEG	$ 64	
	Radionuclide brain scan	$ 190	(460)
Thyroid nodule	Radionuclide thyroid scan	$ 94	(5–35)
	Thyroid ultrasound	$ 87	
	Fine-needle aspiration	$ 190	
Hyperthyroidism	Radionuclide scan with uptake	$ 122	(5–35)
Bone metastases	Whole-body bone scan	$ 218	(23)
	MRI (either chest, abdomen or pelvis)	$ 538	
Osteoporosis	DEXA	$ 141	
	CT quantitative spine	$ 124	
	Ultrasound heel	(not priced by Medicare)	

29

Comparative Cost of Diagnostic Procedures (1999)

Indication	Procedure	Medicare B Payment (Global Fee)	
		Procedure	Radiopharmaceutical
Recurrent lymphoma	Whole-body PET with		
	^{18}F-FDG	$2252	(^{18}F-FDG included)
	Whole-body gallium with SPECT	$ 458	(48)
	MRI chest	$ 588	
	MRI abdomen	$ 588	
	CT chest with contrast	$ 384	
	CT abdomen with contrast	$ 376	
Staging/recurrence, various cancers	Whole-body scan with SPECT (e.g., ^{67}Ga, ProstaScint, Octreo-Scan, OncoScint, CEA-scan)	$ 458	(48–1400)
Therapy, hyperthyroidism	^{131}I therapy (12 mCi)	$ 202	(85–100)
	Propylthiouracil; 1 yr	$ 220	(drug costs alone)
Therapy, painful bone metastases	^{89}Sr	$ 210	(2850)
	External beam radiation, 2 sites	$2225	
Therapy, metastatic thyroid cancer	^{131}I therapy; 150 mCi	$ 240	(590–760)

SPECT, single-photon emission computed tomography; ECG, electrocardiogram; V/P, ventilation-perfusion; CT, computed tomography; ACE, angiotensin-converting enzyme; DMSA, dimercaptosuccinic acid; RBC, red blood cell; MRI, magnetic resonance imaging; WBC, white blood cell; PET, positron emission tomography; FDG, fluorodeoxyglucose; EEG, electroencephalogram; DEXA, dual-energy x-ray absorpitometry; CEA, carcinoembryonic antigen.

Index